DIFFICULTIES IN
TRACHEAL INTUBATION

DIFFICULTIES IN
TRACHEAL INTUBATION

Edited by

I.P. Latto & M. Rosen
FFA RCS   FFA RCS

With contributions from

M. Harmer
FFA RCS

K.R. Murrin
FFA RCS

W.S. Ng
FFA RCS

R.S. Vaughan
FFA RCS

Department of Anaesthetics,
University Hospital of Wales, Heath Park,
Cardiff CF4 4XW, Wales

Baillière Tindall
LONDON · PHILADELPHIA · TORONTO · SYDNEY · TOKYO

Baillière Tindall W.B. Saunders	24–28 Oval Road London NW1 7DX

The Curtis Center
Independence Square West
Philadelphia PA 19106–3399 USA

1 Goldthorne Avenue
Toronto, Ontario M8Z 5T9, Canada

Harcourt Brace Jovanovich Group (Australia) Pty Limited
32–52 Smidmore Street, Marickville, NSW 2204, Australia

Harcourt Brace Jovanovich (Japan) Inc
Ichibancho Central Building, 22–1 Ichibancho
Chiyoda-ku, Tokyo 102, Japan

First published 1985
Reprinted 1989

Typeset by Scribe Design, Gillingham, Kent
Printed and bound in Great Britain by Mackays of Chatham PLC, Letchworth

British Library Cataloguing in Publication Data
Difficulties in tracheal intubation.
  1. Trachea—Intubation
  I. Latto, Ian P.   II. Rosen, M.   III. Harmer, M.
  617'.533   RF517

ISBN 0 7020 1096 0

Contents

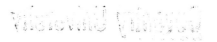

Foreword

The role of tracheal intubation has undergone a complete metamorphosis since it became part of everyday anaesthetic technique less than half a century ago. Intubation has progressed from being a technique for which there were specific indications to an almost routine part of any general anaesthetic. The art of intubation has also changed from being a procedure which was one of the principle skills of the anaesthetist to one which even the humblest tyro is expected to acquire within a very short time of starting training. Intubation now can even be justified as necessary to leave the hands free to fill in the anaesthetic record!

The devaluation of the skill involved in intubation can largely be attributed to the widespread use of muscle relaxants and this in turn has bred a blasé attitude to the problems that may occasionally be associated with the procedure. No anaesthetist of the old school would have recognized a special class of patients as presenting a difficult intubation. To paraphrase Orwell, all intubations were difficult, it was just that some intubations were more difficult than others.

This book, then, is a child of its time and none too soon, some would say. The book tackles more aspects of the subject of intubation than just 'difficulty'. An anaesthetist using good technique will encounter less difficulty than one using sloppy technique and a good knowledge of anatomy will be of primary importance. The expertise of the expert in fact must be rooted in good everyday practice and not sheer eclecticism.

This book brings together into one volume material which is, in fact, already available but diffused over many sources. It attempts to interrelate it in a useful and memorable way. Because memorable it must be: the middle of a life-threatening crisis is no time to be 'looking up the books'. Its style and presentation is testimony to the fact that members of academic departments live in the real world of practical problems and can contribute to the general welfare of their fellow professionals by an academic contribution to a practical problem. I predict this is a book which will come to be regarded as essential for all departments, if not indeed for all serious students of the art and science of anaesthesia.

July 1985   *M.D. Vickers*

Preface

There is one skill above all that an anaesthetist is expected to exhibit and that is to maintain the airway impeccably. Of course it is not always possible to succeed in every attempt at tracheal intubation or to prevent every accident, but most incidents are safely manageable if there has been proper preparation.

The single most pressing impetus for writing this book was the need to bring together knowledge of the problems and solutions to difficult intubations. In obstetric practice problems of intubation figure as a leading cause of maternal mortality. There is no reason to suppose that clinicians are more successful in their management of the airway in less well documented fields of practice. Any individual anaesthetist encounters only a small number of truly difficult intubations in his career and yet as a specialist he must be able to draw on the known methods of management to secure a successful outcome. For instance, local anaesthetic methods can be uniquely helpful, but are under-used by most clinicians, and the range of aids to intubation are not sufficiently well known. Unfortunately, the information is widely disseminated in the world's literature and details are lacking in standard texts. This volume presents not only a comprehensive survey but also supplies sufficient detail to act as a practical guide.

There can be little doubt that widespread adoption of a precise plan for failed or difficult intubation which has been regularly practised should lead to a dramatic improvement in dismal statistics. There is in addition a requirement for regular demonstration and teaching of the more complex techniques.

This book also examines the anatomical and pathophysiological factors which complicate tracheal intubation. The wide-ranging physiological and traumatic consequences of intubation are also dealt with, allied to practical details on their prevention or alleviation.

The aim is to provide a broad survey of tracheal and endobronchial intubation and the problems surrounding the techniques. We hope to give sufficient guidance to the practising, more experienced anaesthetist who has to tackle difficult problems. The text should be useful to the candidate sitting for higher qualifications. Other doctors and paramedic staff who may have to carry out intubation urgently should also find the information helpful.

Acknowledgements

We wish to thank Mr Adrian Shaw and Mrs Janice Sharp for the artwork and the Departments of Medical Illustration at the University Hospital of Wales and Llandough Hospital for photographic assistance.

Dr Paul Baker kindly contributed the case report 'An impossible intubation emergency presentation for a tracheostomy' (see pp. 143–144).

We are indebted to the various editors, authors and publishers for permission to reproduce figures and tables.

Our special thanks go to Miss J.E. Houldey, Miss D.E. Price, Mrs M. Johnson and Mrs H.C. O'Donnell for typing and patiently retyping the manuscript.

CHAPTER 1 Anatomy of the airways

The airways, commencing at the mouth and the external nares, terminate at the entrance to the alveoli. Although there may be considerable variation, congenital or acquired, the applied anatomy in an adult will be described and differences in infants and children indicated.

THE NOSE

The external nares tend to be oval and their shape is used as a guide in selecting an appropriately sized nasotracheal tube. Normally, the adult male accepts a tube of a diameter between 8 and 10 gauge and the adult female between 5 and 8 gauge [1]. The distance from the external nares to the carina in male and female averages 32 cm and 27 cm respectively [1].

The respective diameters and lengths are reduced in children and vary depending upon the size of the head and the length of the trachea. There are several working guides [2–5] which can be used to try and calculate the size of the tracheal tube required to intubate a small child.

The external nares open into the nasal cavity, which is divided into two compartments by the nasal septum. Each compartment has a roof, a floor, a medial wall and a lateral wall. Attached to the lateral walls are three overhanging projections, the conchae, covering three meati which are passages draining the paranasal sinuses and nasolacrimal ducts into the nasal cavities.

The superior and middle conchae arise from the medial aspect of the ethmoid labyrinth while the inferior concha is a separate bone. The medial wall, the nasal septum, is formed from bone and cartilage. In addition, endothelial growths or polypi may project into the cavities between the medial and lateral walls though they may not be visible externally.

The septum is frequently deviated from the mid line so that one nasal cavity is greater in size than the other. If nasal polypi are present, they may cause obstruction and difficulty with instrumentation. It is essential therefore to test the patency of the nasal passages preoperatively in every patient before nasal intubation is contemplated. The floor of the nose slopes upward and backward. However, when the patient is supine, the main part of the floor and its distal portion present a J shape to the anaesthetist with the hook of the J pointing anteriorly (Fig. 1).

The blood supply to the nasal mucosa is generous in order to warm and humidify the inspired air. Consequently, local anaesthetic

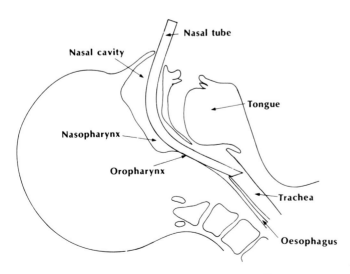

Fig. 1 Nasal intubation (J shape).

1

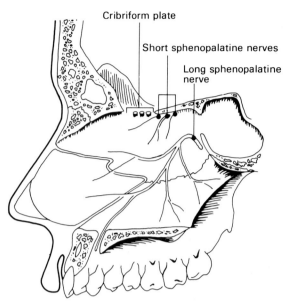

Fig. 2 Nerve supply to the medial wall of nasal cavity. After Macintosh and Ostlere [9], with kind permission of the authors and publisher.

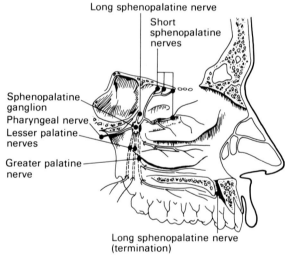

Fig. 3 Nerve supply to lateral wall of nasal cavity. After Macintosh and Ostlere [9], with kind permission of the authors and publisher.

agents can be rapidly absorbed and undue trauma can cause considerable bleeding.

The relevant nerve supply to the nose is derived mainly from the maxillary division of the trigeminal nerve with additional nerves from the ophthalmic division. The nerves supplying both medial and lateral walls of the nose are illustrated in Figs 2 and 3. Although these nerves may be blocked separately, the usual method of producing analgesia in the nasal cavities is by spraying with local analgesic solutions or packing the nose with gauze soaked with cocaine and adrenaline.

Posteriorly, the nasal cavity opens into the nasopharynx through the internal nares or the choanae. These are oval in shape and in the same plane as the external nares. In the erect position the nasopharynx is behind the nasal cavities, above the soft palate, and contains the adenoids. The adenoids are a collection of lymphatic tissue situated on the roof and posterior wall of the nasopharynx. When attempting to pass a nasotracheal tube the adenoids may:

1 prevent passage
2 become dislodged
3 obstruct the lumen of the tube
4 be displaced into the larynx
5 cause severe haemorrhage

The adenoids atrophy around puberty and their presence in children is a relative contraindication to nasal intubation.

THE MOUTH

The mouth (Fig. 4) extends from the lips to the oropharyngeal aperture and encloses the vestibule between the teeth, gums and the inside of the cheeks.

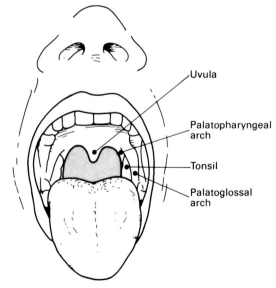

Fig. 4 View of mouth open with tongue depressed. After Ellis and Feldman [8], with kind permission of the publisher, Blackwell Scientific Publications.

The alveolar arches and teeth form the lateral and anterior borders respectively while the oropharyngeal isthmus provides the posterior border. The roof of the oral cavity is formed by the hard and soft palates ending posteriorly in the uvula. Inferiorly, the anterior two-thirds of the tongue and the mucosa on the undersurface forms the floor of the mouth. The tongue is a muscular organ with a large blood supply and is attached to the hyoid bone, styloid process and the back of the mandible. The innervation is derived from the trigeminal, facial, glossopharyngeal, vagus and hypoglossal nerves. However, it is usually the surface of the tongue that is rendered insensitive during awake intubation and is commonly achieved with topically acting local anaesthetic agents.

The mucous membrane covering the dorsal surface of the tongue is thickened posteriorly forming three folds. In the mid line the tongue is attached to the epiglottis by the glossoepiglottic fold. Laterally the mucous membrane combines with the pharyngeal mucous membrane to form the pharyngoepiglottic folds. Between these three folds are two similar depressions called the valleculae. The valleculae are important landmarks during laryngoscopy. The tip of the soft palate, the uvula, hangs freely in the midline and is another important landmark during intubation. Occasionally, however, should the uvula become very swollen, it can cause substantial obstruction to respiration as well as difficulty with nasal and oral intubation.

The oral cavity communicates with the oropharynx through the oropharyngeal isthmus. There are two structures of importance in this area, the tonsils and the tip of the epiglottis. The tonsils are lymphoid tissue and rarely cause difficulty with intubation unless they are considerably enlarged. The tip and the body of the epiglottis come clearly into view during laryngoscopy. These areas are supplied by branches of the trigeminal and glossopharyngeal nerves.

Hence, it is possible to identify a line of structures which can act as landmarks during intubation. The uvula above, the lateral palatopharyngeal arches and the two important inferior areas, the vallecula and the epiglottis. In addition to this imaginary line, three other points must be taken into consideration when attempting to intubate an infant:

1 The infant has a relatively large head [5].
2 The jaw angle is some 20° greater in the infant – 140° compared with 120° in the young adult.
3 The shape of the epiglottis in the newborn is long and thin but, with increasing age, it gradually flattens and widens until it eventually reaches the adult shape (Fig. 5).

THE PHARYNX

The pharynx extends from the base of the skull down to the sixth cervical vertebrae. In shape, it is similar to an ice-cream cone whose walls are mainly derived from the constrictor muscles and fibrous tissue covered by a layer of mucous membrane.

The constrictor muscles are attached above around the base of the skull and below in a wide fan like manner to the mandible, hyoid bone and the larynx. These muscles sweep around into a common insertion posteriorly, the medial raphe of the pharynx. They support the larynx and oesophagus and are important in the deglutition process. Their nerve supply is mainly derived from the vagal and accessory nerves. Trauma either to the constrictor muscles or to the nerve supply can lead to distortion of the position of the larynx [6].

Anatomically, the pharynx is subdivided into three main parts: the oro- and nasopharyngeal areas dealt with earlier and the laryngopharyngeal area.

Laryngopharynx

The laryngopharynx lies at C6 level between the tip of the epiglottis and the lower border of the cricoid cartilage. The relations of the laryngopharynx are more easily understood as one tube being pushed into another (Figs 6–8). On either side, two spaces are formed known as the pyriform fossae through which run the right

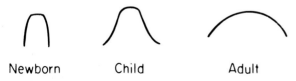

Newborn   Child   Adult

Fig. 5 Changes in the shape of the epiglottis with increasing age. From Brown and Fisk [5], with kind permission of the publisher, Blackwell Scientific Publications.

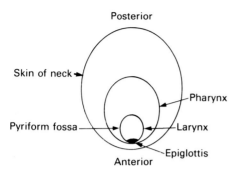

Fig. 6 Three tube concept of the neck.

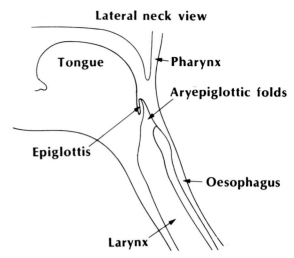

Fig. 7 Lateral view of key areas of the neck.

and left superior laryngeal nerves. As the entrance to the larynx slopes downwards and backwards, the aperture of the larynx faces the laryngopharynx while forming its anterior part. The aryepiglottic folds run from the base of the epiglottis into the arytenoid cartilages. The cricoid cartilage forms the posterior inferior border. Finally the muscular cone, which is the pharynx, terminates at the entrance to the oesophagus below and behind the laryngeal opening. It is this area that is seen at the periphery of the anaesthetist's vision when the laryngoscope has been correctly introduced.

THE LARYNX

The primary function of the tubular larynx is to act as a sphincter to prevent foreign material entering the respiratory tract. It is secondarily adapted for phonation. In the adult, it extends from the fourth to the sixth cervical vertebrae though in the infant the upper boundary is somewhat higher (between C3 and C4). It has a greater anterior inclination in the infant, so backward pressure on the neck brings the larynx into view, facilitating intubation.

The larynx is constructed mainly from cartilages, ligaments and muscles. It commences at the superior laryngeal opening and terminates below the cricoid cartilage where it is attached to the trachea by the cricotracheal membrane.

The cartilages

In the larynx there are single thyroid, cricoid and epiglottic cartilages, and paired arytenoid, corniculate and cuneiform cartilages.

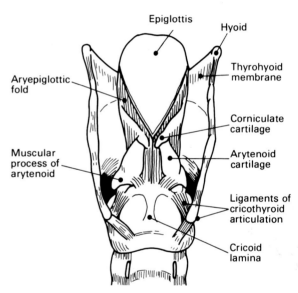

Fig. 8 The cartilages and ligaments of the larynx seen posteriorly. After Ellis and Feldman [8], with kind permission of the publisher, Blackwell Scientific Publications.

The thyroid cartilage

The thyroid cartilage is the largest cartilage and is attached above and below by ligaments. The anatomy is illustrated in Fig. 9.

The laminae meet anteriorly in the mid line but there is a deficiency posteriorly forming the thyroid notch. At the posterior border of each laminae are two projections, the superior and inferior horns.

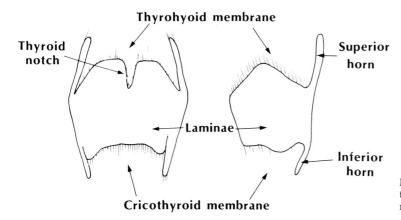

Anterior   **Lateral**

Thyrohyoid membrane

Thyroid notch

Superior horn

Laminae

Inferior horn

Cricothyroid membrane

Fig. 9 Anterior and lateral view of the thyroid cartilage with membranes.

The cricoid cartilage

The cricoid cartilage (Fig. 10) is the only complete cartilage in the laryngeal structure. It has been likened to a signet ring with the wider aspect of the ring facing the oropharynx. The front and sides form the arch but posteriorly there is an expansion of the laminae to form two facets which articulate with both thyroid and arytenoid cartilages. This is the narrowest part of the larynx in a child and consequently determines the size of the tracheal tube. Naturally, oedema of the mucosal surface can reduce the airway diameter considerably. In adult life the narrowest part of the larynx is at the level of the vocal cords.

The arytenoid cartilage

The arytenoid cartilages are pyramidal in shape and are situated on the superior and lateral aspects of the cricoid laminae. The lateral and posterior cricoarytenoid muscles are inserted into two of the three corners of the pyramidal base. The third corner provides the attachment for the vocal ligament. The arytenoid cartilage articulates with the cricoid cartilage forming a synovial joint. This joint may become involved in the general process of rheumatoid arthritis, which could cause hoarseness and some difficulty with intubation.

The epiglottis

The epiglottis is attached inferiorly to the posterior aspect of the thyroid cartilage by the thyroepiglottic ligament. The anterior surface is free and usually visualized at laryngoscopy. The posterior surface of the epiglottis is attached to the hyoid bone. Despite its shape and position, it is interesting to note that deglutition and phonation can occur if the epiglottis is absent.

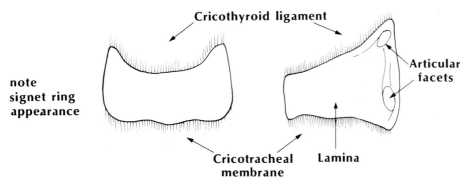

Cricothyroid ligament

note signet ring appearance

Articular facets

Cricotracheal membrane   **Lamina**

Fig. 10 Anterior and lateral views of cricoid cartilage with membranes. Note signet ring appearance.

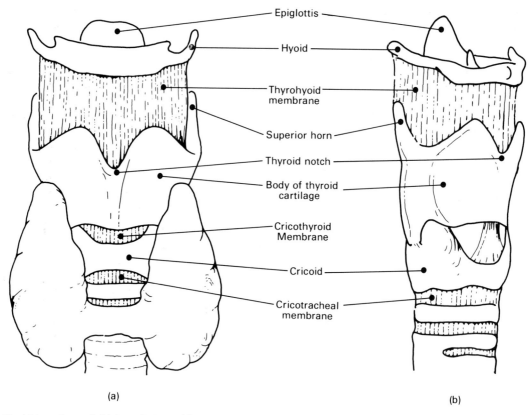

Fig. 11 (a)Anterior and (b) lateral view of larynx: note cricothyroid membrane. After Ellis and Feldman [8], with kind permission of the publisher, Blackwell Scientific Publications.

The corniculate and cuneiform cartilages are very small and are of little importance in the structure of the larynx.

The laryngeal ligaments (Fig. 11)

The thyrohyoid membrane is one of three extrinsic ligaments and runs between the hyoid bone and the upper border of the thyroid cartilage. It is particularly dense medially, forming the median thyrohyoid ligament. Posteriorly this ligament stretches from the greater horn of the hyoid to the upper horn of the thyroid cartilage. Again, these lateral attachments are very dense, forming the lateral thyrohyoid ligaments. These ligaments provide support for the larynx.

The hyoid bone itself is supported superiorly by the hypoglossus and median constrictor muscles. The superior laryngeal blood vessels and the internal branch of the superior laryngeal nerve pass through this membrane to supply the larynx above the vocal cords.

The intrinsic ligaments form the fibrous surroundings of the small synovial joints of the larynx found between the thyroid, arytenoid and cricoid cartilages. They are not as important as the extrinsic ligaments.

The internal fibrous structures are more important. Superiorly, fibrous tissue connects the base of the epiglottis to the arytenoid cartilages and this free upper surface is termed the aryepiglottic fold. Inferiorly, this fibrous tissue thickens to form the vestibular ligament. The mucous membranes run from the medial edge of the aryepiglottic fold down over these fibrous connections and terminate around the vestibular ligament to form the false cords. Below the false cords there is a thin horizontal recess called the sinus of the larynx. Another membrane, the cricovocal membrane, is attached inferiorly to the cricoid cartilage and runs upwards and forwards to be attached anteriorly to the thyroid cartilage and posteriorly to the vocal process of the arytenoid cartilage. The free surface, which is also the lower border of the sinus of the larynx, forms the vocal ligament. The vocal ligaments are covered by mucous membranes and become the vocal cords.

The cricovocal membrane is thickened in front and is termed the median cricothyroid ligament. Laterally it is called the lateral cricothyroid ligament.

The muscles of the larynx are also divided into the extrinsic and intrinsic groups. The extrinsic muscles attach the larynx to nearby structures and are responsible for elevation and depression of the larynx. The intrinsic muscles are important during the respiratory cycle, deglutition and phonation. The posterior cricoarytenoid muscle is important as it is the only abductor of the vocal cords. It is the malfunction or nonfunction of this muscle that can cause problems at intubation and complications following extubation.

The vagus nerve supplies the sensory and motor innervations of the larynx. There are two main branches, namely:

1 The superior laryngeal nerve, which divides into two – the small external and the larger internal branches. The former supplies the cricothyroid muscle while the latter passes through the thyrohyoid membrane into the larynx to provide the sensory supply down to the vocal cords.

2 The recurrent laryngeal nerves, which have different courses, the left looping around the arch of the aorta while the right loops around the right subclavian artery. Both right and left nerves run upwards in the neck in the groove between the oesophagus and the trachea. They provide sensory fibres below the vocal cords and supply all the muscles of the larynx except the cricothyroid. Damage to either of these main nerves may render the larynx incompetent with a potential for aspiration. Such damage may also present clinically as a hoarse voice.

The main relations of the larynx affecting the anaesthetist are found anteriorly and posteriorly.

The posterior aspect of the larynx faces the oropharynx and the oesophagus. Anything that slips out of the posterior aspect of the laryngeal aperture may end up in the oesophagus. Similarly, fluid or solid matter can enter the larynx from the oesophagus with serious consequences.

Anteriorly, the larynx is related to the superficial fascia and the skin of the neck. The thyroid and cricoid cartilages can be palpated relatively easily through the skin and are important landmarks if a cricothyroid puncture is contemplated. It is between these two cartilages that the anaesthetist places the puncturing needle (Fig. 11).

The larynx, however, is most commonly viewed by anaesthetists during intubation and sometimes at extubation. The anatomy seen under normal circumstances is illustrated (Fig. 12). The space between the relaxed vocal cords

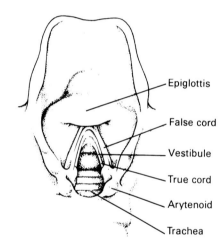

Fig. 12 View of the larynx at laryngoscopy. From Ellis and Feldman [8], with kind permission of the publisher, Blackwell Scientific Publications.

is triangular with the greatest distance posteriorly. The apex disappears into the posterior aspect of the epiglottis.

THE TRACHEA

The trachea commences at the larynx and terminates at the level of the fourth thoracic vertebra where it divides into the two main bronchi. It is approximately 15 cm long, one-third is above and two-thirds below the suprasternal notch. In the newborn the trachea is only 4 cm long, increasing the risks of a tracheal tube entering the right main bronchus. The tracheal architecture consists of a number of horizontal 'C' shaped cartilages which are joined posteriorly by the trachealis muscles. Vertically, these cartilages are joined to each other by fibroelastic tissue. This gives the trachea an appearance similar to that of tyres piled one on top of the other, held together by elastic tissue and both covered by endothelium.

Relations

Although the trachea is usually a midline structure in the neck, the lower aspect is displaced to the right by the aortic arch (Fig. 13). Above the suprasternal notch, the anterior relations of the trachea are two-fold. The isthmus of the thyroid runs across the trachea at the level of the 7th cervical vertebra. Either side of the isthmus are the thyroid lobes which cover the cricoid cartilage and the anterolateral aspect of the trachea. Both the trachea and thyroid are covered anteriorly by two layers of neck fascia and skin. The oesophagus forms the posterior relationship while the recurrent laryngeal nerves are found running laterally in both tracheo-oesophageal grooves.

At the suprasternal notch the trachea enters the superior mediastinum. Anteriorly, the relations include the inferior thyroid veins, the thymus, the arch of the aorta, the brachiocephalic and left common carotid arteries. The oesophagus continues its close posterior relationship into the thorax. However, as the right recurrent laryngeal nerve loops around the right subclavian artery it is not found in the right intrathoracic tracheo-oesophageal groove.

Laterally on the right side, the trachea has a close relationship with the mediastinal pleura, the azygos vein and the vagus nerve. On the left

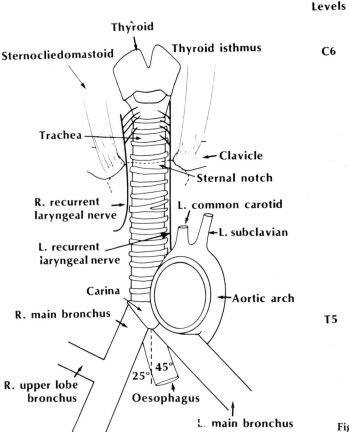

Fig. 13 Trachea and related structures between levels C6 and T5.

side, the aortic arch and the major left sided arteries come between the trachea and pleura. The trachea obtains its blood supply from the inferior thyroid arteries and veins. Large lymph nodes are found either side of the tracheobronchial tree and below the carina. These nodes drain along the paratracheal nodes to the deep cervical nodes. The innervation of the trachea is from the recurrent laryngeal branches of the vagus nerve which also carry sympathetic twigs from the middle cervical ganglion. The trachea divides into the right and left main bronchi but the level of this division varies with the respiratory cycle. During full inspiration, the level may be at the sixth thoracic vertebra. In full expiration it will be at the fourth thoracic vertebra. Where the trachea divides into the bronchi, the lowest tracheal cartilage runs beneath thus forcing up that area, called the carina, which, when

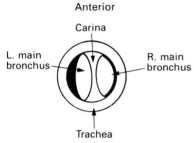

Fig. 14 The carina.

viewed from above, is similar to the keel of a boat. In addition, the mucous membrane covering the carina gives the sharp appearance normally seen at bronchoscopy (Fig. 14).

Bronchi

The left main bronchus is longer and thinner than the right main bronchus with an overall length of approximately 5 cm (Fig. 15). The right bronchus is wider, shorter and conducts more gases as the right lung has a greater volume. At approximately 2.5 cm from the carina, the right main bronchus divides into the right upper and the communal bronchus of the middle and lower lobes. However, in a small percentage of people, the right upper lobe bronchus originates directly from the lower trachea. Such an abnormal origin could have a considerable bearing on anaesthesia utilizing right sided endobronchial tubes for left side pulmonary surgery.

Bronchopulmonary segments

There are usually ten bronchopulmonary segments on the right and eight or nine on the left as illustrated below. An excellent way of remembering the names of these segments is based on the APALM[7] mnemonic. The word 'APALM' is written in a vertical direction then rewritten below, with the 'P' and the 'M' reversed,

Right lung
A–Apical segment
P–Posterior segment   } Right upper lobe
A–Anterior segment
L–Lateral segment   } Right middle lobe
M–Medial segment

A–Apical segment
M–Medial basal segment
A–Anterior basal segment   } Right lower lobe
L–Lateral basal segment
P–Posterior basal segment

Left lung
A–Apical segment
P–Posterior segment   } Left upper lobe
A–Anterior segment
L–Superior segment   } Lingula
M–Inferior segment

A–Apical segment
M–No segment
A–Anterior basal segment   } Left lower lobe
L–Lateral basal segment
P–Posterior basal segment

Occasionally, the left apical and posterior segments combine to form a single segment called the apicoposterior segment. The left upper lobe is then divided into an apicoposterior and anterior lobe hence making eight bronchopulmonary segments. In addition, the L/M of the word APALM become the superior and inferior lobes of the lingula.

The bronchi contain five structural layers, which, working from the outside in are:

1 The outer coat consisting mainly of fibrous tissue containing plates of supporting cartilage.
2 The bronchial muscle which is unstriped and innervated by the autonomic nervous system.
3 The elastic tissue layer which runs along the length of the bronchi and has two important functions. Firstly, it acts as the sub-mucous layer and secondly, contributes significantly to

the recoil of the air-conducting passages during the respiratory cycle.

4 The basement membrane which acts as a support for the mucosal layer.

5 The mucosal layer which has been divided into several layers. Essentially, however, the epithelial lining consists of columnar ciliated cells containing secreting goblet cells.

The bronchi are able to change both length and diameter and assist in the removal of small particles from the bronchial tree. This is achieved by the ciliated columnar cells wafting foreign material trapped in the mucosa towards the trachea forming phlegm which is expelled during coughing.

Anaesthetists in general, and thoracic anaesthetists in particular, should be familiar with the anatomy seen at bronchoscopy as variations can cause difficulty with endobronchial intubation.

Compared with an adult, the level of the carina is higher in infants and also the angles at which the main bronchi divide are different. These differences are illustrated in Figs 15 and 16.

The distal views of bronchial subdivisions are more important to the thoracic surgeon than the anaesthetist: these are illustrated in Figs 17–21.

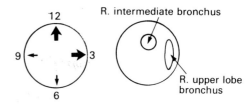

12-hour clock

Fig. 17 Bronchoscopic view at right main bronchus.

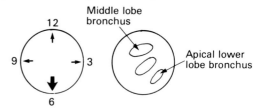

12-hour clock

Fig. 18 Bronchoscopic view after passing right upper lobe orifice.

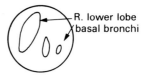

Fig. 19 Bronchoscopic view at right lower lobe basal bronchi.

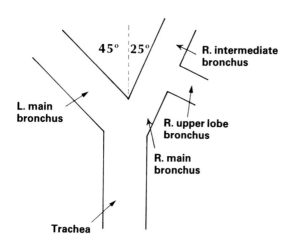

Fig. 15 Bronchial angles in adults.

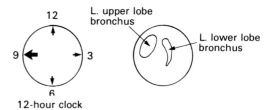

12-hour clock

Fig. 20 Bronchoscopic view at left main bronchus.

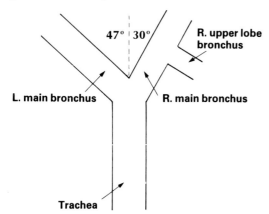

Fig. 16 Bronchial angles in children.

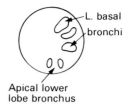

Fig. 21 Bronchoscopic view at left lower lobe bronchi.

The positions of the major bronchial subdivisions on the clockface are included in the illustrations as a 'learn and remember' guide.

Anaesthetists, especially those who practise thoracic anaesthesia, should be familiar with these subdivisions as they are important in diagnosis, anaesthetic techniques, surgery and ultimately prognosis.

REFERENCES

1 Atkinson RS, Rushman GB & Lee JA. *A Symposium of Anaesthesia*, Chap. 13. John Wright, Bristol.

2 Morgan GAR & Steward DJ (1982) A pre-formed paediatric orotracheal tube designed based on anatomical measurements. *Can. Anaesth. Soc. J.* 29:9.

3 Gregory GA (ed.) (1983) *Pediatric Anesthesia*, Vol. 1, p.10. Churchill Livingstone, Edinburgh.

4 Jackson Rees G & Gray TC (eds) (1981) *Paediatric Anesthesia*, p. 6. Butterworths.

5 Brown TCK & Fisk GC (1979) *Anaesthesia for Children*, ch1. Blackwell Scientific Publications, Oxford.

6 Vaughan RS (1971) Anaesthesia for open soft tissue injuries of the neck. *Anaesthesia* 26:225.

7 Last RJ (1984) *Anatomy. Regional and Applied*. Section 4. The Thorax. Churchill Livingstone, Edinburgh.

8 Ellis & Feldman (1983) *Anatomy for Anaesthetists*. Blackwell Scientific Publications, Oxford.

9 Macintosh & Ostlere (1955) *Local Analgesia. Head and Neck*. E.S. Livingstone, Edinburgh.

APPENDIX

Table A.1 Endotracheal tube sizes

Age (y)	Tube size* Magill	Int. diam. (mm)	Length (cm) Oral†	Nasal‡
0–3 months	00	3.0	10	—
	0A	3.5	10–11	—
3–6 months	0	4.0	12	15
6–12 months	1	4.5	12	15
2	2	5.0	13	16
3	2	5.0	13	16
4	3	5.5	14	17
5	3	5.5	14	17
6	4	6.0	15	18
7	4	6.0	15	18
8	5	6.5	16	19
9	5	6.5	16	19
10	6	7.0	17	20
11	6	7.0	17	20
12	7	7.5	18	21
13	7	7.5	18	21
14	8	8.0	21	24
15	8	8.0	21	24
16	8	8.0	21	24
17	9	9.0	22	25
18	9	9.0	22	25
20	10	9.5	23	26
22	10+	10.0+	23	26

*Tube size = $\dfrac{\text{Age (yr)}}{4} + 4.5\,\text{mm}$

†Oral length = $12 + \dfrac{\text{Age (yr)}}{2}\,\text{cm}$

‡Nasal length = $15 + \dfrac{\text{Age (yr)}}{2}\,\text{cm}$

(Reproduced with permission from Dunnill RPH & Colvin MP (1984) *Clinical and Resuscitative Data*. Blackwell Scientific Publications)

Table A.2

Tube size (mm)	Age range (yr)	Weight range (kg)	height range (cm)
8.0	13–15	43–62	154–164
7.5	10–14	31–50	144–154
7.0	8–11	25–40	132–140
6.5	6–9	20–30	121–133
6.0	4–7	18–25	114–122
5.5	3–6	15–22	104–114
5.0	2–4	11–17	87–104
4.5	0.75–2	8–13	74–88
4.0	0.5–1.5	6–11	61–75

(Reproduced with permission from Keep PH & Manford MLM (1974) Endotracheal tube sizes for children. *Anaesthesia* 29:184. The authors concluded that, of the three variables in children, viz age, weight and height, the most accurate correlation was with height.)

CHAPTER 2 Pathophysiological effects of tracheal intubation

INTRODUCTION

Pathophysiological consequences of tracheal intubation are no less important than traumatic and mechanical complications. Many of the body's systems can be affected although the subtle nature of some of the changes remain undetected when only routine monitoring methods are used. Whilst some of these pathological changes may be of little clinical significance to the healthy patient, serious harm can follow when undesirable changes aggravate underlying disease. The possible pathophysiological effects of tracheal intubation are listed in Table 1.

Table 1 Main pathophysiological effects of tracheal intubation

Cardiovascular system
  Dysrhythmias
  Systemic arterial hypertension

Respiratory system
  Hypoxia
  Hypercarbia
  Increased resistance to respiration
  Laryngeal spasm
  Expiratory spasm of respiratory muscles
  Bronchospasm
  Impaired humidification of inspired gases

Central nervous system
  Increased intracranial tension

Eye
  Increased intraocular tension

Alimentary system
  Regurgitation and aspiration of stomach contents

Miscellaneous
  Toxic and side-effects to topical anaesthetic agents
  Postoperative muscle pains
  Malignant hyperpyrexia
  Increased plasma endorphins

CARDIOVASCULAR SYSTEM

When tracheal intubation is performed under light general anaesthesia cardiovascular changes occur in response to both laryngoscopy and insertion of the tube. The changes can occur with an easy atraumatic intubation in the absence of coughing, straining, hypoxaemia or hypercarbia.

Observations of acute cardiac dysrhythmias [1] were followed by numerous other reports of cardiac disturbances accompanying tracheal intubation. The reported incidence of dysrhythmias has varied between 0 and 90%; the differences can be attributed to variations in patients, anaesthetic agents, the varying definitions of dysrhythmia and the technique of recording dysrhythmias [2].

These observations of ECG changes were followed by a spate of reports in which investigators noted the marked increase of heart rate and arterial blood pressure associated with intubation [3–15] (Fig. 1).

The earliest workers soon recognized that reflex cardiovascular disturbances occurred more readily when light anaesthesia was used; deep anaesthesia minimized or eliminated the changes [3,5]. With the introduction of direct and continuous arterial blood pressure measurement in clinical practice confirmation was obtained that changes occurred as soon as laryngeal stimulation commenced and prior to actual intubation [5]. These changes occurred in lightly anaesthetized healthy patients. Both systolic and diastolic pressures rose within 5 s of laryngoscopy, reaching a peak in 1–2 min and returning to prelaryngoscopy levels within 5 min. The average elevation of systolic and diastolic pressures were more than 53 and 34 mmHg respectively. Heart rate increased on average by 23 beats per minute. Laryngoscopy alone produced a variable response in rate, elevations occurring in only half the cases. No electrocardiographic changes occurred with laryngoscopy alone but extrasystoles and premature ventricular contractions were noted in a small number of patients during intubation. These observations are typical of those described by many other workers (Fig. 1).

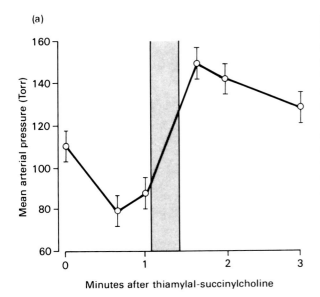

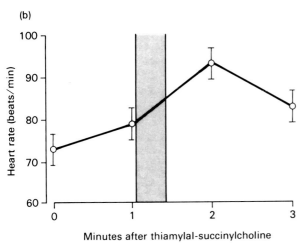

Fig. 1 Changes in arterial blood pressure (a) and heart rate (b) with laryngoscopy and tracheal intubation. Shaded area represents duration of laryngoscopy and tracheal intubation. After Stoelting [55], with kind permission of the International Anesthesia Research Society.

Clinical significance

Transient hypertension and tachycardia are probably of little or no consequence in healthy subjects.

Patients with hypertension

Hypertensive patients often show an exaggerated increase of blood pressure in response to stress including that induced by laryngoscopy and intubation. Previous drug treatment modifies the response towards the normal but changes occur even when the individual is taking antihypertensive drugs and is apparently well controlled [13–15]. Increases of mean arterial pressure exceeding 100 mmHg have been described in such patients [13].

In spite of the very large number of hypertensive patients who undergo surgery, reports of severe circulatory complications following tracheal intubation are rare. It may well be that the changes are so short lived remaining undetected in most cases, that subsequent cardiovascular sequelae are attributed to other causes. There are many investigators who report ECG evidence of ischaemic changes at intubation occurring in hypertensive patients [16]. However, only two cases of severe complications have been reported in relation to a hypertensive episode following laryngoscopy and intubation. In one case, pulmonary oedema was precipitated and in another (pre-eclamptic) patient a cerebral aneurysm ruptured. Both patients were markedly hypertensive before the start of anaesthesia [17].

Patients with ischaemic heart disease

The balance between oxygen demand and supply is critical in patients with coronary artery disease. Increased blood pressure and heart rate elevate myocardial oxygen demand so circulatory changes at intubation can lead to myocardial ischaemia and infarction [18, 19] as well as depressed left ventricular function [20]. In a large and detailed study of patients who had had a previous myocardial infarction, the incidence of reinfarction after operation was significantly higher in those patients who developed intraoperative hypertension and tachycardia (as well as hypotension). The investigation showed that prompt treatment of haemodynamic aberrations could result in a reduced morbidity and mortality [21].

The product of heart rate and systolic arterial pressure (rate pressure product) has been used as a measure of myocardial oxygen demand. Whilst there is unanimity in recommending the close control of blood pressure and heart rate in these patients there is no agreement as to the level at which these variables should be kept. Recommendations of maximum permitted rate pressure product range from 12 000 [22] to

23 000 [23]. The patient's preoperative levels should serve as a useful baseline.

Sudden death has followed intubation [11].

Pathophysiology

Sensory impulses from the root of the tongue, epiglottis and trachea are carried in the vagal nerve. The effector system has been in doubt. An early view was that cardiovascular changes following intubation were produced by a sudden increase of vagal tone [1]. This has not been supported by other workers who found that atropine (3 mg), which is sufficient to block vagal action, did not prevent the pressor response [7]. Later workers have suggested the effector limb to be reflex stimulation of the cardiac accelerator nerves [3, 4]. However, the pressor response is not accompanied by the usual reflex cardiac slowing so this mechanism is unlikely. Another suggested mechanism was that the cardiovascular changes resulted from an overall increase of sympathetic preponderance as a consequence of an increased sympathetic and sympathoadrenal activity [5].

The current view, based on measurements of plasma catecholamine levels, is that stimulation of laryngeal and tracheal tissues at laryngoscopy and intubation cause a reflex increase of both sympathetic and sympathoadrenal activity [24]. Significant increase of plasma noradrenaline level was found to parallel elevation of blood pressure at intubation [25]. In addition to confirming this finding, studies by another investigator demonstrated a large increase of plasma adrenaline at intubation, especially when suxamethonium was included in the induction sequence in which cases a particularly marked pressure response occurred; smaller blood pressure changes followed intubation when pancuronium was used and a smaller increase in adrenaline level occurred [24]. This author suggests that similar levels of increased plasma adrenaline would occur when intubation was carried out under any light general anaesthetic.

These findings are supported by studies in which intubation was carried out under deep halothane anaesthesia. The pressor response did not materialize and plasma catecholamine levels remained unchanged [26, 27].

Other workers have failed to demonstrate changes in plasma catecholamine levels at intubation following conventional intravenous induction techniques even when a marked pressor response took place [28].

These findings are helpful when selecting drugs to prevent cardiovascular complications of intubation. β-blocking agents alone may inhibit tachycardia and arrhythmias but an α-blocking drug is needed as well to counter the hypertensive response.

Prevention of cardiovascular effects of intubation

Numerous methods have been advocated to prevent undesirable cardiovascular disturbances at intubation (Table 2). The efficacy of

Table 2 Methods of preventing or attenuating cardiovascular effects of intubation

Deep anaesthesia
   Inhalation anaesthesia
   Fentanyl
   Alfentanil

Topical anaesthesia
   Direct spraying of larynx and trachea
   Transtracheal spraying
   Mouthwash and gargle with viscous lignocaine
   Inhalation of nebulised lignocaine

Intravenous lignocaine

Drug prevention of sympathoadrenal responses
   Atropine
   Vasodilators
   Alpha-adrenergic blockers
   Beta-adrenergic blockers
   Precurarization when suxamethonium used

Avoidance of mechanical stimulation of the larynx
   Awake intubation
   Blind nasal intubation
   Fibreoptic nasotracheal intubation

depth of anaesthesia was recognized early on and deep inhalation anaesthesia has been replaced by intravenous agents, notably fentanyl. Prevention of noxious stimuli by topical anaesthesia applied to the larynx and trachea in a variety of ways remains a popular method used alone or in conjunction with other techniques. Blind nasal and fibreoptic techniques have been used in an attempt to reduce the mechanical stimulation of conventional laryngoscopy. Lastly, a large group of techniques involves intravenous administration of antivagal and antisympathetic drugs to suppress the autonomic effects of intubation.

The large number of different methods advocated speaks for itself. No method is without serious drawbacks and no one technique is appropriate to every case.

Deep anaesthesia

(a) Inhalation anaesthesia. Deep anaesthesia minimizes cardiovascular changes in laryngoscopy and intubation [3, 5, 13]. However, this approach may be inappropriate to patients with severe cardiovascular disease. Other investigations have found that moderately deep anaesthesia such as inhalation of halothane 1% for 5–10 min is not wholly effective in preventing the pressor response [14].

(b) Fentanyl (conventional dose). Moderate doses of fentanyl to supplement thiopentone induction can minimize the cardiovascular effects of intubation in healthy adults [29, 30]. In one study involving patients with no cardiovascular disease [30] a dose of 6 µg/kg was sufficient to abolish both pressor and heart rate changes. Indeed, the blood pressure fell gradually to 18% below base levels. A smaller dose of 2 µg/kg prevented any significant change of heart rate and the systolic pressure never rose by more than 20 mmHg.

The fall of pressure with the 6 µg/kg dose was of no clinical concern in these healthy patients but it is possible that much greater falls could occur in the more labile hypertensive subject.

Several mechanisms could be at play to account for the way in which fentanyl attenuates the pressor response to intubation. The analgesic effect could block the nociceptive stimuli of intubation, centrally mediated depression of sympathetic tone [31], and activation of vagal tone. The stable heart rate with fentanyl, even in the lower dose, would seem to put the technique at an advantage over other regimes in which control of the heart rate is more difficult than control of the pressure. The mode of action again possibly includes fentanyl's analgesic effect but also results from parasympathetic activity in the presence of sympathoadrenal stimulation by laryngoscopy and intubation [32]; lastly fentanyl is known to cause bradycardia [33–35].

The main disadvantage of using fentanyl in this way, especially if the 6 µg/kg dose is used, is the increased risk of postoperative respiratory depression especially after short procedures. If this danger is borne in mind then the technique would seem to be a useful one in patients with significant cardiovascular disease. Similar results were found in another investigation [30] in which nitrous oxide and fentanyl (4 µg/kg) were used prior to intubation in patients with minimal cardiovascular disease. With this drug regime heart rate, arterial systolic and mean pressure and cardiac output were all significantly reduced, peripheral vascular resistance remaining unchanged. However, tracheal intubation aided by suxamethonium did not result in any further alteration of these cardiovascular parameters.

(c) Fentanyl (high dose). Low dose fentanyl following conventional thiopentone induction or when used in conjunction with nitrous oxide satisfactorily attenuates circulatory responses to tracheal intubation in normal subjects as well as those with minimal circulatory disease. It is uncertain whether these regimes would be equally effective in patients with serious cardiovascular disease. A higher dose of fentanyl was used in a series of cases undergoing mitral valve replacement [36]. Prior to administration of suxamethonium and intubation, fentanyl (8–15 µg/kg) was given in sufficient dosage to produce loss of responsiveness to verbal commands and pin-prick stimulation. The average dose administered was 660 µg equivalent to a dose of 11 µg/kg. Apart from diazepam no other drugs were used. Respiration was invariably depressed and necessitated manual assistance. Injection of suxamethonium, laryngoscopy and intubation produced no significant alteration of cardiovascular variables. Similar results were found in an investigation in the definite 'at risk' group of patients – those undergoing coronary artery surgery [37]. The average dose of fentanyl needed to induce loss of consciousness was 18 µg/kg. A further infusion of fentanyl to make a total of 50 µg/kg was administered before suxamethonium was given and intubation accomplished. No significant changes occurred in either arterial blood pressure or heart rate. This finding contrasts sharply with the lack of protection from cardiovascular changes at intubation conferred by morphine. Morphine was commonly used as the main anaesthetic agent in patients undergoing cardiac surgery in doses ranging between 1 and 3

mg/kg, supposedly equipotent with the fentanyl dosages described above. However, with the morphine regime, heart rate and blood pressure are consistently elevated even when used in conjunction with other anaesthetic agents [38, 39, 40]. Equipotency with fentanyl may apply to analgesia but it has been suggested that fentanyl is more than 100 times as potent as morphine in the suppression of laryngotracheal reflexes [29].

The main disadvantage of these higher dose regimes of fentanyl is the significant increase of postoperative respiratory depression. Prolonged respiratory depression ranged from 2 to 8 h [37] to 8 to 12 h [38]. Furthermore, as fentanyl is administered in such large doses respiration rapidly diminishes so that assisted respiration with a facemask becomes necessary. Difficulty may result if the rigid chest wall syndrome develops and gastric distension may also be produced. The method does not appear to be suitable for those patients with a full stomach.

(d) Alfentanil. Alfentanil has been shown to reduce the cardiovascular changes of intubation with the advantage over fentanyl of a shorter duration of action so that undue postoperative respiratory depression is avoided [40].

A dose of 15 µg/kg (equivalent to 4–5 µg/kg of fentanyl) prevents the pressor response but a higher dose of 30 µg/kg is needed to prevent increases of heart rate as well. No cardiac arrhythmias were observed in patients treated with alfentanil.

Topical anaesthesia

(a) Direct spray with topical anaesthesia. Spraying of the larynx and trachea with lignocaine 4% is commonly practised to prevent coughing and cardiovascular responses to intubation although reports on the efficacy of the technique vary. The first study of the method was carried out on normotensive cardiac surgery patients using lignocaine 4% (3 ml/70 kg) sprayed under direct vision at laryngoscopy. Significant increases of systolic blood pressure followed the spraying itself but never increasing by more than 20 mmHg (mean 13 mmHg) even after intubation. This compared favourably with increases of up to 78 mmHg in a control group. The effect on

controlling heart rate increases was less successful [41].

Other workers have found the technique to have no effect on the magnitude of blood pressure and heart rate increases although these changes were more transient when a spray had been used [42]. The undesirable effects of the laryngoscopy thus appear to largely cancel out the value of topical anaesthesia [9, 43, 44].

Plasma levels of lignocaine due to absorption from the mucous membrane probably never reach therapeutic concentrations sufficient to suppress ventricular arrhythmias [45].

Care should be exercised when spraying the larynx in children. Severe bradycardia occurs in many healthy children in the 6–7 year age group. Routine preoperative intramuscular atropine or glycopyrrolate does not prevent the changes although intravenous administration of either drug is effective in controlling the bradycardia. In a comparable adult group bradycardia was not observed [46].

(b) Transtracheal spraying. Transtracheal injection of lignocaine (2 ml of 4%) has been used to prevent circulatory responses to intubation [47]. Injection was performed 3 min after induction of anaesthesia with thiopentone and halothane. Suxamethonium preceded intubation. The treated patients were largely protected from the pressor response to intubation whereas 72% of a control group had a rise of mean arterial pressure averaging 65 mmHg lasting for 1–5 min. No significant heart rate or rhythm changes occurred in treated and untreated patients.

However, in the treated cases a transient hypertension (mean rise of 78 mmHg lasting for 10–60 s) always followed the tracheal injection itself. In one patient suffering from hypertension blood pressure rose with tracheal injection from 185 to 280 mmHg systolic.

Whilst there is some benefit in reducing the pressor response to intubation because of the hypertension produced by transtracheal injection there would seem to be little indication to administer topical anaesthesia in this way.

(c) Mouthwash and gargle with viscous lignocaine. In order to avoid the stimulation of laryngoscopy, topical anaesthesia has been attempted by mouthwash and gargling with viscous lignocaine. This method has been used in normal [44]

and coronary artery surgery patients [43]. Two 12.5 ml doses of 2% viscous lignocaine were given 10 min prior to induction of anaesthesia: the patient was in the sitting position. Any residual lignocaine was swallowed. In both studies the pressor response was attenuated but no effect on the heart rate was noted. A recent study has shown that the haemodynamic disturbance produced by the stimulating effect of gargling with viscous lignocaine exceeds that produced by spraying [44].

(d) Inhalation of nebulized lignocaine. This method is another attempt to arrest the cardiovascular responses to instrumentation in the laryngeal area [48]. Whilst in the sitting position the patient inhales between 6 and 8 ml of a mixture of one-third 2% viscous lignocaine and two-thirds 4% aqueous lignocaine. The viscous lignocaine is added to increase the droplet size in order to enhance drop out in the upper airways. The solution is nebulized with a Bird nebulizer modified to ensure coarser droplet size, again to improve drop out in the upper airways. Compared with a control group nebulized lignocaine treatment significantly reduced but did not abolish all the changes due to laryngoscopy. Blood pressure rose on average by 10% compared to a 56% rise in the control group and heart rate increased by 16% compared to a 38% rise in the control group. No arrhythmias occurred in those inhaling the aerosol compared with an incidence of 40% in controls. However, the changes following intubation were not as well suppressed, probably because the mist did not effectively anaesthetize the trachea.

The elimination of arrhythmias can be accounted for partly by systemic absorption of the lignocaine which was found to reach over 2 µg/ml in some patients in this study; 2–5 µg/ml is sufficient to treat premature ventricular contractions [49]. Systemic absorption of lignocaine could also contribute to dampening of the reflex response to laryngoscopy since intravenous lignocaine is known to obtund the cough reflex [50].

Although the method appears effective, the technique requires a cooperative patient. The technique is unsuitable in patients with a full stomach and those who are hypersensitive to local anaesthetics.

A commercially available metered dose of lignocaine spray has been used to give patients inhalations of local anaesthetic [44]. With the patient supine the tongue and pharynx were sprayed with 10 doses of lignocaine 10% (Xylocain 10 mg dose, Astra, Sweden). Subsequently 10 doses were sprayed into the mouth whilst the patient was taking deep breaths. Some patients complained of the bitter taste but generally accepted the technique.

Moderate attenuation of the pressor response to laryngoscopy and intubation was obtained but the aerosol was ineffective in suppressing tachycardia.

Intravenous lignocaine

Intravenous lignocaine has been found to be effective in reducing cardiovascular responses to intubation by several workers [41, 51, 52]. The usual dose of 1.5 mg/kg given prior to induction and laryngoscopy results in only minimal increases in blood pressure and heart rate and an absence of arrhythmias. Lower doses of intravenous lignocaine, in the order of 0.7 mg/kg, are ineffective and some studies suggest that intravenous lignocaine is less reliable than inhalation of nebulized lignocaine [48].

There is some controversy as to whether the beneficial effect of topically applied lignocaine is due to systemic absorption with its subsequent depressant effect on the circulatory system. In most cases plasma concentrations are unlikely to reach therapeutic levels. Even the intravenous lignocaine technique, which results in levels approaching the therapeutic level needed to suppress arrhythmias, is not sufficient to produce suppression of the typical blood pressure and heart rate increases seen at intubation [172]. It is likely that some of the beneficial effects of intravenous lignocaine are due to a direct action of the drug on the mucous membrane of the airways.

Intravenous lignocaine (1 mg/kg) administered 2 min before tracheal extubation prevents coughing, blood pressure and heart rate changes during and after removal of the tube. This technique has been recommended in patients with ischaemic heart disease [53]. However, other workers have noted the need to use larger doses (2 mg/kg) to produce suppression of coughing at extubation.

Although intravenous lignocaine appears to be fairly reliable in its suppression of cardiovascular responses to intubation caution should be exercised when substantial doses are administered to patients with a serious cardiovascular disease for fear of producing excessive depression.

Drug prevention of sympathoadrenal responses

(a) *Atropine.* Following the suggestion that circulatory responses to intubation could be mediated by 'vasovagal' pathways, the use of large doses of atropine sufficient to block vagal transmission was studied [7].

Atropine (3 mg) was given intravenously prior to intubation in healthy subjects. The customary increase in blood pressure was prevented. There was no further increase in heart rate but this was already significantly elevated following the injection of atropine. Some of the patients developed transient cardiac arrhythmias. In a more recent study, conventional doses of atropine appeared to be potentially harmful [54]. Atropine (0.6 mg) was given either intramuscularly 30 min preoperatively or intravenously 5 min before induction to patients free of cardiovascular disease. Compared to patients who received only normal saline, atropine was associated with significantly greater increases of heart rate and incidence of arrhythmias at intubation. The greatest increase in heart rate and the incidence and severity of the abnormal rhythms were seen in patients given intravenous atropine. Neither atropine regimes had any influence on the typical hypertension produced by intubation. There seems no basis, therefore, for using atropine to prevent cardiovascular responses to intubation. Indeed the enhanced pulse rate could increase the danger of intubation in patients at risk.

(b) *Vasodilators.* Sodium nitroprusside, used in a dose of 1–2 µg/kg administered by rapid intravenous injection about 15 s before laryngoscopy, attenuates but does not fully prevent, the pressor response [55]. The timing of injection is made so that its peak effect coincides with the maximum hypertensive effect of intubation. The technique does not prevent the increased heart rate.

(c) *Alpha-adrenergic blockers.* Phentolamine in doses of 5 mg given intravenously has been shown to effectively block both heart rate and

pressor response to intubation [7]. Surprisingly, no fall of blood pressure occurred in healthy subjects anaesthetized and lying supine. A 5 mg dose of phentolamine is substantial and normally causes a rapid fall of blood pressure. Caution should therefore be used when administering this drug in patients with unstable cardiovascular systems.

(d) *Beta-adrenergic blockers.* Many authorities have advocated the use of beta-adrenergic blocking agents to inhibit the reflex sympathoadrenal discharges following intubation [15, 56, 57]. There is unanimity in the recommendation that patients receiving beta-blockers preoperatively in the treatment of their cardiovascular disease should continue to do so up to the time of surgery [58–62]. Patients with coronary artery disease are protected to some extent from the circulatory effects of intubation when preoperative beta-receptor antagonists are not stopped compared to similar patients in whom therapy has been discontinued. Of equal importance is the finding by these workers that continuation of beta-blockade does not lead to adverse haemodynamic function during anaesthesia in patients with coronary artery disease. Whilst beta-blockers should therefore be continued, techniques that are of proven value in attenuating undesirable consequences of intubation should always be used in such patients [63].

The use of intravenously administered beta-blocking agents prior to the induction of anaesthesia in patients not previously taking these drugs is controversial. Their use must be based on the careful assessment of all the relevant details of the patient's condition. The use of beta-blockers to attenuate the pressor response to intubation led to circulatory collapse and cardiac arrest in a 80 kg patient who was probably hypovolaemic [64]. The drug employed was practolol (12 mg injected over 4 min) preceded by atropine (0.9 mg). This latter dose of atropine produced an increase in heart rate from 88 to 157 bpm but fell to 112 bpm after practolol administration.

Beta-blockers have proved useful in reducing the heart rate and incidence of arrhythmias but not the pressor response to rapid (crash) intubation sequence (induction agent with suxamethonium followed by immediate intubation). Both acebutolol (0.5 mg/kg) and propranolol (0.04

mg/kg) which represent subclinical doses proved effective [65].

(e) Pretreatment with non-depolarizing muscle relaxants when suxamethonium used. This is commonly practised to prevent some of the undesirable side-effects of suxamethonium, such as muscle fasciculation. Pretreatment has also been shown to have some stabilizing effect on cardiac rhythm during intubation [66].

In this study patients free of cardiorespiratory disease were premedicated with pethidine and atropine and induced with thiopentone. The cardiovascular effects at intubation were compared in groups receiving either d-tubocurarine (0.05 mg/kg), alcuronium (0.03 mg/kg), pancuronium (0.008 mg/kg) or no pretreatment at all.

Whilst the systolic and diastolic pressures increased in all patients following intubation the tubocurarine treated patients showed only small increases of less than 45 mmHg except in one case. Attenuation was least with pancuronium which exhibited no improvement from the control group in which blood pressure rose by more than 50 mmHg. The alcuronium group was intermediate in reducing pressure increases. Heart rate increased in all groups and was maximal immediately after intubation except in the alcuronium group where the greatest rise occurred rather later. There was no difference between the groups, the rises lying between 20 and 30 beats per minute. Comparison of heart rate changes in the control group was difficult to assess because many of the patients in the control group had high starting pulse rates. Some changes in cardiac rhythm occurred at the time of laryngoscopy and intubation, the highest incidence occurring in the pancuronium group and the lowest in the alcuronium patients.

The beneficial effect of reducing blood pressure changes found with d-tubocurarine, and to a lesser extent with alcuronium is mirrored by their ability to abolish muscle fasciculations produced by suxamethonium whereas pancuronium pretreatment prevented fasciculation in less than half of the subjects and was correspondingly less successful in protecting against blood pressure elevations.

Thus, when using suxamethonium to aid intubation it is useful to know that pretreatment with d-tubocurarine (and alcuronium) reduce blood pressure changes but it should be remembered that supplementary measures are needed to guarantee effective control of blood pressure changes in high risk cases.

Avoidance of mechanical stimulation of the larynx

(a) Awake intubation

This technique does not appear to confer any advantage over general anaesthesia. However, neither does it produce more adverse circulatory response when skilfully carried out in healthy subjects [69]. These 'awake' patients were, in fact, sedated with intravenous diazepam, fentanyl, lignocaine (1.5 mg/kg) administered i.v. over a 20 min period whilst topical anaesthesia was applied. Both oral and blind nasal techniques were employed.

(b) Blind nasal intubation

Another approach to minimize stretching of the tissues of the laryngopharynx with a rigid laryngoscope is to insert the tracheal tube by blind nasal intubation. This technique successfully avoided hypertension and tachycardia in four patients undergoing dental surgery, although in two of the patients, previous laryngoscopy had produced a marked pressor response [14]. However, these patients were anaesthetized with nitrous oxide with 10% carbon dioxide and intubation was successful at the first attempt. The lack of circulatory changes is surprising in view of the use of carbon dioxide.

(c) Awake fibreoptic nasotracheal intubation

Pressure on the laryngeal tissues precipitates cardiovascular reflexes. Pressures of up to 2.5 kg have been recorded in routine laryngoscopy and up to 4 kg in difficult intubations [70]. One study set out to see whether avoiding laryngoscopy with a rigid laryngoscope and the use of suxamethonium would reduce cardiovascular effects [72]. Patients were sedated with a mixture of diazepam and fentanyl after premedication with combinations of diazepam, opiates and atropine. Sedation was taken to the point at which the patient could still obey commands. Before laryngoscopy was started topical anaesthesia was secured. Between 1 and 1.5 ml of cocaine (6%) was applied to the nasal passage using cotton tipped swabs. Anaesthesia of the larynx and trachea was achieved by transtracheal injection of 3 ml of lignocaine (4%). These steps would leave out the oropharynx and posterior portion of the tongue. A well lubricated nasal tube was passed over the fibreoptic scope when the latter had been successfully inserted. The average changes in the group of 200 subjects appeared very satisfactory. Even during application of topical anaesthesia no significant change of mean arterial pressure occurred. The greatest increase of mean pressure was a modest 10 mmHg above the baseline when the tube passed through the nasal passage. Although alterations in heart rate occurred progressively through the whole process the change was again modest. The maximum rise of 14 beats per minute occurred when the tube entered the trachea. However, in 32% of cases mean arterial pressure rose by more than 20 mmHg and by more than 30 mmHg in 11% of patients. Heart rate increased by more than 20 beats in 30% of cases and more than 30 beats in 12% of patients. More than half the patients coughed, some severely, when transtracheal puncture was carried out. Half the patients were aware of the intubation process although only a few found it very unpleasant.

Fibreoptic nasotracheal intubation appears, therefore, to offer a means of achieving the goal with only moderate cardiovascular disturbance. This supports the finding that blind nasotracheal intubation causes no significant increases in heart rate or blood pressure [14]. Skill is of course needed in fibreoptic techniques and awake intubation is not always appropriate in patients with severe cardiovascular disturbance. It is probably not the method of choice in such high risk patients because it is not entirely reliable in suppressing vascular responses.

(d) Laryngoscope design

Traditional teaching suggests that straight bladed (e.g. Magill or Forreger) laryngoscopes produce a greater change in heart rate and rhythm than the Macintosh type. The straight blade is inserted posterior to the epiglottis, an area innervated by the superior laryngeal nerve which is a branch of the vagus nerve. The Macintosh blade, on the other hand, is positioned in front of the epiglottis which is supplied by the glossopharyngeal nerve. Contrary to this teaching, some studies showed that the Macintosh blade produced a greater effect on heart rate than the straight blade [8, 9]. However not all these patients were fully anaesthetized and some were suffering from pulmonary tuberculosis.

In fact, when healthy subjects were fully anaesthetized prior to intubation, no difference in cardiovascular response could be demonstrated between the patients intubated with a straight laryngoscope blade and those intubated with a curved blade [72].

RESPIRATORY SYSTEM

Hypoxaemia and hypercarbia

There are two ways in which undesirable effects on respiration may complicate tracheal intubation. Firstly, whatever technique is used, impairment of blood gas exchange will result from hypoventilation, apnoea, respiratory obstruction or expiratory muscle spasm. Secondly, when muscle relaxants are used to facilitate intubation a period of hypoventilation leading to apnoea normally occurs. If ventilation is not artificially maintained a further period of apnoea occurs before intubation is completed, and connection to a breathing system and inflation of the lungs have taken place. The time interval between injection of the induction agent and laryngoscopy has been reported to be 124 ± 10 s and the time from laryngoscopy to intubation 43 ± 6 s [73]. The further time interval between intubation and inflation of the lungs does not appear to have been studied. All these times may be considerably prolonged when intubation is difficult or if the operator is inexperienced.

Fall of arterial oxygen

When oxygen is not administered prior to induction and paralysis secured with suxamethonium, arterial oxygen saturation falls rapidly to a mean value of about 75% in 1 min after administration of these drugs [74, 75]. This finding has recently been confirmed [76]. The danger of hypoxaemia during laryngoscopy has long been recognized and the need to elevate the arterial oxygen by denitrogenation prior to induction has been advocated by many authorities [74, 75, 77–82, 86].

Clinical practice varies. Some anaesthetists do not routinely administer oxygen whilst others employ one of a variety of techniques:

1 Preoxygenation with a facemask with tidal breaths over a period varying between 2 and 10 min.
2 Preoxygenation with a facemask with three or four vital capacity breaths over a period of 30 s.
3 Combination of (1) and (2).
4 Manual inflation of the lungs with oxygen after the onset of hypoventilation or apnoea following induction.
5 Both preoxygenation and post induction oxygenation

(1) Preoxygenation with tidal breaths (Fig. 2). Several recommendations have been made as to the duration of preoxygenation, varying between 2 and 10 min [83]. The reasons for these differing recommendations are not wholly clear. Normal subjects breathing 100% oxygen achieve over 98% denitrogenation after 7 min [84]. Different times would therefore be advocated depending on the degree of denitrogenation thought advisable. However, reducing the alveolar nitrogen concentration to 4% is a satisfactory level to aim for and gives 5–6 min of

apnoea without hypoxaemia [83]. The difference in oxygen store in the lungs when completely denitrogenated and at 4% levels of nitrogen is very small, 2.53 and 2.65 l respectively.

Another reason for the various times recommended is that studies have involved the use of different breathing systems. Circuits using low fresh gas flows take longer to complete denitrogenation of the lungs. Most studies, though, show that rapid nitrogen washout is easily accomplished with non-rebreathing systems [83].

Three minutes of breathing has been recommended with the Magill (Mapleson A) system using an 8 l oxygen flow rate [83]. One minute of oxygen breathing with a Magill system using a 10 l gas flow gives 3 min of apnoea time before the arterial oxygen saturation falls more than 6% [76]. When a circle system is used with a 5 l oxygen flow, an adequate level of denitrogenation is reached within 5 min [73]. However, these times are based on administration of oxygen with leak proof facemasks, a proviso not always achieved in clinical practice because of inadequate technique or awkward facial anatomy. When there is a leak, preoxygenation may be far from satisfactory and desaturation of arterial blood exceeding 10% can easily occur at intubation [76]. Even when a close fit is achieved the recommendations may be inadequate in certain types of patient (see below).

(2) Preoxygenation with vital capacity breaths (Fig. 3). An alternative to the traditional method of preoxygenation has recently been advocated [73]. These workers showed that four voluntary maximal deep breaths of 100% oxygen over a period of 30 s produced a similar level of oxygenation to 5 min of tidal breathing of oxygen. Very deep inhalations lead to more rapid denitrogenation of the inspiratory reserve volume and the functional residual capacity than the shallower tidal breathing. It would appear that this technique would require a non-breathing system with a large reservoir bag and a large fresh gas flow rate. Nevertheless, satisfactory results are obtained with a circle system employing a 5 l fresh gas flow. Similarly satisfactory oxygenation has been obtained using a Magill (Mapleson A) system with a fresh gas flow rate of 8 l. The patient is encouraged to inhale slowly so that the reservoir bag does not completely collapse [76].

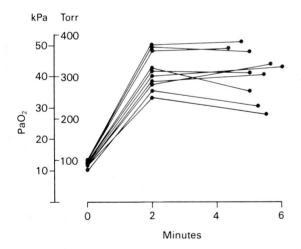

Fig. 2 Pre-oxygenation with tidal breaths and changes in PaO_2 during induction and intubation. Pre-oxygenation started at time 0, thiopentone at 2 min; termination of intubation represented by the last point on each graph. After Gabrielsen and Valentin [91], with kind permission of the editor of *Acta Anaesthesiologica Scandinavica*.

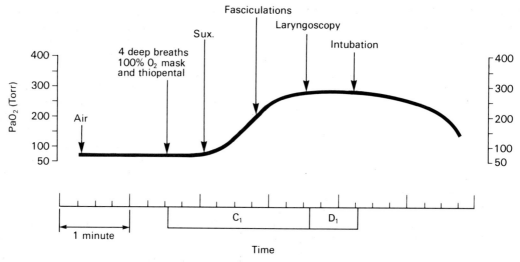

Fig. 3 Pre-oxygenation with deep breaths and changes in PaO_2 during induction and intubation. C_1 = time from induction of anaesthesia to end of laryngoscopy; D_1 = time from laryngoscopy to end of intubation. After Gold and Muravchick [73], with kind permission of the International Anesthesia Research Society.

(3) Oxygenation after induction. This technique is commonly practised in routine intubations and is even used when patients have been adequately preoxygenated, during the period whilst awaiting full paralysis and satisfactory intubating conditions. The technique is invariably used when non-depolarizing muscle relaxants have been administered and where the onset of full action is delayed for at least 2 min. When preoxygenation is adequate post induction hyperventilation and oxygenation is superfluous in most patients. However, the presence of oxygen in the respiratory passages slows down the fall of arterial oxygen tension even in the absence of ventilation [75] so adds a safety margin in those intubations which prove to be unexpectedly prolonged. Most anaesthetists employ oxygenation after induction routinely in elective cases where easy intubation is anticipated.

Oxygen administration after induction is thought to be significantly less effective than preoxygenation because the volume of manual inflation is limited by the volume of the reservoir bag. Functional residual capacity is less under anaesthesia and only the inspiratory reserve volume is used [84]. On the other hand, workers elsewhere could demonstrate no difference between arterial oxygen levels 3 min after induction with either the post induction oxygenation or preoxygenation technique [73]. However, post induction oxygenation was found to be less effective than four deep breaths of oxygen before induction in that arterial oxygen tension was lower at the moment of laryngoscopy than in preoxygenated patients although in neither group did hypoxaemia ensue [73]. Post induction oxygenation alone therefore gives adequate cover if intubation follows without undue delay.

(4) Preoxygenation and post induction oxygen administration. When preoxygenation has been carried out with either tidal breathing or deep breaths, further oxygenation after induction does not significantly increase oxygen stores. However, where preoxygenation has been less than perfect, it offers an additional reserve of available oxygen and is of value in patients at risk. In patients who have potentially full stomachs, extra care is needed to ensure adequate preoxygenation as inflation of the lungs after induction is contraindicated.

Whilst the regimes described above appear to be satisfactory for most patients, greater attention is necessary in obese and pregnant patients. Other groups at risk are those with deficient oxygen carrying capacity, poor lung function, patients with full stomachs and those in whom difficult intubation is likely.

Obese patients. In these patients lung volume is decreased in the supine anaesthetized state [85] so arterial saturation falls more rapidly during apnoea. Careful preoxygenation is therefore obligatory.

Pregnant women. In these patients lung volume is again small and in labour oxygen consumption is high so that arterial oxygen tension falls more rapidly during apnoea than in non pregnant women [86]. Maternal oxygen tension has been observed to fall below 100 mmHg following difficult intubation [87]. The pregnant woman is particularly at risk during intubation for emergency operations whilst in labour. Supplementation of preoxygenation by manual inflation after induction is usually avoided to reduce the chance of regurgitation. Three minutes of preoxygenation or four deep breaths of oxygen over 30 s before induction have both been shown to provide adequate maternal and fetal oxygenation at Caesarean section [88]. However, additional preoxygenation in excess of these minimum recommendations for routine operations is probably an advantage [76].

Poor lung function. Complete denitrogenation in these patients takes longer because of the larger functional residual capacity, small vital capacities and poor alveolar mixing which impairs oxygen wash-in. In one study, complete filling of the lungs with oxygen took nearly 3 min in normal subjects whilst in those with moderate or serious lung disease complete filling took over 4 min and 7 min respectively. However, there was not much difference in the time required to reach 90% filling of the lungs: 1 min in normal subjects against up to 1.5 min in the diseased groups [89].

Relatively routine periods of preoxygenation can, therefore, produce adequate saturation of the lungs with oxygen in patients with pulmonary pathology. However, when lung volume is reduced by disease absolute oxygen content is smaller and this limits the maximum time during which arterial oxygen levels remain adequate during intubation. In practice in patients with serious lung disease a longer period of preoxygenation is probably beneficial to complete denitrogenation and this should be supplemented by post induction oxygenation to increase the safety margin.

Patients with full stomachs or anticipated difficult intubation. In both these groups careful preoxygenation is essential since manual inflation after induction cannot be safely carried out in those with full stomachs and may be difficult in those with anatomical problems. Prolonged intubation may also be a feature of the latter type of patient.

Elevation of arterial carbon dioxide tension (see Fig. 4)

The rate at which the arterial carbon dioxide tension rises in apnoea has been investigated by numerous workers and has been reviewed [90]. In a study conducted by that reviewer eight lightly anaesthetized subjects were subjected to apnoeic oxygenation for periods of up to 53 min. In six of these individuals arterial PCO_2 levels reached between 130 and 160 mmHg. The mean average rise of carbon dioxide tension was 3 mmHg per min (range 2.7–4.9 mmHg). Onset of ventricular arrhythmias terminated the period of apnoea in two patients. In more recent studies, involving elderly patients with serious cardiac disease, the rate of rise of carbon dioxide tension in one group below the age of 60 was 2.2 mmHg and 3.5 mmHg per min in another group

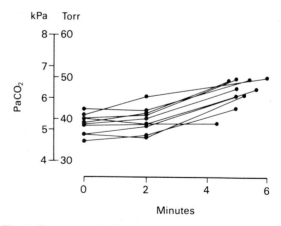

Fig. 4 Changes in $PaCO_2$ during anesthesia and tracheal intubation. Thiopentone at 2 min; termination of intubation represented by the last point on each graph. After Gabrielsen and Valentin [91], with kind permission of the editor of *Acta Anaesthesiologica Scandinavica*.

over 60. The period measured was that between induction, which included administration of a muscle relaxant, and intubation. Although respiration decreased rapidly after induction true apnoea was not present for the entire time interval [91].

Interestingly enough, in one study when intubation was preceded by a 'slow' inhalation induction using cyclopropane and ether until the patient was sufficiently relaxed to intubate, carbon dioxide levels rose rapidly and markedly from the onset of anaesthesia until intubation. The average rise was 15 mmHg (range 7–35 mmHg). Depression of respiration caused by the inhalation induction agent was responsible. This technique, which is sometimes used in the poor risk patient, is therefore less safe than might be thought [79].

In most cases the small increase of arterial CO_2 tension is unlikely to be of any clinical significance when the conventional intravenous induction and muscle relaxant technique precedes intubation. Hyperventilation during the period of preoxygenation reduces this potential danger further in those patients with pre-existing elevations of arterial CO_2 tension. Furthermore, unless contraindicated by complications such as a full stomach, manual ventilation whilst awaiting optimum intubating conditions is a further safeguard in those patients in whom intubation is likely to be prolonged.

Resistance to breathing

Tracheal intubation bypasses the upper airways which normally contribute about one-third of the total airway resistance when spontaneously breathing through the mouth. The tracheal tube does, however, substitute its own mechanical resistance to spontaneous respiration.

Recent work suggests that tracheal intubation imposes a further resistance to respiration in the airways distal to the tube [92]. Significant increases of airway resistance, up to 210%, were reported in awake healthy subjects. Intubation was preceded by topical anaesthesia only. Reflex bronchoconstriction reduced by irritation of the airway by the tube was thought to be the cause. These findings suggest that increased bronchoconstriction might result if adequate general anaesthesia is not deep enough or if topical anaesthesia to the trachea is not used.

Patients with chronic obstructive pulmonary disease showed an enhanced response to tracheal irritation by demonstrating an even greater increase in airway resistance.

Impairment of humidification

The normal warming and humidifying of inspired gases is lost when the upper airways are bypassed by tracheal tube. Any humidifying of dry medical gases falls entirely to the lower respiratory tract. Earlier workers showed that inhalation of dry gases is harmful to the normal function of the respiratory mucous membrane [93] and this has been confirmed by more recent studies. Inhalation of dry gases produces drying of the mucous membrane and damages the ciliated cells so that ciliary movement virtually ceases in the tracheobronchial tree extending as far as the pulmonary alveoli [94, 95]. These changes have been correlated with an increase in postoperative pulmonary complications, notably when exposure to dry gases exceeds 1 h. Conversely, complications can be reduced if gases are adequately humidified [95].

Longer term inhalation of dry gases through a tracheal tube leads to fibrous exudation and crusting of the mucous membranes of the trachea and larger bronchi. All these changes can be effectively prevented by adequate humidification of inspired gases.

INTRACRANIAL CHANGES

Hypoxia, hypercarbia and respiratory obstruction associated with increased venous pressure can all increase brain volume. This effect is sometimes easily seen in the cerebral congestion and swelling of the brain in intracranial operations. These changes are accompanied by elevations of cerebrospinal fluid pressure which reflects intracranial tension. Changes in cerebrospinal fluid pressure have been demonstrated at laryngoscopy and tracheal intubation [96]. Similar observations have been described by other workers (Fig. 5). The rise of intracranial tension can be as much as 10 mmHg [97] although most other authors found changes of a lesser degree [98–102]. Increases of intracranial pressure have been related to a number of factors which could be associated with tracheal intubation: the use of succinylcholine [103], increased arterial blood

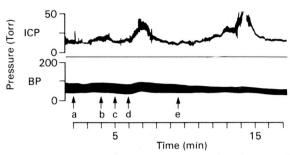

Fig. 5 Changes in intracranial tension with induction of anaesthesia, laryngoscopy and intubation in patients with pre-existing raised intracranial pressure. a, b = increments of thiopentone; c = suxamethonium; d = laryngoscopy and intubation; e = halothane on. After Shapiro et al [98], with kind permission of the editor and J.B. Lippincott Co., publishers of *Anesthesiology*.

pressure [96, 102] and increased venous pressure [102, 104] (Fig. 5).

Of equal importance to changes in intracranial pressure produced at the time of intubation are the changes in cerebral blood flow which can result. Cerebral perfusion pressure is the difference between mean arterial blood pressure and intracranial pressure. Whilst an increase in arterial pressure may mitigate the effect of an increase in intracranial pressure, by the same token a fall of blood pressure would aggravate an increase in brain tension and lead to a reduction of cerebral perfusion. Even more subtle changes may take place. If cerebral blood flow is marginally adequate in a patient with cerebrovascular disease a rise of venous pressure could lead to cerebral insufficiency especially if the arterial blood pressure were to fall at the same time. In some situations an intracerebral 'steal' can occur: when local brain disease is associated with local acidosis, and therefore a state of maximal local vasodilation already exists, cerebral vasodilation due to any cause could increase blood flow to normal brain tissue at the expense of the diseased area.

Limited and transient increases of intracranial tension and alterations of cerebral blood flow are unlikely to be of any clinical significance in the healthy. However, such changes may be of crucial importance in patients with pre-existing raised intracranial pressure, due to a tumour or other space occupying lesions, in whom increases of intracranial pressure are much more marked [98, 101]. These increases produce pressure gradients across intracranial compartments which can lead to dangerous brain shifts

[98], precipitate cerebral oedema, or impair an already inadequate cerebral blood flow.

Whilst numerous factors can contribute to alterations in intracranial pressure, intubation itself, drugs used to facilitate intubation and the consequent physiological changes have all been incriminated. These are listed below:
1 laryngoscopy and intubation;
2 suxamethonium;
3 hypercarbia and hypoxia;
4 elevated venous pressure produced by coughing and straining;
5 inhalation anaesthetic agents and ketamine.

(1) Laryngoscopy and intubation

When these manoeuvres are performed faultlessly the change of intracranial pressure can be very slight even in patients with pre-existing raised intracranial tension with papilloedema. Even packing the pharynx produced no alteration [102].

However, laryngoscopy and intubation can produce a rise in arterial blood pressure. In healthy patients, if other contributing factors are kept within the normal range, cerebral blood flow does not alter greatly between systolic blood pressures of 60–150 mmHg over a whole range of intracranial pressures [99]. However, it has been suggested that the acute hypertension seen at laryngoscopy can induce rapid cerebral swelling in patients with a brain tumour or acute cerebrovascular disease [105]. In patients with pre-existing raised intracranial tension, a further large rise in pressure may result from the raised arterial pressure. Cerebral perfusion pressure is aided by this hypertension but, on the other hand, the raised intracranial pressure can lead to undesirable brain shifts. So whilst the arterial pressure should be controlled it should not be allowed to fall excessively thus compromising cerebral perfusion [98, 99].

(2) Suxamethonium

The use of suxamethonium is a common factor in many studies in which patients exhibited elevations of intracranial pressure [98, 101]. Indeed, the greatest changes in intracranial tension with intubation occurred in those series where suxamethonium was employed with increases of up to 100 mmHg reported [97, 100]. Elevation of brain tension was much smaller in those series where intubation was facilitated by non-depolarizing relaxants. Pancuronium and tubocurarine gave rise to less changes compared with suxamethonium [99, 102]. However, the anaesthetic techniques were not always comparable in individual cases. Patients receiving non-depolarizing relaxants still showed a marked rise in intracranial pressure [102]. Why suxamethonium should be associated with raised intracranial pressure is not entirely clear. Administration of suxamethonium without subsequent intubation produces elevation of spinal fluid pressure in healthy subjects and this has been attributed to increased cerebral blood flow [103]. Others have suggested that the raised pressure is related to muscle fasciculations, the direct action of the drug or because the period of hyperventilation before intubation is shorter than when non-depolarizing relaxants are used. In the latter cases the longer period of hyperventilation produces a lower level of carbon dioxide which can restore defective autoregulation of the cerebral circulation [106].

(3) Hypercarbia and hypoxia

The depressed respiration and apnoea associated with induction of anaesthesia and the use of muscle relaxants preceding intubation must result in a fall of oxygen tension and a rise of carbon dioxide level which are of clinical importance when intubation is not carried out immediately. Hypoxia can be reliably prevented by preoxygenation but the increase of carbon dioxide tension goes on until ventilation is resumed. Hypercarbia results in increased cerebral blood flow. It has been shown that for every 1 mmHg elevation of arterial PCO_2 over the range between 20 and 60 mmHg, cerebral blood flow increases by 1 ml/min/100 g brain tissue [107]. Normal cerebral blood flow is 44 ml/min/100 g brain tissue. However in a well conducted intubation any small rise in PCO_2 is unlikely to contribute significantly to raising intracranial tension [101]. On the other hand, when intubation is prolonged the increase of intracranial pressure can be significant [99]. In one report, intracranial pressure rose above 27 mmHg when the level of carbon dioxide rose by 8.25 mmHg to reach a level of only 39 mmHg at the time of intubation [102].

Hyperventilation immediately after induction is commonly practised not only to prevent hypercarbia but deliberately to reduce PCO_2 as a protective measure. The maximal decrease in cerebral blood flow can be obtained by reducing carbon dioxide levels to the range 10–20 mmHg [108] but this results in extreme cerebral vasoconstriction and possible cerebral hypoxaemia. Therefore levels between 30 and 35 mmHg should be aimed for [99]. Another advantage of hyperventilation before intubation is that the low PCO_2 may protect against the increased cerebral blood flow as a consequence of the acute elevation of arterial blood pressure that occurs with laryngoscopy and intubation; hypocarbia possibly restores defective autoregulation of cerebral blood flow [106].

Hypoxia has a marked effect on cerebral blood flow. A fall in inspired oxygen concentration of 10% results in an increased cerebral blood flow of 30% [109]. Cerebral oedema is a well recognised complication of severe hypoxaemia.

(4) Elevated venous pressure due to coughing and straining

Coughing and straining increase intracranial pressure substantially. In one study in patients with intracranial pathology, where induction and intubation were carried out with great care, only one patient showed a marked increase in intracranial tension and this was due to straining on the tube; the intracranial pressure rose by 13 mmHg [102].

An abrupt increase of venous pressure, especially if associated with a fall of arterial pressure, may further compromise cerebral blood flow.

(5) Inhalation anaesthetics and ketamine

Adequate depth of anaesthesia is desirable before attempting laryngoscopy because it helps to prevent the arterial hypertension that follows intubation. Unfortunately, most volatile halogenated agents produce cerebral vasodilatation which can lead to increased intracranial tension. This can be marked with pre-existing elevated intracranial pressure [110, 111]. Ketamine is also a cerebral vasodilator and has the same danger in patients at risk [109]. Enflurane and isoflurane are the exceptions in that they do not increase intracranial pressure. Inhaling enflurane at concentrations between 0.85 and 3.2% has no effect on cerebral blood flow [99].

Agents which are advisable for induction of anaesthesia in high risk patients prior to intubation are those which are potentially vasoconstricting, such as thiopentone [112] and a combination of fentanyl and droperidol.

Elevation of intracerebral pressure in patients can be successfully minimized by employing a very careful technique in intubating patients at risk [99, 102]. Helpful measures include the use of liberal amounts of intravenous induction agent; the use of long acting non-depolarizing muscle relaxants, rather than suxamethonium; and awaiting full muscle relaxation before laryngoscopy and intubation.

THE EYE—INCREASED INTRAOCULAR TENSION

There are several ways in which tracheal intubation may result in an undesirable elevation of intraocular pressure (Table 3). Whatever anaesthetic technique is employed, insertion of the

Table 3 Causes of raised intraocular tension during tracheal intubation

Increased venous pressure
coughing
straining
respiratory obstruction
Suxamethonium
Hypoxaemia
Hypercarbia

tube itself may increase the tension. The use of suxamethonium to facilitate intubation is a well demonstrated cause of increased intraocular pressure. During the process of intubation, tension will be grossly increased by coughing, straining or any obstruction to venous return. Furthermore, any hypoxia and hypercarbia may increase eye tension.

Laryngoscopy and intubation

There appear to be no reports on the effects of laryngoscopy on ocular pressure. Passage of a tracheal tube may produce a reflex rise of intraocular tension even in the absence of coughing and straining and even when intubation is preceded by topical analgesia applied to the airways.

Suxamethonium (see Fig. 6)

Since the original report [116] that suxamethonium raised the intraocular pressure in conscious volunteers as well as in anaesthetized subjects numerous investigators have studied this relationship. The original findings were soon confirmed [117] and subsequently seen by many other workers [113, 118. 119]. The normal intraocular tension lies between 15 and 20 mmHg [120]. An average rise of 7.8 mmHg after suxamethonium occurred in one series [117]. In some cases the tension rose by up to 15 mmHg.

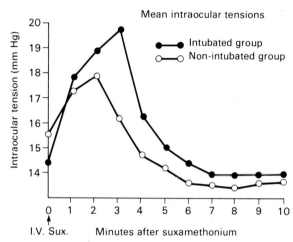

Fig. 6 Graph showing mean pre- and post-suxamethonium intraocular tensions in intubated and non-intubated patients. Arrow marked 'I.V.SUX' indicates time of administration of suxamethonium. After Pandey et al [124].

In another series rises of up to 30 mmHg occurred with an average rise of 19 mmHg. Similar rises were found by other workers in the 60s [114, 121] as well as by recent workers [115, 122]. Suxamethonium administered by intravenous drip in adults likewise produced elevation of intraocular tension in about half the patients. Increases were also found in infants and small children in whom intramuscular suxamethonium with hyaluronidase was administered [121]. No elevation of intraocular tension occurred if suxamethonium was injected in patients moderately deeply anaesthetized [117, 123]. Glaucomatous patients do not seem to be at a greater risk than normal patients [119].

Suxamethonium followed by intubation

Much of the literature on suxamethonium and intraocular tension relates to the effects of the drug itself, measurements being made prior to passage of the tracheal tube. However, some investigators have shown that the elevation of ocular pressure following suxamethonium was further increased when intubation followed [113]. The time course of intraocular hypertension produced by suxamethonium has been studied in patients devoid of systemic or ophthalmic disease [124]. The peak action occurred between 2–4 min after suxamethonium was given and had subsided by 6 min. Topical anaesthesia with lignocaine (4%) was applied to the larynx and trachea before intubation. Tracheal intubation produced a further significant rise but this had vanished within 1 min (fig.1). The increase of pressure was usually below 10 mmHg rising by 13 mmHg in one case. In none of these patients did the pressure exceed the upper level of the normal range.

Recent studies [115, 122] show a similar pattern of change of intraocular tension. Intubation after suxamethonium produced a further significant peak of pressure in over half the patients in one series and in 80% in another series. However, elevation of eye tension never exceeded 10 mmHg. Again in all these patients, topical analgesia preceded intubation.

Other workers [114] failed to show a further rise of eye pressure when a tube was inserted in patients who had received suxamethonium.

How suxamethonium increases intraocular tension remains uncertain. Fasciculation and contracture of the external ocular muscles is an important factor [117, 118] but elevation of tension still occurs when the extraocular muscles are cut [121]. Another mechanism may be a vascular one, transient dilatation of the choroidal blood vessels [125].

Several specific techniques to reduce or prevent the elevation of ocular tension created by suxamethonium have been advocated.

Pretreatment with non-depolarizing muscle relaxants

Drugs which prevent fasciculation might be expected to be at least partly effective. Unfortunately, the evidence is conflicting.

Many workers have found these drugs effective. Hexafluorenium has been effectively employed [126]. Gallamine (20 mg) or d-tubocurarine (3 mg) given 3 min prior to suxamethonium was successful in both normal and glaucomatous eyes [127, 128]. In these studies, however, intubation was not carried out.

Other workers have found opposing results. Ocular tension rose in spite of pretreatment with d-tubocurarine in one study [129] whilst others found the effect of pretreatment to be inconsistent albeit with very small rises of tension [130].

Recent studies [115, 122] compared the effect on intraocular pressure between control groups and groups pretreated with gallamine (20 mg), d-tubocurarine (3 mg), and pancuronium (1 mg). No significant difference was found between any of the groups as regards the incidence or severity of elevated intraocular pressure.

Suxamethonium self taming

Pretreatment with small sub-paralysing doses of suxamethonium prior to administration of the main bolus of the drug reduces muscle fasciculation. However, a small dose of suxamethonium can itself produce elevation of intraocular tension and furthermore does not prevent the usual rise of eye tension associated with full doses of suxamethonium. This technique, therefore, offers no solution to the problem in the patient where the integrity of the eye is lost or threatened [131].

Topical analgesia of larynx and trachea

Surface analgesia is effective in reducing the further increase of pressure from suxamethonium which actual intubation imposes [113, 114, 136].

Acetazolamide (Diamox)

This carbonic anhydrase inhibitor has been advocated to prevent elevation of intraocular tension [132] but needs further evaluation [125].

Propranolol (Inderal)

The usefulness of this drug [133] has been proposed but remains to be confirmed.

Haemodynamic changes

Arterial blood pressure

Endotracheal intubation often results in marked

elevation of arterial blood pressure. Fortunately, these changes are relatively unimportant since any rise of arterial blood pressure leads to displacement of aqueous humour from the anterior chamber and blood from the choroidal vessels [134]. It has been shown [125] that in normal eyes intraocular pressure remains constant over a fairly wide range of normal blood pressures but once mean arterial pressure falls to below 90 mmHg then intraocular tension also falls.

Venous pressure

If the stimulation of intubation results in an increased venous pressure, such as is produced by cough or straining or respiratory obstruction, then this is transmitted immediately to the globe [117]. The choriocapillaries distend and back pressure is produced on the aqueous veins draining the canal of Schlemm. The highest elevations of intraocular pressure measured have occurred in venous obstruction produced by coughing [136] although they returned to normal levels very quickly after relief of venous obstruction. Obstructed respiration may increase intravenous tension by up to 60% whilst a slight cough may elevate the pressure.

Hypoxaemia and hypercarbia

Hypoxaemia and hypercarbia may easily arise during intubation especially when apnoea is produced by muscle relaxants. In dogs hypoventilation elevates the intraocular tension and 5% carbon dioxide added to the inspired mixture produces a marked rise. The ocular pressure can be lowered by hyperventilation [134]. Similar changes have been found in man [125]. Hypoxaemia may also tend to elevate intraocular tension [134].

Conclusion

Suxamethonium greatly facilitates tracheal intubation and it should not necessarily be withheld in most ophthalmic surgical cases because of its tendency to produce modest increases of intraocular tension. In any case increases vanish within minutes, which is a sufficient interval between induction and incision of the eye.

However, suxamethonium alone should not be used for the first time whilst the eye has been opened and is definitely contraindicated in penetrating eye injuries. Unfortunately, it is in these very cases that suxamethonium is indicated to facilitate intubation when the patient has a full stomach. Pretreatment with non-depolarizing relaxants has been shown to be unreliable in preventing a rise of pressure. Nevertheless, the sequence of pretreatment with d-tubocurarine or gallamine before induction of anaesthesia with adequate barbiturate dosage and suxamethonium prior to intubation, has not been associated with a single published report of loss of intraocular contents. The safety of this method in emergency surgery for penetrating eye injury is supported by extensive practical experience [135]. The non-depolarizing rapidly acting relaxant fazadinium has been proposed as an alternative to suxamethonium in producing rapid full paralysis but experience suggests that this claim is not fully met.

An alternative to using suxamethonium in patients with full stomachs and penetrating eye injuries is to use high dose pancuronium (0.15 mg/kg) prior to intubation [137]. However, using this technique in conjunction with light general anaesthesia in children (2 months to 10 years) with no eye disease, increases of intraocular pressure were found at intubation to be no different from those increases seen after injection of suxamethonium, so the value of the method appears dubious [138].

PULMONARY ASPIRATION OF STOMACH CONTENTS

A cuffed tracheal tube eliminates the danger of aspiration of gastric contents but the actual process of tracheal intubation is fraught with the risk of aspiration of stomach contents before the tube is safely inserted. During this critical period pulmonary aspiration occurs when regurgitated gastric contents reach an airway in which the normal protective reflexes are depressed or eliminated by anaesthesia or paralysed by relaxant drugs. Pulmonary aspiration and resultant chemical pneumonitis is a major cause of mortality and morbidity in obstetric and surgical anaesthetic practice [139–142].

Loss of protective reflexes

The normal cough reflexes which protect the airways can be attenuated or eliminated by both topical and general anaesthesia as well as by muscle paralysis. All three of these measures are used to facilitate tracheal intubation and therefore pose a definite risk in patients with gastric residue before the tube is inserted. Intubation, without the use of any form of anaesthesia, should overcome this risk but is unreasonable and may be impossible in the adult patient.

Regurgitation

Suxamethonium

Fasciculations following intravenous administration of suxamethonium have been found, in some cases, to be associated with marked increases of intragastric pressure [143–147]. A direct correlation has been demonstrated between the magnitude of abdominal muscle fasciculation (measured by integrated electromyography) and acute elevation of intragastric pressure after injection of suxamethonium [148]. It has been suggested that this increase of intragastric pressure predisposes to regurgitation of gastric contents [146]. However, it is now known that the force producing regurgitation is not the intragastric pressure itself but the difference between the lower oesophageal sphincter pressure and the intragastric pressure [149]. This gradient is referred to as the *barrier pressure* and it is a reduction of this pressure which will increase the tendency to regurgitation. In comparison with the barrier pressure, other mechanisms independent of the lower oesophageal sphincter are thought to be of minor importance in preventing gastric reflux. These other mechanisms include the pinchcock action of the diaphragm, the flap valve effect of the angle of entry of the oesophagus into the stomach and the mucosal rosette at the gastro-oesophageal junction [150]. Some studies show that suxamethonium, whilst consistently increasing intragastric pressure, always increases the lower oesophageal pressure even more and therefore increases the barrier pressure by a small and significant amount. These findings apply to both normal patients and patients with gastroduodenal disease. The conclusion reached was that there is no increased tendency to regurgitate when the gastric pressure is elevated in response to fasciculations induced by suxamethonium. However, these findings may

not apply to those patients with an abnormality in the gastro-oesophageal region such as hiatus hernia [151]. Similar reservations apply to pregnant patients where the oesophagogastric fundal angle is less acute, or in gross gastric distension which may reduce the competence of the cardia [148]. No significant deterioration of barrier pressure with suxamethonium fasciculations has been noted by others [152]. Even if intragastric pressure does rise with suxamethonium, it is transient and any tendency to regurgitation should be easily controlled by cricoid pressure.

Pretreatment with a non-depolarizing muscle relaxant is controversial [153]. Indeed, the reduced efficacy of suxamethonium preceded by non-depolarizing relaxant could result in less than perfect relaxation, turning an easy intubation into a more difficult one. A further contraindication to pretreatment may be that the barrier pressure is lowest during the period of flaccid paralysis that follows the fasciculation of suxamethonium [154]. Pretreatment with non-depolarizing relaxants antagonizes the depth of paralysis produced by suxamethonium, delays the onset of paralysis [155] and may be associated with a significant incidence of coughing and difficulty with tracheal intubation unless the dose of suxamethonium is substantially increased [156]. Coughing during intubation in patients with full stomachs has been shown to produce marked rises of intragastric pressure [145, 157, 158] as well as subsequent aspiration of gastric contents [159]. It would seem, therefore, that pretreatment with non-depolarizing relaxants is unnecessary and might be dangerous practice in emergency cases.

Suxamethonium in children

Intragastric pressure changes when suxamethonium is given to infants and children have been studied. Unlike adults, no increase of intragastric pressure was noted in either infants or children up to the age of 12 years. Pressure fell in most patients. Fasciculations were absent or minimal in all infants and young children, only being marked in those above 5 years where they were too incoordinate to increase intragastric pressure. However, straining and coughing at the time of intubation produced abrupt and marked rises of intragastric pressure [158].

Other adjuvant drugs given prior to intubation

Many drugs used in anaesthetic practice may influence gastro-oesophageal sphincter function.

Atropine and hyoscine

The administration of atropine prior to induction and intubation has been recommended to reduce the chance of gastric reflux in patients at risk [160, 161]. This followed the finding that atropine (0.6 mg) given intravenously markedly increases lower oesophageal sphincter tone [162]. However, in contrast, several more recent studies have shown that atropine administration significantly decreases lower oesophageal sphincter pressure [150, 152, 163, 164] so that pre-treatment with atropine would seem to be undesirable. Other studies have shown that lower oesophageal sphincter pressure is similarly reduced by both hyoscine and morphine [166].

Metoclopramide

Not only does metoclopramide increase the tone of the lower oesophageal sphincter [150, 152] (the mode of action remains in doubt) but it also has the advantages of being a potent anti-emetic and speeds up gastric emptying [167]. The routine use of metoclopramide in at risk patients has therefore been recommended [150, 152] but atropine, if given, should be administered after metoclopramide as the latter drug fails to increase the lower oesophageal tone which has been already depressed by atropine [152].

Apomorphine

This has been used to induce vomiting prior to induction of anaesthesia [168] and rapid 'crash' intubation, but this method has never become widely used.

Antacids

Pretreatment with antacids has been recommended to minimize the harmful effects of pulmonary aspiration. Magnesium trisilicate is commonly used but oral cimetidine has been condemned as unreliable unless administered some time before operation [169, 170].

MISCELLANEOUS EFFECTS

Many other undesirable pathophysiological consequences could be indirectly attributed to tracheal intubation. The use of suxamethonium is associated with a host of unwanted effects which include postoperative muscle pain, elevation of serum potassium level and malignant hyperpyrexia. Detailed examination of these subjects is dealt with in other texts.

Unusual physiological effects of tracheal intubation continue to be reported. A recent study indicates that plasma beta-endorphin level is activated by intubation. Release of endorphins is thought to play a part in the endocrine response to surgical stress. Since endorphin release can be prevented by topical anaesthesia to the airways or deeper levels of anaesthesia it suggests that ascending neurological pathways exist analogous to those that mediate cardiovascular responses to tracheal intubation [171].

REFERENCES

1 Reid LC & Brace DE (1940) Irritation of the respiratory tract and its reflex effect on the heart. *Surg Gynecol Obstet* 70:157.
2 Katz RL & Bigger JT (1970) Cardiac arrhythmias during anesthesia and operation. *Anesthesiology* 33:193
3 Burstein CL, LoPinto FJ & Newman W (1950) Electrocardiographic studies during endotracheal intubation. 1. Effects during usual routine technics. *Anesthesiology* 11:224.
4 Burstein CL, Woloshin G & Newman W (1950) Electrocardiographic studies during endotracheal intubation. 11. Effects during general anaesthesia and intravenous procaine. *Anesthesiology* 11:229.

5 King BD, Harris LC, Greifenstein FE, Elder JD & Dripps RD (1951) Reflex circulatory responses to direct laryngoscopy and tracheal intubation performed during general anesthesia. *Anesthesiology* 12:556.
6 Noble MJ & Derrick WS (1959) Changes in electrocardiogram during endotracheal intubation and induction of anaesthesia. *Can Anaesth Soc J* 6:276
7 DeVault M, Greifenstein FE & Harris LC (1960) Circulatory responses to endotracheal intubation in light general anesthesia – the effect of atropine and phentolamine. *Anesthesiology* 21:360.
8 Wycoff CC (1960) Endotracheal intubation: effects on blood pressure and pulse rate. *Anesthesiology* 21:153.

9 Takeshima K, Noda K & Higaki M (1964) Cardiovascular response to rapid anesthesia induction and endotracheal intubation. *Anesth Analg* 43:201.

10 Sagarminaga J & Wynands JE (1963) Atropine and electrical activity of the heart during induction of anaesthesia in children. *Can Anaesth Soc J* 10:328.

11 Gibbs JM (1967) The effects of endotracheal intubation on cardiac rate and rhythm. *NZ Med J* 66:465.

12 Dottori O, Lof B, Axelson & Ygge H (1970) Heart rate and arterial blood pressure during different forms of induction of anaesthesia in patients with mitral stenosis and constrictive pericarditis. *Br J Anaesth* 42:849.

13 Forbes AM & Dally FG (1970) Acute hypertension during induction of anaesthesia and endotracheal intubation in normotensive man. *Br J Anaesth* 42:618.

14 Prys-Roberts C, Greene LT, Meloche R & Foex P (1971) Studies of anaesthesia in relation to hypertension. 11 Haemodynamic consequences of induction and endotracheal intubation. *Br J Anaesth* 43:531.

15 Prys-Roberts, C, Foex P, Biro GP & Roberts JG (1973) Studies of anaesthesia in relation to hypertension. V: Adrenergic beta-receptor blockade. *Br J Anaesth* 45:671.

16 Bedford RF & Feinstein B (1980) Hospital admission blood pressure: a predictor of hypertension following endotracheal intubation. *Anesth Analg* 59:367.

17 Fox EJ, Sklar GS, Hill CH, Villanueva R & King BD (1977) Complications related to the pressor response to endotracheal intubation. *Anesthesiology* 47:524

18 Roy LW, Edelist G & Gilbert B (1979) Myocardial ischemia during non-cardiac surgical procedures in patients with coronary artery disease. *Anesthesiology* 51:393.

19 Prys-Roberts C & Meloch R (1980) Management of anesthesia in patients with hypertension or ischemic heart disease. *Int Anesthesiol Clin* 18:181.

20 Barash PG, Kopriva CJ, Giles RW et al (1980) Global ventricular function and intubation: Radionuclear profiles. *Anesthesiology* 53: S-109.

21 Rao TLK, Jacobs KH & El-Etr AA (1983) Reinfarction following anesthesia in patients with myocardial infarction. *Anesthesiology* 59:499.

22 Kaplan JA (1979) (ed) Hemodynamic Monitoring in Cardiac Anesthesia, p.109. Grune and Stratton, New York

23 Cokkinos DV & Voridis EM (1975) Constancy of rate-pressure product in pacing induced angina pectoris. *Br Heart J* 38:39.

24 Derbyshire DR, Chmielewski A, Fell D, Vater M, Achola K & Smith G (1983) Plasma catecholamine response to tracheal intubation. *Br J Anaesth* 55:855.

25 Russell WJ, Morris RG, Frewin DB & Drew SE (1981) Changes in plasma catecholamine concentrations during endotracheal intubation. *Br J Anaesth* 53:837.

26 Stanley TH, Berman L, Green O & Robertson D (1980) Plasma catecholamine and cortisol responses to fentanyl-oxygen anesthesia for coronary artery operations. *Anesthesiology* 53:250.

27 Hoar PF, Nelson NT, Mangano DI, Bainton CR & Hickey RF (1981) Adrenergic responses to morphine diazepam anesthesia for myocardial revascularization. *Anesth Analg* 60:406.

28 Zsigmond EK & Kumar SM (1980) Endotracheal intubation and catecholamines after anesthesia induction. *Proceedings of the 7th World Congress of Anaesthesiologists*, p.447. Excerpta Medica, Amsterdam.

29 Bennett GM & Stanley TH (1980) Human cardiovascular responses to endotracheal intubation during morphine-N_2O and fentanyl-N_2O anesthesia. *Anesthesiology* 52:520.

30 Kautto U-M (1982) Attenuation of the circulatory response to laryngoscopy and intubation by fentanyl. *Acta Anaesthesiol Scand* 26:217.

31 Laubie M, Schmitt H, Canellas J, Roquebert J & Demichel P (1974) Centrally mediated bradycardia and hypotension induced by narcotic analgesics: dextromoramide and fentanyl. *Eur J Pharmacol* 21:66.

32 Tomori Z & Widdicombe JG (1969) Muscular bronchomotor and cardiovascular reflexes elicited by mechanical stimulation of the respiratory tract. *J Physiol* 200:25.

33 Tammisto T, Takki S & Toikka P (1970) A comparison of the circulatory effects in man of the analgesics fentanyl, pentazocine and pethidine. *Br J Anaesth* 42:317.

34 Graves CL, Downs NH & Browne, AB (1975) Cardiovascular effects of minimal quantities of Innovar, fentanyl and droperidol in man. *Anesth Analg* 54:15.

35 Reitan JA, Stengert KB, Wymore ML, Martucci BW. Central vagal control of fentanyl-induced bradycardia during halothane anaesthesia. *Anesth Analg* 57:411.

36 Stanley TH & Webster LR (1978) Anesthetic requirements and cardiovascular effects of fentanyl-oxygen and fentanyl-diazepam-oxygen anesthesia in man. *Anesth Analg* 57:411.

37 Lunn JK, Stanley TH, Eisele J, Webster L & Woodward A (1979) High dose fentanyl anesthesia for coronary artery surgery: plasma fentanyl concentrations and influence of nitrous oxide on cardiovascular responses. *Anesth Analg* 58:390.

38 Arens JF, Benbow BP & Ochsner JL (1972) Morphine anesthesia for aorto-coronary bypass procedures. *Anesth Analg* 51:901.

39 Kistner JR, Miller ED, Lake CL et al (1979) Indices of myocardial oxygenation during coronary revascularization in man with morphine versus halothane anesthesia. *Anesthesiology* 50:324.

40 Black TE, Kay B & Healy TEJ (1984) Reducing the haemodynamic responses to laryngoscopy and intubation. A comparison of alfentanil with fentanyl. *Anaesthesia* 39:883.

41 Denlinger JK, Ellison N & Ominsky AJ (1974) Effects of intratracheal lidocaine on circulatory responses to tracheal intubation. *Anesthesiology* 41:409.

42 Stoelting RK & Peterson C (1976) Circulatory changes during anesthetic induction: impact of d-tubocurarine pretreatment, thiamylal, succinylcholine, laryngoscopy and tracheal lidocaine. *Anesth Analg* 55:77

43 Stoelting RK (1977) Circulatory changes during direct laryngoscopy and tracheal intubation: Influence of duration of laryngoscopy with or without prior lidocaine. *Anesthesiology* 47:381.

44 Kautto U-M & Heinonen J (1982) Attenuation of circulatory response laryngoscopy and tracheal intubation: a comparison of two methods of topical anaesthesia. *Acta Anaesthesiol Scand* 26:599.

45 Rosenberg PH, Heinonen J & Takasari M (1980) Lidocaine concentration in blood after topical anesthesia of the upper respiratory tract. *Acta Anaesthesiol Scand* 24:125.

46 Mirakhur RK (1982) Bradycardia with laryngeal spraying in children. *Acta Anaesthesiol Scand* 26:130.

47 Ward RJ, Allen GD, Deveny LJ & Green HD (1965) Halothane and the cardiovascular response to endotracheal intubation. *Anesth Analg* 44:248.

48 Abou-Madi M, Keszler H & Yacoub O (1975) A method for prevention of cardiovascular reactions to laryngoscopy and intubation. *Can Anaesth Soc J* 22:316.

49 Gianelly R, von der Groeben JO, Spivack AP et al (1967) Effects of lidocaine on ventricular arrhythmias in patients with coronary artery disease. *N Engl J Med* 277:1215.

50 Bromage R & Robson J (1961) Concentrations of lignocaine in the blood after intravenous, intramuscular, epidural and endotracheal administration. *Anaesthesia* 16:461.

51 Abou-Madi MN, Keszler H & Yacoub JM (1977) Cardiovascular reactions to laryngoscopy and tracheal intubation following small and large intravenous doses of lidocaine. *Can Anaesth Soc J* 24:12.

52 Hamill JF, Bedford RF, Weaver DC & Colohan AR (1981) Lidocaine before endotracheal intubation: intravenous or laryngotracheal. *Anesthesiology* 55:578.

53 Bidwai AV, Bidwai VA, Rogers CR & Stanley TH (1979) Blood pressure and pulse-rate responses to endotracheal extubation with and without prior injection of lidocaine. *Anesthesiology* 51:171.

54 Fassoulaki A & Kaniaris P (1982) Does atropine premedication affect the cardiovascular response to laryngoscopy and intubation? *Br J Anaesth* 54:1065.

55 Stoelting RK (1979) Attenuation of blood pressure response to laryngoscopy and tracheal intubation with sodium nitroprusside. *Anesth Analg* 58:116.

56 Siedlecki J (1975) Disturbances in the function of cardiovascular system in patients following endotracheal intubation and attempts of their prevention by pharmacological blockade of sympathetic system. *Anaesth Intensive Care* 3:107.

57 Greenbaum R, Cooper R, Hulme A & Mackintosh JP (1975) The effect of induction of anaesthesia on intracranial pressure. In: *Recent Advances in Anesthesiology and Resuscitation* p.794. Excerpta Medica, Amsterdam.

58 Kaplan JA, Dunbar RW, Bland JW, Sumpter R & Jones EL (1975) Propranolol and cardiac surgery: a problem for the anesthesiologist? *Anesth Analg* 54:571.

59 Kaplan JA & Dunbar RW (1976) Propranolol and surgical anesthesia. *Anesth Analg* 55:1.

60 Kopriva CJ, Brown ACD & Pappas G (1978) Hemodynamics during general anesthesia in patients receiving propranolol. *Anesthesiology* 48:28.

61 Slogoff S, Keats AS & Ott E (1978) Preoperative propranolol therapy and aortocoronary by pass operation. *JAMA* 240:1487.

62 Prys-Roberts C (1981) Beta-receptor blockade and tracheal intubation. *Anaesthesia* 36:803.

63 McCammon RL, Hilgenberg JC & Stoelting RK (1981) Effect of propranolol on circulatory responses to induction of diazepam-nitrous oxide anesthesia and to endotracheal intubation. *Anesth Analg* 60:579.

64 Farnon D & Curran J (1981) Beta-receptor blockade and tracheal intubation. *Anaesthesia* 36:803.

65 Takahashi T, Sakai T, Nakajo N et al (1978) Clinical use of acebutolol (beta blocking agent) during induction of anesthesia accompanied with crash intubation technique. *Jap J Anaesthesiol* 27:37.

66 Karhunen U, Heinoen J & Tammisto T (1972) The effects of tubocurarine and alcuronium on suxamethonium induced changes in cardiac rate and rhythm. *Acta Anaesthesiol Scand* 16:3.

67 Mathias JA, Evans-Prosser CDG & Churchill-Davidson HC (1970) The role of the non-depolarizing drugs in the prevention of suxamethonium bradycardia. *Br J Anaesth* 42:609.

68 Kautto U-M (1981) Effects of precurarization on the blood pressure and heart rate changes induced by suxamethonium facilitated laryngoscopy and intubation. *Acta Anaesthesiol Scand* 25:391.

69 Long US, Zebrowski ME & Graney WF (1982) Awake vs. anesthetized intubation: a comparison of hemodynamic responses. *Anesthesiology* 57:A30.

70 Scheck PAE (1982) Measurements of the pressure of the laryngoscope during tracheal intubation. *Anaesthesia* 37:370.

71 Ovassapian A, Yelich SJ, Dykes MHM & Brunner EE (1983) Blood pressure and heart rate changes during awake fibreoptic nasotracheal intubation. *Anesth Analg* 62:951.

72 Cozanitis DA, Nuuttila K, Merrett JD & Kala R (1984) Influence of laryngoscope design on heart rate and rhythm changes during intubation. *Can Anaesth Soc J* 31:155.

73 Gold MI & Muravchick S (1981) Arterial oxygenation during laryngoscopy and intubation. *Anesth Analg* 60:316.

74 Weitzner SW, King 3D & Ikezono E (1959) The rate of arterial oxygen desaturation during apnea. *Anesthesiology* 20:624.

75 Heller ML & Watson TR (1961) Polarographic study of arterial oxygenation during apnea in man. *N Engl J Med* 264:326.

76 Drummond GB & Park GR (1984) Arterial oxygen saturation before intubation of the trachea. *Br J Anaesth* 56:987.

77 Hamilton WK & Eastwood DW (1955) A study of denitrogenation with some inhalation anesthetic systems. *Anesthesiology* 16:861.

78 Dillon JB & Darsi ML (1955) Oxygen for acute respiratory depression due to administration of thiopental sodium. *JAMA* 159:1114.

79 Lachman RJ, Long JH & Krumperman LW (1955) The changes in blood gases associated with various methods of induction for endotracheal anesthesia. *Anesthesiology* 16:29.

80 Bartlett RG Jr, Brubach HF & Specht H (1959) Demonstration of aventilatory mass flow during ventilation and apnoea in man. *J Appl Physiol* 14:97.

81 Downes JI, Wilson JF & Goodson D (1961) Apnea, suction and hyperventilation: effect on arterial oxygen saturation. *Anesthesiology* 22:29.

82 Heller ML, Watson TR & Imredy DS (1964) Apneic oxygenation in man: polarographic arterial oxygen tension study. *Anesthesiology* 22:25.

83 Berthoud M, Read DH & Norman J (1982) Preoxygenation – how long? *Anaesthesia* 38:96.

84 Fowler WS & Comroe JH (1948) Lung function studies. I. The rate of increase of arterial oxygen saturation during the inhalation of 100% O_2. *J Clin Invest* 27:327.

85 Don HF, Wahba WM & Craig DB (1972) Airway closure, gas trapping and the functional residual capacity during anesthesia. *Anesthesiology* 36:533.

86 Archer GW Jr & Marx GF (1974) Arterial oxygen tension during apnoea in parturient women. *Br J Anaesth* 46:358.

87 Marx GF & Mateo CV (1971) Effects of different oxygen concentrations during general anaesthesia for elective caesarean section. *Can Anaesth Soc J* 18:587.

88 Norris MC & Dewan DM (1984) Preoxygenation for caesarean section: a comparison of two techniques. *Anesthesiology* 61:A400.

89 Braun U & Hudjetz W (1980) The duration of preoxygenation in patients with normal and impaired pulmonary function. *Anaesthetist* 29:125.

90 Frumin MJ, Epstein RM & Cohen G (1959) Apneic oxygenation in man. *Anesthesiology* 20:789.

91 Gabrielsen J & Valentin N (1982) Routine induction of anaesthesia with thiopental and suxamethonium: apnoea without ventilation? *Acta Anaesthesiol Scand* 26:59.

92 Gal TJ & Suratt PM (1980) Resistance to breathing in healthy subjects following endotracheal intubation under topical anesthesia. *Anesth Analg* 59:270.

93 Burton JDK (1962) Effects of dry anesthetic gases on the respiratory mucous membrane. *Lancet* i:235.

94 Marfia S, Donahoe PK & Hendren WH (1975) Effect of dry and humidified gases on the respiratory epithelium in rabbits. *J Pediatr Surg* 10:583.

95 Chalon J, Patel C, Mahgul A et al (1979) Humidity and the anesthetized patient. *Anesthesiology* 50:195.

96 Stephen CR, Woodhall B, Golden JB, Martin R & Nowill WK (1954) The influence of anesthetic drugs and techniques on intracranial tension *Anesthesiology* 15:365.

97 Greenbaum R, Cooper R, Hulme A & Mackintosh IP (1975) The effect of induction of anaesthesia on intracranial pressure. In: *Recent Advances in Anaesthesiology and Resuscitation* (ed. A.Arias), p. 794 Excerpta Medica, Amsterdam.

98 Shapiro HM, Wyte SR, Harris AB & Galindo A (1972) Acute intraoperative intracranial hypertension in neurosurgical patients. *Anesthesiology* 37:399.

99 McLeskey CH, Cullen BF, Kennedy RD & Galindo A (1974) Control of cerebral perfusion pressure during induction of anesthesia in high risk neurosurgical patients. *Anesth Analg* 53:985.

100 Misfeldt BB, Jorgensen PB & Rishoj M (1974) The effect of nitrous oxide and halothane upon the intracranial pressure in hypocapnic patients with intracranial disorders. *Br J Anaesth* 46:853.

101 Burney RG & Winn R (1975) Increased cerebrospinal fluid pressure during laryngoscopy and intubation for induction of anesthesia. *Anesth Analg* 54:687.

102 Moss E, Powell D, Gibson RM & McDowall DG (1978) Effects of tracheal intubation on intracranial pressure following induction of anaesthesia with thiopentone or althesin in patients undergoing neurosurgery. *Br J Anaesth* 50:353.

103 Halldin M & Wahlin A (1959) Effect of succinylcholine on the intraspinal fluid pressure. *Acta Anaesthesiol Scand* 3:155.

104 Hunter AR (1952) Present position of anaesthesia for neurosurgery. *Proc R Soc Med* 45:427.

105 Alexander SC & Lassen NA (1970) Cerebral circulatory response to acute brain disease. *Anesthesiology* 32:60.

106 Paulson OB, Olesen J & Christensen MS (1972) Restoration of autoregulation of cerebral blood flow by hypocapnia. *Neurology* 22:286.

107 Kety SS, Shenkin H & Schmidt CF (1948) The effects of increased intracranial pressure on cerebral circulatory function in man. *J Clin Invest* 27:493.

108 Wollman H, Alexander SC, Cohen PJ et al (1965) Cerebral circulation during general anesthesia and hyperventilation in man. *Anesthesiology* 26:329.

109 Atkinson RS, Rushman GB & Lee JA (1982) *A Synopsis of anaesthesia*, 9th edn, p. 420. John Wright, Bristol.

110 Christensen MS, Hoedt-Rasmussen K & Lassen NA (1967) Cerebral vasodilatation by halothane anaesthesia in man and its potentiation by hypotension and hypercarbia. *Br J Anaesth* 39:927.

111 McDowall DG, Jennett WB & Barker J (1968) The effect of halothane anaesthesia on cerebral perfusion and metabolism and on intracranial pressure. *Prog Brain Res* 28:83.

112 Pierce EC, Lambertsen CJ, Deutsch S, Chase PE, Linde HW, Dripps RD et al (1962) Cerebral circulation and metabolism during thiopental anesthesia and hyperventilation in man. *J Clin Invest* 41:1664.

113 Wynands JE & Crowell DE (1960) Intraocular tension in association with succinylcholine and endotracheal intubation: a preliminary report. *Can Anaesth Soc J* 7:39.

114 Goldsmith E (1967) Succinylcholine and gallamine as muscle relaxants in relation to intraocular tension. *Anesth Analg* 46:557.

115 Bowen DJ, McGrand JC & Hamilton AG (1978) Intraocular pressures after suxamethonium and endotracheal intubation. *Anaesthesia* 33:518.

116 Hofmann H, Holzer H, Bock J & Spath F (1953) Die Wirkung von Muskelrelantien auf den introklaren Druck. *Klin Monatsbl Augenheilkd* 123:1.

117 Lincoff HA, Breinin GM & DeVoe AG (1957) Effect of succinylcholine on extraocular muscles. *Am J Ophthalmol* 43:440.

118 Dillon JB, Sabawala P, Taylor DB & Gunter R (1957) Action of succinylcholine on extraocular muscles and intraocular pressure. *Anesthesiology* 18:44.

119 Taylor TH, Mulcahy M & Nightingale DA (1968) Suxamethonium chloride in intraocular surgery. *Br J Anaesth* 40:113.

120 Duke-Elder S (1955) *Glaucoma, a Symposium*. 1st edn, p. 309. Blackwell Scientific Publications, Oxford.

121 Craythorne NWB, Rottenstein HS & Dripps RD (1960) The effects of succinylcholine on intraocular pressure in adults, infants and children during general anaesthesia. *Anesthesiology* 59:63.

122 Bowen DJ, McGrand JC & Palmer RJ (1976) Intraocular pressures after suxamethonium and endotracheal intubation in patients pretreated with pancuronium. *Br J Anaesth* 48:1201.

123 Macri FJ & Grimes PA (1957) The effects of succinylcholine on intraocular pressure. *Am J Ophthalmol* 44:221.

124 Pandey K, Badola RP & Kumar S (1972) Time course of intraocular hypertension produced by suxamethonium. *Br J Anaesth* 44:191.

125 Adams AK & Barnett KC (1966) Anaesthesia and intraocular pressure. *Anaesthesia* 21:202.

126 Sobel AM (1962) Hexafluorenium, succinylcholine and intraocular tension. *Anesth Analg* 41:399.

127 Miller RD, Way WL & Hickey RF (1968) Inhibition of succinylcholine-induced increased intraocular pressure by non-depolarising muscle relaxants. *Anesthesiology* 29:123.

128 Dickman P, Goecke M & Wiemars K (1969) Beeinflussung der intraocularen Drucksteigerung nach Succinylcholin durch depolarisationshemmende Relaxantien. *Anaesthetist* 18:370.

129 Wahlin A (1960) Clinical and experimental studies on effects of succinylcholine. *Acta Anaesthesiol Scand* (Suppl) 5:1.

130 Smith RB & Leano N (1973) Intraocular pressure following pancuronium. *Can Anaesth Soc J* 20:742.

131 Meyers EF, Singer P & Otto A (1980) A controlled study of the effect of succinylcholine self-taming on intraocular pressure. *Anesthesiology* 53:72.

132 Carballo AS (1965) Succinylcholine and acetazolamide (Diamox) in anaesthesia for ocular surgery. *Can Anaesth Soc J* 12:486.

133 Kaufman L (1967) General anaesthesia in ophthalmology. *Proc R Soc Med* 60:1280.

134 Duncalf D & Weitzner SW (1963) The influence of ventilation and hypercapnia on intraocular pressure during anesthesia. *Anesth Analg* 42:232.

135 Libonati MM, Leahy JJ & Ellison N (1985) The use of succinylcholine in open eye surgery. *Anesthesiology* 62:637.

136 Bain WES & Maurice DM (1959) Physiological variations in the intraocular pressure. *Trans Ophthalmol Soc UK* 79:249.

137 Brown EM, Krishnaprasad D & Smiler BG (1979) Pancuronium for rapid induction technique for tracheal intubation. *Can Anaesth Soc J* 26:489.

138 Lerman J (1984) Effects of high-dose pancuronium and endotracheal intubation on intraocular pressure in children. *Anesthesiology* 61:434.

139 Harrison GG (1968) Anaesthetic contributory death – its incidence and causes. *S Afr Med J* 42:514.

140 Scott DB (1978) Mendelson's syndrome (editorial). *Br J Anaesth* 50:977.

141 Department of Health and Social Security (1975) *Report of Confidential Enquiry into Maternal Deaths in England and Wales, 1970–1972*. HMSO, London.

142 Lunn JN & Mushin WW (1982) *Mortality Associated with Anaesthesia*. Nuffield Provincial Hospital Trust, London.

143 Andersen N (1962) Changes in intragastric pressure following the administration of suxamethonium. *Br J Anaesth* 34:363.

144 Roe RB (1962) The effect of suxamethonium on intragastric pressure. *Anaesthesia* 17:179.

145 Spence AA, Moir DD & Finlay WE (1967) Observations on intragastric pressure. *Anaesthesia* 22:249.

146 La Cour D (1969) Rise in intragastric pressure caused by suxamethonium fasciculations. *Acta Anaesthesiol Scand* 13:255.

147 Miller RD & Way WL (1971) Inhibition of succinylcholine-induced increased intragastric pressure by non-depolarizing muscle relaxants and lidocaine. *Anesthesiology* 34:185.

148 Muravchick S, Burkett L & Gold MI (1981) Succinylcholine-induced fasciculations and intragastric pressure during induction of anesthesia. *Anesthesiology* 55:180.

149 Cohen S & Harris LD (1971) Does hiatus hernia affect competence of the gastroesophageal sphincter? *N Engl J Med* 284:1053.

150 Brock-Utne JG, Rubin J, Downing JW, Dimopoulos GE, Moshal MG & Naicker M (1976) The administration of metoclopramide with atropine (a drug interaction effect on the gastro-oesophageal sphincter in man). *Anaesthesia* 31:1186.

151 Smith G, Dalling R & Williams TIR (1978) Gastro-oesophageal pressure gradient changes produced by induction of anaesthesia and suxamethonium. *Br J Anaesth* 50:1137.

152 Laitinen S, Mokka REM, Valanne JVI & Larmi TKI (1978) Anaesthesia induction and lower oesophageal sphincter pressure. *Acta Anaesthesiol Scand* 22:16.

153 Smith G (1982) Pretreatment with non-depolarizing muscle relaxant does not decrease gastric regurgitation following succinylcholine. *Anesthesiology* 56:408.

154 Smith G, Dalling R & Williams TIR (1978) Gastro-oesophageal pressure gradient changes produced by induction of anaesthesia and suxamethonium. *Br J Anaesth* 50:1137.

155 Cullen DJ (1971) The effect of pretreatment with non-depolarizing muscle relaxants on the neuro-muscular blocking action of succinylcholine. *Anesthesiology* 35:572.

156 Takki S, Kauste A & Kjellberg M (1972) Prevention of suxamethonium induced fasciculations by prior dose of d-tubocurarine. *Acta Anaesthesiol Scand* 16:230.

157 La Cour D (1970) Prevention of rise in intragastric pressure due to suxamethonium fasciculations by prior dose of d-tubocurarine. *Acta Anaesthesiol Scand* 14:5.

158 Salem MR, Wong AY & Lin YH (1972) The effect of suxamethonium on the intragastric pressure in infants and children. *Br J Anaesth* 44:166.

159 Snow RG & Nunn JF (1959) Induction of anaesthesia in the foot-down position for patients with a full stomach. *Br J Anaesth* 31:493.

160 Lee JA & Atkinson RS (1973) *A Synopsis of Anaesthesia*, 7th edn, p. 125. John Wright, Bristol.

161 McCleavi DJ & Blakemore WB (1975) Anaesthesia for electroconvulsive therapy. *Anaesth Intensive Care* 3:250.

162 Clark CG & Riddoch ME (1962) Observations on the human cardia at operation. *Br J Anaesth* 34:875.

163 Skinner DB & Camp TF (1968) Relation of oesophageal reflux to lower oesophageal sphincter pressures decreased by atropine. *Gastroenterology* 54:543.

164 Lind JF, Crispin JS & McIver DK (1968) The effect of atropine on the gastroesophageal sphincter. *Can J Physiol Pharmacol* 46:233.

165 Brock-Utne JG, Rubin J, McAravey R, et. al. (1977) The effect of hyoscine on the lower oesophageal sphincter in man (a comparison with atropine). *Anesth Intensive Care* 5:233.

166 Hall AW, Moossa AR, Clark J, Cooley GR & Skinner DB (1975) The effects of premedication drugs on the lower oesophageal high pressure zone and reflux status of Rhesus monkeys and man. *Gut* 16:347.

167 Howard FA & Sharp DS (1973) Effects of metoclopramide on gastric emptying during labour. *Br Med J* 1:446.

168 Burns THS (1982) Apomorphine and obstetric anaesthesia. *Anaesthesia* 37:346.

169 Crawford JS (1981) Cimetidine in elective Caesarean section. *Anaesthesia* 36:641.

170 Farquharson S (1982) Cimetidine in elective Caesarean section ineffective again. *Anaesthesia* 37:346.

171 Lehtinen A-M, Hovorka J, Leppaluoto J, Vuolteenaho O & Widholm O (1984) Effect of intratracheal lignocaine, halothane and thiopentone on changes in plasma beta-endorphin immunoreactivity in response to tracheal intubation. *Br J Anaesth* 56:247.

172 Thomas DV (1975) Intratracheal lidocaine – local anesthesia or direct cardiac effect? *Anesthesiology* 42:517.

CHAPTER 3 Complications of tracheal intubation

INTRODUCTION

Tracheal intubation confers many advantages for patient, anaesthetist and surgeon. In most patients, the technique is easily performed and relatively free from serious complications. Nevertheless, both minor and occasionally very serious sequelae occur following laryngoscopy and intubation. Equally important are the undesirable consequences arising from drugs and procedures used for intubation such as the side-effects of depolarizing muscle relaxants. Although the incidence of complications is related, as with all procedures, to the experience and expertise of the clinician, it is advisable even in experienced hands to confine tracheal intubation to those instances in which clear cut indications exist.

The undesirable consequences of tracheal intubation can be classified in a number of ways: topographically relating lesions to lips, teeth or larynx; aetiologically relating complications to trauma, reflexes, chemical reactions; but probably the most useful classification for the practising anaesthetist is chronological order with complications being related to laryngoscopy, the act of intubation, the period of intubation, extubation and the postextubation period.

Laryngoscopy and intubation are associated with trauma and also acute, but transient, physiological disturbances whilst the possibility of respiratory obstruction and other respiratory accidents and disturbances dominate the period.

Complications whilst intubated generally relate to equipment problems or failure.

Table 1 Classification of complications associated with tracheal intubation.

At intubation	At extubation
Direct trauma to teeth, lips, tongue, pharynx, larynx, nose	Difficult or impossible extubation
Fracture-luxation of cervical spine	Tracheal collapse
Haemorrhage	Airway obstruction
Trauma to eye	Aspiration of stomach contents and foreign bodies
Mediastinal emphysema	
Retropharyngeal dissection and abscess	*Post intubation*
Aspiration of gastric contents and foreign bodies	
Accidental intubation of the oesophagus	*Early (0–24 h)*
Distension of the stomach due to oesophageal intubation	Sore throat
Misplacement of tube	Damage to lingual nerve
	Glottic oedema
Whilst intubated	Vocal cord paralysis
Obstruction of the airway	
From outside the tube:	*Medium (24–72 h)*
biting on tube	Infections
bevel abutting against tracheal wall	
By the tube itself:	*Late (72 h)*
kinking of tube	Laryngeal ulcer and granuloma
herniation of cuff	Synechia of vocal cords
From within the tube:	Laryngotracheal membranes and webs
blockage by blood, secretions, etc	Laryngeal fibrosis
internal herniation of cuff	Tracheal fibrosis
Rupture of trachea or bronchus	Stricture of nostril
Aspiration of stomach contents	
Displacement of tube	
Ignition of tube	

At extubation, physiological disturbances mirror those found at intubation but traumatic consequences are now much less common. Acute respiratory embarrassment may attend extubation, and this period is again one of great anxiety to all anaesthetists.

Short-term complications after extubation may be either immediate serious problems related to respiratory exchange or later unpleasant, but less severe, problems such as sore throat and muscle pains. Late sequelae result from the progression of pathological changes initiated during intubation and are particularly prevalent following long-term intubation. Table 1 presents the complications and sequelae of intubation.

PREDISPOSING FACTORS

The patient

(a) Age. Infants have smaller and more delicate airways than adults so that injury is more likely, especially with an inexperienced operator. It is also easier for malposition to occur. Infants have a higher incidence of oedema of the glottis as well as subglottic stenosis following intubation [1].

Adults on the other hand are more prone to develop granulomatous reactions to intubation [1].

Elderly patients have a more easily damaged and less elastic trachea. Perforation of the trachea is thus a greater hazard.

(b) Sex. Post intubation sore throat [2], granulomatous lesions [3] and post suxamethonium pains are more common in women.

(c) Adverse anatomical features. Facial or cervical abnormalities as well as short neck, receding chin or obesity make intubation more difficult and are associated with a higher incidence of traumatic complications [1]. Congenital or acquired anomalies of the larynx (laryngeal webs [4], bands, cysts, tumours) are predisposing factors to difficulty in intubation and hence laryngotracheal sequelae.

(d) Adverse pathophysiological features. Upper airway infection may produce difficulty with intubation and therefore be liable to further sequelae.

The operation or procedure

(a) Surgery of the neck. As expected neck surgery is responsible for most cases of laryngeal nerve damage with consequent postoperative hoarseness or respiratory obstruction [5].

(b) Duration of intubation. There is a direct correlation between the duration of intubation and the extent of laryngotracheal complications. The maximum permissible time for safe tracheal intubation is not agreed and many variables are involved (age, tube calibre, underlying pathology). Safe permissible times suggested in the literature range in adults from 8 h to 1 week and in children from 48 h to 3 weeks. The maximum safe period of intubation is until the incidence of sequelae increases significantly and this will vary from centre to centre.

(c) Route of intubation. Nasal intubation is associated with a higher incidence of injury than oral, most problems relating to epistaxis although acute airway obstruction may occur from dislodged adenoidal tissue or nasal polyps. In 13% of neonates intubated by the nasal route acute otitis media occurs [6].

Apparatus

(a) Size of tube. Placing a tube with an excessively large external diameter in the trachea is associated with a higher incidence of postoperative sore throat, laryngeal damage and tracheal stenosis [1].

(b) Cuff pressure. A high intracuff pressure is a major factor in the occurrence of tracheal wall complications, although intracuff pressure must be sufficient to prevent aspiration. For further details of cuff design and its effects see Chapter 4.

(c) Excessive movement. Allowing excessive movement of the tracheal tube on vocal cords and tracheal wall increases the risk of sequelae. This is true during both spontaneous and controlled ventilation.

(d) Tube material. Plastic tubes are favoured over red rubber for long-term intubation. However, additives used in the manufacture of plastic tubes may act as irritants and produce tissue

damage [7]. Vocal cord paralysis has been associated with tubes sterilized with ethylene oxide [8].

(e) Stylet. This accessory can be useful but a sharp rigidly tipped stylet protruding through the bevel of the tracheal tube is a serious hazard to the larynx and tracheal wall.

Experience of the operator

Even using accepted techniques, an inexperienced operator is more likely to be associated with a traumatic intubation.

COMPLICATIONS AT INTUBATION

Direct trauma

Laryngoscopy and intubation inevitably produce an incidence of trauma depending on the skill of the operator and the difficulties encountered during intubation. These injuries include bruised or lacerated lips and tongue, chipped or inadvertent extraction of teeth, lacerations of the pharynx, submucosal haemorrhage and tears of the vocal cords. In nasal intubation, it is more difficult to avoid trauma and epistaxis is easily produced unless preliminary local application of cocaine or phenylephrine is used to shrink the mucosa. Dislodgement of nasal polypi has been reported [9]. In addition to these commoner complications, subcutaneous emphysema and pneumothorax have been described usually originating from a small mucosal tear during intubation [10].

The incidence and nature of laryngeal trauma after intubation was investigated in 1000 patients by Kambic & Radsel [11]. Laryngoscopy was performed immediately after extubation and revealed an incidence of injuries of 6.2%. Haematoma of the vocal cord was the most common (4.5%), whilst haematoma of the supraglottic region occurred in 0.7% of patients. Injury to the left vocal cord predominated. Haematoma occurred more commonly in patients suffering from allergic laryngitis with local oedema or when the cords were not fully relaxed at intubation, or if intubation was not carefully performed. Laceration of the mucosa of the vocal cord occurred in 0.8% whilst there was only one case (0.1%) each of deeper laceration of the vocal cord including muscle, and of

subluxation of the arytenoid. Most patients suffered no long-term serious disability. A more recent study [12] has confirmed these data with similar patterns of injury and has shown that recovery is generally prompt with conservative management.

Injuries of the laryngeal muscles and suspensory ligaments have been described [13]. They follow severe flexion of the head during intubation when distortion of the whole larynx occurs. If movement of the cricothyroid muscle is affected, serious impairment in singing ability may result.

Injury to teeth upsets the patient and can result in litigation against the anaesthetist. Wright & Manfield [14], officers of a medical defence organization, reported that injuries to teeth most commonly occurred during laryngoscopy for tracheal intubation although the use of an oropharyngeal airway and incorrect use of mouth openers, props and gags also contributed. The risk of injury is greatly increased in the presence of dental disease, crowns, bridges or heavily restored teeth, and in the very young and the elderly. In the young, both deciduous teeth and the permanent teeth (at first) have little support. Avoiding damage to the permanent incisors between 5 and 9 years of age is important. With increasing age, teeth become more brittle and are more easily damaged. Persisting with instrumentation in difficult cases is more likely to lead to damage. If a tooth is lost then its whereabouts must be ascertained by radiology and if it is in the respiratory tract it must be removed.

Fracture-luxation of cervical spine

Careless movement of the head may produce serious lesions such as fracture-luxation of the cervical spine with spinal cord compression or section [1]. This problem is more likely in the vulnerable patient whose muscle tone has been abolished by curarizing drugs. Potential cervical cord damage must be particularly borne in mind in patients with existing fractures of the cervical spine, congenital weaknesses or malformations of the cervical spine (Morquio's syndrome) and the elderly and those with pathological fragility of the cervical spine (connective tissue disorders, lytic bone tumours and osteoporosis). The act of intubation can be particularly fraught with risk in patients with an acutely injured spine where cervical stabilization must be maintained during intubation [15]. In these circumstances it is advisable to have the head held in a safe position by the surgeon during intubation.

Haemorrhage

Minor haemorrhage is common following intubation by the nasal route. This may be prevented, or at least reduced in severity, by spraying cocaine or phenylephrine in the nose prior to intubation. Extensive haemorrhage requiring repeated blood transfusion has been reported due to dislocation of the middle turbinate along with a mucosal flap [16]. In addition, laceration to the nasal canal has occurred as a result of silver foil wrapped around a tube inserted for laser surgery to the larynx [17]. The passage of the tube can also be guided past potential haemorrhagic obstructions by means of a finger inserted above the soft palate [18].

Haemorrhage caused during oral intubation is sometimes related to a stylet that protrudes from the end of the tracheal tube.

Trauma to eye

Trauma to the eye may be caused by inadvertently rubbing the cornea with the operator's hand or the catheter mount attached to a tracheal tube. During head and neck surgery, the eyes should be covered carefully with soft eyepads to prevent corneal damage by the surgeon or from surrounding sterile covers. Minor corneal abrasions, although painful, usually heal well.

Great care should be taken in patients with penetrating eye injuries not to aggravate the condition by traumatic intubation or the use of depolarizing muscle relaxants. The pathophysiological effects of intubation on the eye are discussed in Chapter 2.

Mediastinal emphysema

Tearing of the mucosa lining the pyriform fossae may lead to surgical emphysema of the neck and mediastinum when the lungs are inflated prior to intubation. This is a potential problem in the patient who is difficult to intubate and requires several attempts to position the tracheal tube. Although this complication usual-ly settles following intubation it may lead to tension pneumothorax.

Retropharyngeal dissection

Nasal intubation may lead to damage and perforation of the nasopharyngeal mucosa with the creation of a false passage. Such injury, in addition to causing haemorrhage, may lead to the formation of a retropharyngeal abscess or mediastinitis. A classical case of retropharyngeal abscess has been reported [19] which developed 1 week after a difficult oral intubation using a stylet.

Aspiration of gastric contents and foreign bodies

The risk of aspiration of stomach contents is particularly high in patients with a full stomach, poorly functioning cardiac sphincter or loss of protective reflexes. The pregnant mother is the patient most often requiring the administration of a general anaesthetic with these predisposing factors. Deaths from aspiration of stomach contents during obstetric general anaesthesia are a constant finding in the Confidential Reports into Maternal Mortality. A large proportion of the reported cases of aspiration are associated with difficulty in intubation and it is essential that all anaesthetists have a plan of management for failed intubation in obstetrics. This topic is covered in detail in Chapter 9.

Other patients at risk are those with acute intestinal obstruction and the mainstays of prevention remain the recognition of the risk, preoperative drainage of the full stomach and the use of a smooth rapid sequence induction technique with applied cricoid pressure.

In addition to stomach contents the aspiration of foreign bodies such as teeth, parts of laryngoscopes and dentures has been reported. If it is suspected that such an item has been inhaled the patient must have a chest radiograph and if necessary endoscopic removal.

Accidental intubation of the oesophagus

An anaesthetist may accidently insert a tracheal tube into the oesophagus. It is obvious that this error must be recognized rapidly and remedied. However, there are reports of accidental oesophageal intubation, even in experienced hands, in which the mistake has remained un-detected. This topic is discussed in detail in Chapter 7.

Distension of stomach due to oesophageal intubation

The respiratory consequences of accidental in-tubation of the oesophagus are of paramount importance, but other complications may result. Excessive distension of the stomach follows vigorous manual inflation whilst testing for cor-rect placement of the tube. Severe gastric dis-tension can be readily relieved by passage of a gastric tube. If the cardio-oesophageal sphincter is closed whilst inflation continues through a tube placed in the oesophagus, gross distension of the oesophagus is a potential hazard.

Misplacement of tube

The most common site for tube misplacement is in a main bronchus, usually the right. This easily happens if the tube is cut too long and advanced its whole length rather than just through the vocal cords. However tubes have been misplaced in other less obvious sites. One such instance followed attempted nasal intuba-tion in a patient with severe fractures of the face and base of skull where the tube found a tract intracranially [20].

COMPLICATIONS WHILST INTUBATED

Obstruction of the airway

Obstruction of the airway must be the com-monest serious complication of tracheal intuba-tion. The possible causes are numerous but can be divided into those circumstances where the tube may be obstructed from outside, the tube itself may result in obstruction or the lumen of the tube can become obstructed.

Obstruction from outside the tube

Biting on the tube by the patient just prior to extubation is not an uncommon occurrence but inadequate anaesthesia during maintenance may also lead to biting. This has been reported even with a wire reinforced tube which re-mained pinched when the bite was released

[21]. This problem can be prevented either by maintaining an adequate depth of anaesthesia or by the use of an oropharyngeal airway to act as a 'bite-block'.

The end of the tube may become obstructed by abutting against the tracheal wall. The siting of a hole in the tube wall near the tip helps to prevent this problem. An unusual example of this complication involved the use of an Endo-trol tube which has a tip adjustable by a pull-cord. When such a tube was inserted nasally the loop on the pull-cord abutted against the nares causing the tip of the tube to bend and obstruct against the tracheal wall. The problem was solved by cutting the pull-cord [22].

Obstruction by the tube

Kinking of the tube, once a common occurrence with the use of recycled tubes which become old and weakened, is now unusual unless the tube is carelessly inserted so as to cause acute angulation. This can occur when a tube inserted from the right side of the mouth is transferred to the left side without ensuring that the entire tube has been moved to the left of the tongue. Armoured latex tubes offer a degree of protec-tion against kinking but this may still occur between the proximal termination of the spiral reinforcement and the non-reinforced section into which the connector is placed. The cuff may herniate over the distal orifice of the tube resulting in airway obstruction and is a well known hazard. In addition cuff herniation may occur internally and may not be so obvious when the tube is tested prior to use [23].

Obstruction within the tube

Complete or partial blockage can result from blood clot, tissue [24], dried secretions [25], dried tube lubricants [26], loosened parts of a faultily manufactured tube [27] and foreign bodies (including such unlikely articles as in-sects and cigarette tips). Acute obstruction of the tube has been reported after aluminium foil covering a tube during carbon dioxide laser surgery broke loose [28].

A recent report [29] has highlighted the potential hazard of oral premedication where a tablet has been inhaled and later caused tracheal tube blockage.

Airway obstructions may be partial, and so unnoticed, or complete. The signs of tube obstruction are a high inflating pressure, absent or impaired chest excursion, marked inspiratory and expiratory efforts with paradoxical movements in spontaneously breathing patients, accompanied by cyanosis and venous congestion. Lesser degrees of obstruction may go unnoticed.

If airway obstruction is noticed in the intubated patient:
1 Check by direct observation and with a finger that there is no kinking.
2 Check the patency of the tube by passing a suction catheter down it.
3 If still in any doubt change the tube.

Rupture of trachea or bronchus

Rupture of the trachea or a main bronchus is a rare, but very serious, complication of tracheal intubation. Rupture is usually reported posteriorly in the membranous portion, unsupported by cartilaginous bands. The membranous portion is more fragile and less elastic in infants, the elderly and in patients suffering from chronic obstructive airway disease [30].

This complication can usually be traced back to faulty or careless intubation technique. The following factors have been implicated:
1 sharply bevelled tubes or sharp tipped stylets protruding beyond the end of the tube;
2 the use of excessive force or repeated attempts at intubation [30];
3 overinflation of the cuff [31, 32].

Onset of signs of this complication may be delayed some hours such as may occur when the distending force of an overinflated cuff is responsible for airway rupture. Bronchial rupture has been reported in the absence of any trauma or gross airway disease [33]. In one of the few case reports of this complication in neonates, delayed appearance of surgical emphysema resulted in a missed diagnosis and death [34]. More rapid recognition produced a favourable result in another neonate [35].

The clinical diagnosis may be confirmed by a chest radiograph and prompt endoscopy should reveal a tracheal or bronchial tear. Conservative management may suffice but chest drainage and open surgical correction may prove necessary [33].

Aspiration of stomach contents

Silent regurgitation occurs in an appreciable proportion of intubated patients [36] and leakage past the cuff may occur particularly during prolonged intubation. This topic is discussed in more detail in Chapter 4.

Displacement of tube

The tracheal tube may be displaced downwards into one or other main bronchi or upwards into the hypopharynx. Displacement most commonly occurs when there is movement of the head and neck to accommodate the surgical requirements. Therefore particular care should be taken in securing tracheal tubes for head and neck surgery.

Ignition of tube

Since the 1970s, the carbon dioxide laser has become increasingly used for laryngeal surgery. The surgical laser may cause ignition of a tracheal tube, whether made of rubber or plastic, with serious burns of the airways. There have been several reports of fires precipitated in this way [37]. In addition it is possible for a fire to be started from flaming tissues that are being treated [38].

Several methods have been suggested to avoid this bizarre complication of tracheal intubation. A ventilating laryngoscope eliminates the need for a tracheal tube [39] but it is not always convenient or possible. The tube can be wrapped with aluminium foil tape [28], or moistened muslin, or protected by coating the exterior with dental acrylic [40]. However, these precautions have also led to complications by detachment of aluminium foil which may lead to airway obstruction [28] and severe epistaxis from damage by a sharp edge of a foil cover [17]. A flexible jointed metal tracheal tube has been produced [41] which is not yet generally available and a non-flammable plastic tube is under development [37].

Should a fire occur whilst using a laser the damage to the patient will be influenced by the material from which the tube is made. PVC tubes cause more damage and red rubber appears to cause less damage [42].

COMPLICATIONS AT EXTUBATION

Difficult or impossible extubation

Difficulty in removing a tracheal tube at the end of an operation is a rare but alarming experience. The possible causes are failure to deflate the cuff, adhesion of the tube to the tracheal wall due to lack of lubricant [43] or transfixation of the tube by a suture to a nearby organ [44, 45]. A rare instance has been reported of obstruction of the cuff inflating tube by a nasogastric tube [46].

In most cases the cause is failure to deflate the cuff. This can be inadvertently omitted when a patient suddenly regains his reflexes and makes vigorous attempts to expel the tracheal tube. In other cases the cause is failure of the cuff deflating mechanism. A common example of the latter occurs when the cuff inflating tube of an armoured latex tube has been clipped off by an artery forceps, and the walls of the tube remain crimped. Persistent cuff inflation can result in difficulty in extubation.

Inability to deflate a cuff was the cause of difficulty in removing a self-inflatable spongy cuffed (Bivona) tube [47], in which the cuff inflating tube was accidentally pulled out. Using direct laryngoscopy the tube had to be pulled back to the larynx, the point at which the cuff inflating tube had been dislodged identified and deflation then achieved after the insertion of a suitable plastic cannula. If these manoeuvres had failed forceful removal could have damaged the vocal cords. It has been suggested that if attempts to remove a tube with a persistently inflated cuff fail, then deflation of the cuff could be achieved by puncturing the cuff with a needle passed through the cricothyroid membrane [47].

In one case, a Carlens double lumen catheter was accidentally stitched into the airway by a suture extending from the pulmonary artery into the trachea and through the tube wall just above the level of the hook on the Carlens tube. Vigorous attempts to remove the tube resulted in rupture of the pulmonary artery and sudden death of the patient [44].

Another example of accidental fixation of the tube occurred during an operation to reduce fractures of the facial bones. The nasotracheal tube used was accidentally transfixed to the bony structures by a Kirschner wire. Repeated attempts to extubate failed. The tube was removed only after a lengthy and complex additional operation. These authors recommended that whenever the possibility of fixation of the tube during surgery exists, the tube should be moved up and down slightly to ensure that it is not accidentally fixed [45]. A similar problem occurred during fixation of the maxilla using a Kirschner wire even though the tube could be freely moved up and down but at extubation it was discovered that the wire had passed between the tube and the pilot balloon. Extubation was impossible until the pilot tube was cut off [48].

An unusual case involved a rubber tracheal tube which had been repeatedly boiled resulting in a flabby non-elastic cuff [46]. During extubation the loose cuff folded in on itself at its distal attachment thereby causing a valvular obstruction to passage through the vocal cords during extubation. Attempts to remove the tube were only successful after reinsertion, rotation and traction.

Direct laryngoscopy should always be carried out to assess any laryngeal damage if attempts to remove a tracheal tube have been forceful and repeated.

Tracheal collapse

Tracheomalacia can be congenital or secondary (to tumours of the neck and thyroid) and may produce respiratory obstruction only at extubation. Blanc & Tremblay [1] described a case of tracheomalacia in a child with Pott's disease of the spine. Obstruction occurred on removing the tube 4–5 cm from the carina and was corrected by reinserting the tube to within 1–2 cm from the carina.

In such cases extubation must be slow and careful. Should obstruction occur, the tube should be left in place, in a good position, until the lesion can be surgically corrected.

An identical situation is possible in Morquio's disease with malformation of the tracheal cartilages. Such patients should undergo thorough radiological investigation prior to intubation.

Airway obstruction

The most common cause of postextubation airway obstruction is laryngeal spasm. Many methods have been proposed to prevent or treat this complication including extubation in a deep plane of anaesthesia, intravenous lignocaine [49] and intravenous doxapram [50]. In general, airway obstruction due to laryngeal spasm may be treated by applying positive pressure oxygen via a facemask but may require reintubation. Pulmonary oedema following laryngeal spasm has been reported both in children [51] and adults [52].

Other causes of airway obstruction at extubation largely relate to foreign bodies such as throat packs, dentures or blood clot. These require urgent removal to relieve the obstruction.

Aspiration of gastric contents and foreign bodies

Aspiration of stomach contents at extubation may follow passive regurgitation or active vomiting at a time when the protective laryngeal reflexes are still depressed. Regurgitation is more likely to follow a difficult tracheal or oesophageal intubation as there will be gaseous distension of the stomach. The most commonly inhaled foreign bodies are blood clot and secretions though teeth, and dentures may be occasionally inhaled.

The best protection can be obtained by good pharyngeal suction under direct vision followed by extubation in the semi-prone lateral position with head-down tilt.

POST INTUBATION COMPLICATIONS

Early (0–24 h)

Sore throat

This is a common and reasonably benign sequel of tracheal intubation, whose incidence varies between 6% [53] and 90% [54]. However it may not be due entirely to intubation and Conway [55] reported an incidence of 10.2% in patients who had not even been intubated. The use of lubricant on the tube had no effect on the incidence of sore throat [56], though humidification of the inspired gases seemed beneficial. Symptomatic treatment is usually all that is necessary. This topic is dealt with in more detail in Chapter 4.

Damage to hypoglossal or lingual nerves

These rarer sequelae may be due to pressure from a Macintosh laryngoscope blade in the vallecula region behind the tongue. Right sided lingual nerve damage is more common [57, 58] and recovery usually occurs over a few months.

Glottic oedema

Children are the most frequently afflicted by this complication [1]. The oedema may occur in the supraglottic, retroarytenoidal or subglottic regions.

Supraglottic oedema. Oedema commonly occurs in the loose areolar connective tissue on the anterior surface of the epiglottis and aryepiglottic folds. The epiglottis may be squeezed back by the swelling, blocking the glottic aperture on inspiration and hence causing severe respiratory obstruction.

Retroarytenoidal oedema. The submucous connective tissue on the vocal cords is dense and therefore not prone to development of oedema, but it may occur in the loose connective tissue just below the cords and behind the arytenoid cartilages, limiting abduction of the vocal cords on inspiration.

Subglottic oedema. This is most serious and frequently requires urgent reintubation or tracheostomy, especially in infants and children. The degree of severity in the young is from the small internal cross-sectional area of the larynx of the newborn which is no greater than 14 mm^2. A 1 mm thick layer of oedema in the subglottis reduces the opening to 5 mm^2 (35.7% of normal). Expansion outwards is limited by the cricoid cartilage encircling the subglottic region [1]. Moreover, the subglottic region has fragile respiratory epithelium with loose submucosal connective tissue that is easily traumatized and oedema prone.

Glottic oedema persisting beyond 24 h is often associated with more serious permanent lesions.

Vocal cord paralysis

Vocal cord paralysis following tracheal intubation is not a common finding. One or both cords may be paralysed, usually following head and neck surgery where direct or indirect injury to the recurrent laryngeal nerves has occurred. For instance, 19 of 25 cases followed thyroidectomy [5]. However, vocal cord paralysis has occurred unexpectedly after abdominal and other non head and neck surgery [59–61].

In addition to damage to the recurrent laryngeal nerves it is possible to cause lasting voice changes from damage to the external laryngeal nerves. Although more commonly associated with thyroidectomy, permanent voice changes have been reported following intubation in 3% of patients undergoing non-head and neck surgery [62].

Unilateral vocal cord paralysis is the more benign condition. Clinical features are limited to hoarseness, usually immediately postoperatively or soon after. Apparent recovery takes place within a few weeks although laryngoscopy has in some of these cases revealed that partial unilateral cord paralysis of some degree persists, with compensation by the other vocal cord [60].

Bilateral vocal cord paralysis following tracheal intubation is a much more serious condition. The complication has also occurred unexpectedly where surgery was remote from the head and neck [5, 59, 63, 64]. In this situation the cause of the palsy has been attributed to neuropraxia from pressure on the recurrent laryngeal nerve by the cuff of the tracheal tube [64].

Bilateral vocal cord paralysis causes signs of increasing upper airway obstruction which may follow immediately after extubation or be delayed for some hours. The patient particularly has increasing difficulty in vocalizing the letter 'E'. Auscultation over the larynx reveals inspiratory and expiratory vibrations [63]. As the respiratory obstruction progresses stridor appears together with paradoxical respiration and eventually complete obstruction supervenes. The usual methods of relieving respiratory obstruction – extension of the neck, insertion of an oropharyngeal airway or manual protraction of the jaw – do not help. The administration of a steroid, such as dexamethasone, is also ineffective. Obstruction may be relieved by positive pressure ventilation through a facemask. However, the condition is immediately eliminated by re-insertion of a tracheal tube. Laryngoscopy reveals motionless vocal cords which

lie adducted with a very narrow glottic chink (2–3 mm). Most cases of bilateral vocal cord paralysis recover but may take up to 34–36 days. Tracheostomy is often required to tide the patient over this period.

Medium (24–72 h)

Infection

Infection may occur at any point along the route of the tube. This may be minor, little more than an inconvenience to the patient, or may lead to the development of life-threatening abscess formation. Most severe infections, such as retropharyngeal abscess, follow a difficult intubation with mucosal damage. It is known that nasotracheal intubation can be followed by sinusitis [1].

aAirway infection is less common with prolonged tracheal intubation than after tracheostomy although pulmonary infection may still occur secondary to retained secretions.

The treatment of infections from intubation ranges from management of local problems by the use of mouthwashes to the use of parenteral antibiotic therapy.

Late (72 h +)

Laryngeal ulcer, granuloma and polyp

Clausen [65] first reported a polypoid growth of granulation tissue on the vocal cord after tracheal intubation. The incidence is low, from about 1:1000 cases of tracheal anaesthesia [66] to 1:10 000–20 000 [67]. Females are usually affected (80–90%) and no cases have been reported in children.

Granulomata related to tracheal intubation most commonly lie on the posterior third of the vocal process of the arytenoid cartilages [68] and least commonly on the anterior and middle thirds of the vocal process. Less than half the lesions are bilateral.

The aetiology of granulomata is almost certainly due to trauma to a vocal cord. Injury may also result from pressure of the tube when the head and neck are excessively flexed or extended which may explain the high incidence of granuloma following surgery of the head and neck [67] or thyroidectomy [69]. Excessive movement of the tube in the larynx or of the larynx against the tube and allergic reaction to the lubricant are also possible contributing factors.

The development of a granuloma does not seem to be related to the type of tube, the route of intubation, or the duration of intubation [66].

The initial damage is ulceration which usually heals but if there is excessive granulation tissue then a small granulomatous nodule forms, sessile at first and then pedunculated. Rarely, a pedunculated granuloma can cause acute airway obstruction [68].

Granuloma should be suspected if a patient complains of persistent hoarseness more than 1 week postoperatively. Other symptoms include fullness or discomfort in the throat, the feeling of the presence of a foreign body or even pain radiating to the ear.

Although granulomata occur in spite of prophylactic measures, the avoidance of intubation trauma, excessively large tube, extreme positions of the head and neck and excessive movements during intubation would all seem to be worthwhile preventative measures.

Pedunculated granulomata require surgical removal.

Synechia of vocal cords

The posterior third of the vocal cords may stick and fuse together following necrosis of the free edges of the vocal cords. The same may occur with the arytenoid vocal processes, leaving only a small laryngeal aperture [70]. Clinically there is aphonia and respiratory obstruction and with early diagnosis, surgical correction is satisfactory [43].

Laryngotracheal membranes and webs

Laryngeal and subglottic webs were found by Stein in 3 out of 42 postmortems performed on previously intubated patients [1]. The membrane formed may be extensive and occupy some two-thirds of the glottic opening. These sequelae are particularly dangerous as a portion of the membrane may become detached leading to sudden respiratory obstruction. Surgical removal of webs can be difficult, as they epithelialize in continuance with the laryngotracheal mucosa.

Laryngeal fibrosis

This is the gravest of the postintubation sequelae, since surgical correction is limited. Fibrous tissue formation leads to ankylosis of the cricoarytenoid joints, laryngeal stenosis and hence narrowing of the subglottic region. The result is always respiratory obstruction [71]. Symptoms come late (45 to 60 days post extubation) and children are more susceptible than adults [43].

Tracheal fibrosis

A minor area of mucosal insult as a result of excessive cuff pressure or tube tip erosion may be followed by spontaneous resolution, or a devastating sequence of events may produce stenosis, tracheomalacia or even tracheo-oesophageal fistula. The reported incidence of tracheal stenosis following long-term intubation varies from 19% where patients have been studied with tomography [15] to another report of only 1% [70].

A number of factors act alone or together to influence the frequency and severity. These include size of tube relative to the size of the trachea, duration of intubation, shape and composition of the tube and cuff, chemical irritants used in cleaning reusable tubes, movement of the tube in the trachea, inflation pressure of the cuff and intubation trauma. In addition patient factors such as infection, diabetes, anaemia and hypotension may influence the vulnerability of the mucosa [71].

The most frequent single cause is the inflation pressure of the cuff. Cuff pressures in excess of 30 mmHg produce a deficit in capillary perfusion, and this level is often exceeded during shorter and longer term intubation.

In severe cases it may be necessary to resect the affected portion of trachea although this procedure may lead to stitch granuloma formation especially if non-absorbable suture material is used [72]. This may lead to further stenosis. The management of such a restenosis is presented in Chapter 8.

Further details concerning the cuff and its effect on the trachea may be found in Chapter 4.

Stricture of nostril

Long-term nasal intubation may lead to damage

to the alar rim which is followed by fibrosis and stricture formation. In addition necrosis can occur to the nasal septum leading to fistula formation. Stricture of the nostril may cause airway problems in small children.

REFERENCES

1 Blanc VF & Tremblay NAG (1974) The complications of tracheal intubation. A new classification with a review of the literature. *Anesth Analg* 53:202.

2 Wolfson B (1958) Minor laryngeal sequelae from endotracheal intubation. *Br J Anaesth* 30:326.

3 Howland WS & Lewis JS (1965) Post intubation granulomas of the larynx. *Cancer* 9:1244.

4 Capistrano-Baruh E, Wenig B, Steinberg L, Stegnjajic A & Baruh S (1982) Laryngeal web: a cause of difficult endotracheal intubation. *Anesthesiology* 57:123.

5 Gorman JB & Woodward FD (1965) Bilateral paralysis of the vocal cords. *South Med J* 58:34.

6 Halac E, Indiveri DR, Obregon RJ, Begue E & Casanas M (1983) Complication of nasal endotracheal intubation. *J Pediatr* 103:166.

7 Stetson JB & Guess WL (1970) Causes of damage to tissues by polymers and elastomers used in the fabrication of tracheal devices. *Anesthesiology* 33:635.

8 Jones GOM, Hale DE, Wasmuth CE, Homi J, Smith ER & Biljoen J (1968) A survey of acute complications associated with endotracheal intubation. *Cleve Clin Q* 35:23.

9 Binning R (1974) A hazard of blind nasal intubation. *Anaesthesia* 29:366.

10 Dripps RD, Eckenhoff JE & Vandam LD (1979) *Introduction to Anesthesia. The Principles of Safe Practice* 5th ed. W.B. Saunders, Philadelphia.

11 Kambic V & Radsel Z (1978) Intubation lesions of larynx. *Br J Anaesth* 50:587.

12 Peppard SB & Dickens JH (1983) Laryngeal injury following short-term intubation. *Ann Otol Rhinol Laryngol* 92:327.

13 Paparella MM & Shumrick DA (1973) *Otolaryngology*, Vol. 13. W.B. Saunders, Philadelphia.

14 Wright RB & Manfield FF (1974) Damage to teeth during the administration of general anesthesia. *Anesth Analg* 53:405.

15 Stauffer JL, Olson DE & Petty TL (1981) Complications and consequences of endotracheal intubation and tracheostomy: a prospective study of 150 critically ill adult patients. *Am J Med.* 70:65.

16 Scamman FL & Babin RW (1983) An unusual complication of nasotracheal intubation. *Anesthesiology* 59:352.

17 Brightwell AP (1983) A complication of the use of the laser in ENT surgery. *J. Laryngol Otol.* 97:671.

18 Vellacott WN (1962) Nasal intubation: some postnasal obstructions and how they may be overcome. *Br J Anaesth* 34:115.

19 Majumdar B, Stevens RW & Obara LG (1982) Retropharyngeal abscess following tracheal intubation. *Anaesthesia* 37:67.

20 Horrelou MF, Mathe D & Feiss P (1978) A hazard of nasotracheal intubation. *Anaesthesia* 33:73.

21 McTaggart RA, Shustack A, Noseworthy T & Johnston R (1983) Another cause of obstruction in an armoured endotracheal tube. *Anesthesiology* 59:164.

22 Glinsman D & Pavlin EG (1982) Airway obstruction after nasal tracheal intubation. *Anesthesiology* 56:229.

23 Famewo CE (1983) A not so apparent cause of intraluminal tracheal tube obstruction. *Anesthesiology* 58:593.

24 Barat G, Ascorve A & Avello F (1976) Unusual airway obstruction during pneumonectomy. *Anaesthesia* 31:1290.

25 Torres LE & Reynolds RC (1980) A complication of use of a microlaryngeal surgery endotracheal tube. *Anesthesiology* 53:355.

26 Uehira A, Tanaka A, Oda M & Sato T (1981) Obstruction of an endotracheal tube by lidocaine jelly. *Anesthesiology* 55:598.

27 Harrington JF (1984) An unusual cause of endotracheal tube obstruction. *Anesthesiology* 61:116.

28 Kaeder CS & Hirshman CA (1979) Acute airway obstruction: a complication of aluminium tape wrapping of tracheal tubes in laser surgery. *Can Anaesth Soc J* 26:138.

29 Ehrenpreis MB & Oliverio RM (1984) Endotracheal tube obstruction secondary to oral preoperative medication. *Anesth Analg* 63:867.

30 Thompson DS & Read RC (1968) Rupture of the trachea following endotracheal intubation. *JAMA* 204:995.

31 Tornvall SS, Jackson KH & Oyanedel ET (1971) Tracheal rupture, complications of cuffed endotracheal tube. *Chest* 59:237.

32 Smith BAC & Hopkinson RB (1984) Tracheal rupture during anaesthesia. *Anaesthesia* 39:894.

33 Patel KD, Palmer SK & Phillips MF (1979) Mainstem bronchial rupture during general anesthesia. *Anesth Analg* 58:59.

34 Serlin SP & Daily WJR (1975) Tracheal perforation in the neonate: a complication of endotracheal intubation. *J Pediatr* 86:596.

35 Finer NN & Stewart AR (1976) Tracheal perforation in the neonate: treatment with a cuffed endotracheal tube. *J Pediatr* 89:510.

36 Blitt CD, Gutman HL, Cohen DD, Weisman H & Dillon JB. 'Silent' regurgitation and aspiration with general anesthesia. *Anesth Analg* 49:707.

37 Wainwright AC, Moody RA & Carruth JA (1981) Anaesthetic safety with the carbon dioxide laser. *Anaesthesia* 36:411.

38 Hirshman CA & Smith J (1980) Indirect ignition of the endotracheal tube during carbon dioxide laser surgery. *Arch Otolaryngol* 106:639.

39 Oulton JL & Donald DM (1971) A ventilating laryngoscope. *Anesthesiology* 35:540.

40 Kumar A & Frost E (1981) Prevention of fire hazard during laser microsurgery. *Anesthesiology* 54:350.

41 Norton ML & Devos P (1978) New endotracheal tube for laser surgery of the larynx. *Ann Otol Rhinol Laryngol* 87:554.

42 Ossoff RH, Eisenman TS, Duncavage JA & Karlan MS (1983) Comparison of tracheal damage from laser-ignited endotracheal tube fires. *Ann Otol Rhinol Laryngol* 92:333.

43 Debain JJ, LeBrigand H & Binet JB (1968) Quelques incidents et accidents de l'intubation tracheale prolongue. *Ann Otolaryngol Chir Cervicofac* 85:379.

44 Dryden GE (1977) Circulatory collapse after pneumonectomy (an unusual complication from the use of a Carlens catheter): case report. *Anesth Analg* 56:451.

45 Lee C, Schwartz S & Mok MS (1977) Difficult extubation due to transfixation of a nasotracheal tube by a Kirschner wire. *Anesthesiology* 46:427.

46 Lall NG (1980) Difficult extubation. *Anaesthesia* 35:500.

47 Tavakoli M & Corssen G (1976) An unusual case of difficult extubation. *Anesthesiology* 45:552.

48 Hilley MD, Henderson RB & Giesecke AH (1983) Difficult extubation of the trachea. *Anesthesiology* 59:149.

49 Gefke K, Andersen LW & Friesel E (1983) Lidocaine given intravenously as a suppressant of cough and laryngospasm in connection with extubation after tonsillectomy. *Acta Anaesthesiol Scand* 27:111.

50 Owen H (1982) Post extubation laryngospasm abolished by doxapram. *Anaesthesia* 37:1112.

51 Lee KWT & Downes JJ (1983) Pulmonary edema secondary to laryngospasm in children. *Anesthesiology* 59:347.

52 Melnick BM (1984) Postlaryngospasm pulmonary edema in adults. *Anesthesiology* 60:516.

53 Hartsell CJ & Stephen CR (1964) Incidence of sore throat following endotracheal intubation. *Can Anaesth Soc J* 11:307.

54 Loeser EA, Stanley TH, Jordan W & Machin R (1980) Postoperative sore throat: influence of tracheal tube lubrication versus cuff design. *Can Anaesth Soc J* 27:156.

55 Conway CM, Miller JS & Sugden FLH (1960) Sore throat after anaesthesia. *Br J Anaesth* 32:219.

56 Stock M & Downs JB (1982) Lubrication of tracheal tubes to prevent sore throat from intubation. *Anesthesiology* 57:418.

57 Loughman E (1983) Lingual nerve injury following tracheal intubation. *Anaesth Intensive Care* 11:171.

58 Jones BC (1971) Lingual nerve injury: a complication of intubation. *Br J Anaesth* 43:730.

59 Yamashita T, Harada Y & Ueda N (1965) Recurrent laryngeal nerve paralysis associated with endotracheal anesthesia. *Nippon Jibiinkoka Gakkai Kaiho* 68:1452.

60 Hahn FW, Martin JT & Lillie JC (1970) Vocal cord paralysis with endotracheal intubation. *Arch Otolaryngol* 92:226.

61 Cox RH & Welborn SG (1981) Vocal cord paralysis after endotracheal anesthesia. *South Med J* 74:1258.

62 Kark AE, Kissen MW, Auerbach R & Meikle M (1984) Voice changes after thyroidectomy: role of the external laryngeal nerve. *Br Med J* 289:1412.

63 Holley HS & Gildea JE (1971) Vocal cord paralysis after tracheal intubation. *JAMA* 215:278.

64 Gibbin KP & Eggiston MJ (1981) Bilateral vocal cord paralysis following endotracheal intubation. *Br J Anaesth* 53:1091.

65 Clausen RJ (1932) Unusual sequelae of tracheal intubation. *Proc Roy Soc Med* 25:1507.

66 Howland WS & Lewis JS (1965) Post intubation granulomas of the larynx. *Cancer* 9:1244.

67 Snow JC, Harano M & Balogh K (1966) Post intubation granuloma of the larynx. *Anesth Analg* 45:425.

68 Balestrieri F & Watson CB (1982) Intubation granuloma. *Otolaryngol Clin North Am* 15:567.

69 Campkin V (1959) Postintubation ulcer of the larynx. *Br J Anaesth* 31:561.

70 Lindolm DE (1969) Prolonged endotracheal intubation (a clinical investigation with specific reference to its consequences for the larynx and the trachea and to its place as an alternative to intubation through a tracheostomy). *Acta Anaesthesiol Scand* (Suppl) 33.

71 Keane WM, Denneny JC, Rowe LD & Atkins JP (1982) Complications of intubation. *Ann Otol Rhinol Laryngol* 91:584.

72 Grillo HC (1979) Surgical treatment of postintubation tracheal injuries. *J Thorac Cardiovasc Surg* 78:860.

CHAPTER 4 **The cuff**

Functions of the cuff

The inflatable cuff has two main functions. It should seal the airway thus preventing aspiration of pharyngeal contents into the trachea and it should ensure that there are no leaks past the cuff during positive pressure ventilation. At the same time the pressure exerted by the inflated cuff on the trachea should not be so high that capillary circulation is compromised. A 'high' cuff pressure prevents aspiration into the trachea and ventilatory leaks but can result in tracheal damage; a 'low' cuff pressure minimizes tracheal damage but may result in aspiration past the cuff. The ability to meet these conflicting requirements depends both on the design and the management of the cuff. The early thick walled rubber cuffs frequently caused major trauma when used for more than a few hours. Modern plastic cuffs with thin walls and high volume, low pressure characteristics can if properly managed provide an adequate seal without significant tracheal damage. However there is room for improvement both in cuff design and the accurate control of cuff pressures.

Early tracheal tubes did not have cuffs and a throat pack was used both to prevent aspiration and also to ensure relatively leak free positive pressure ventilation. Young children are commonly managed with uncuffed tubes but this can result in a high incidence of silent aspiration. Ten out of thirteen such children who were being ventilated showed evidence of silent tracheal aspiration 10 min after dye had been placed on the back of the tongue [114].

History

The development of cuffed tubes is closely linked with the development of tracheal tubes and the associated anaesthetic techniques [1].

In 1871 Friedrich Trendelenburg described a tube which was inserted into the trachea through a tracheostomy [2] (Fig. 1). The tube

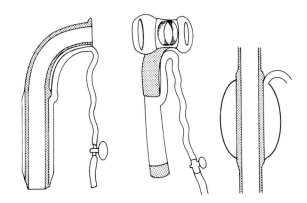

Fig. 1 Trendelenburg's Cuff catheter which was inserted through a tracheostomy. After Trendelenburg [2].

had a small, thick-walled, low volume, inflatable rubber cuff which made watertight contact with the tracheal wall. This tube was widely used for clinical anaesthesia during the last three decades of the 19th century [1]. In 1880, William Macewen, a Glasgow surgeon, sought an alternative to Trendelenburg's tracheostomy tube and described the use of a tracheal tube passed blindly through the mouth [3]. This tube was used to relieve airway obstruction as well as for anaesthesia and was introduced in conscious patients without the use of local anaesthesia. The technique employed manual palpation in the throat. A finger depressed the epiglottis onto the tongue and the tube was guided over the back of the finger into the larynx. A sponge was then placed at the upper end of the larynx to prevent aspiration of blood. In 1893 Eisenmenger in Vienna described the first tracheal tube with an inflatable high volume cuff [4]. A large pilot balloon signalled the tension in the cuff and intracuff pressure could be limited. In 1910, Dorrance described a tube with an inflatable cuff similar to those in use today (Fig. 2). In 1921, Rowbotham & Magill reported their experience with tracheal anaesthesia using to-and-fro breathing through uncuffed rubber tubes in managing cases for head

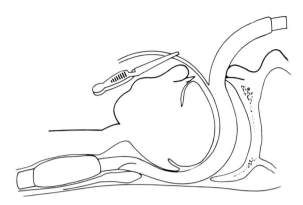

Fig. 2 Dorrance's cuffed catheter with cuff inflated. After Dorrance [8].

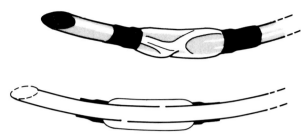

Fig. 3 Self inflating cuff described by Macintosh in 1943. Redrawn from Macintosh [9], with kind permission of the author and the *British Medical Journal*.

and neck surgery [5]. In 1930, Magill published a description of his experience with blind nasal intubation using uncuffed curved soft rubber catheters [6]. The pharynx was packed with gauze both to reduce the risk of aspiration past the uncuffed catheter and to help obtain a gas tight fit.

In 1928, Guedel & Waters described a cuffed tracheal tube designed for closed circuit intra-tracheal administration of anaesthesia using a carbon dioxide absorption technique [7]. This tube was similar to the earlier cuffed tube described by Dorrance [8]. It had a thin rubber cuff, 1½ inches long and with a diameter of ⅝ of an inch when the rubber was just starting to stretch. The cuff was cemented to the tube. When deflated the rubber cuff lay in folds close to the catheter wall. They showed the effective-ness of the cuff in preventing aspiration in a dog anaesthetized with ethylene which survived total immersion in water for 1 h. The cuffed tube was then tested in two patients whose mouths and noses were filled with water. Only a very small drop in the level of the water was observed at the end of 5 min [7]. In 1943, Macintosh described a tube with a self inflating cuff designed by Mushin [9] (Fig. 3). This cuff facilitated controlled ventilation for thoracic anaesthesia. Holes were cut in the tube under-neath the cuff. The cuff thus inflated only on inspiration. The holes, however, sometimes became blocked by plugs of mucus.

Although the first cuffed tracheal tube had been described in 1893 non-cuffed tubes were more commonly used until the 1950s. In 1952 during the polio epidemic in Copenhagen cuffed tubes were used [10, 11]. After that

experience it became standard clinical practice to use cuffed tubes during anaesthesia. The use of plain tubes is now largely restricted to children and neonates.

Early tubes were made of red rubber with rigid thick walled cuffs and high cuff and tracheal wall pressures were required to effect a seal. When these cuffed tubes were left in situ for long periods it soon became apparent that major complications could result from the high pressure exerted on the tracheal wall. Increased understanding of cuff related tracheal patholo-gy has led to improved design of cuffs and techniques for limiting intracuff pressure.

An important development was the introduc-tion of disposable plastic tubes which are increasingly being used in preference to rubber tubes. Several reasons support this trend. The high pressure on the tracheal wall that can occur with the use of rubber cuffs is undesirable. The cuffs of red rubber tubes frequently inflate eccentrically resulting in the tip being pushed against the tracheal wall introducing the risk of distal tracheal erosion. Rubber can release toxins and irritants resulting in allergic reactions especially when used long-term. There is also the potential hazard of cross infection associ-ated with repeated sterilization. Finally rubber deteriorates on repeated autoclaves.

Manufacturers are continually improving and refining the design of plastic cuffs. There has been a move towards high volume, low pressure cuffs for long-term use. One design objective here is to eliminate wrinkles which can occur in these sometimes bulky cuffs. It is important to recognize however that any cuff, even a so called low pressure cuff, can be overfilled in vivo resulting in high intracuff and tracheal wall pressures. Even 'ideal' cuffs require careful management.

Position of the cuff and the tip of the tracheal tube

Malposition of a tracheal tube can result in an increase both in morbidity and mortality especially in those patients in respiratory failure [12]. The position of the cuff and tube tip are therefore often identified with a chest X-ray in patients in the intensive care unit. In critically ill patients endobronchial intubation is particularly harmful; the potential for intubation of the right main bronchus is clearly increased, if long uncut tubes are used. An alternative less commonly used method is to assess the position of the tip of the tube in relation to the carina with a fibreoptic laryngoscope [13].

Such precautions are not usually taken to confirm the proper placement of a tube during general anaesthesia. The cuff is usually seen passing through the cords at intubation and can then easily be placed in the required position. In one study it was shown that the distance from the cricothyroid membrane to the carina was approximately 11 cm and from the vocal cords to the cricothyroid membrane was 1 cm [14]. Their tracheal tube measured 5.5 cm from the proximal end of the cuff to the tip. Thus if the proximal end of the cuff was placed 1 cm below the cords the tip of the tube was approximately 5 cm from the carina.

On rare occasions, however, the tube is not seen passing through the cords at induction of anaesthesia and there is doubt about the length of tube in the trachea. Under these circumstances a chest radiograph enables the position of the tube to be determined accurately. It is important to auscultate the chest to confirm that there is bilateral air entry and that the tip of the tube is not in the right main bronchus; it is well known however that, although usually unequivocal, this technique can be misleading [15]. Difficulty may be encountered in patients with limited chest movement or quiet breath sounds. In these circumstances it is important also to listen over the trachea and left hypogastrium. A case was reported in which intubation of the right main bronchus resulting in massive atelectasis did not give rise to cyanosis, tachycardia or other changes in vital signs during general anaesthesia [15].

Fluid can accumulate in the trachea above the cuff of a tube. Pharyngeal suction may not remove this fluid and aspiration may occur when the cuff is deflated. To prevent this it has been recommended that the inflated cuff be withdrawn until resistance is felt which signals that the upper end of the cuff is impinging on the lower surface of the vocal cords [16]. The patient is extubated in a 10° head down position and aspiration is performed through the tube before removal. In the United States, where the use of uncut disposable tracheal tubes is routine, in some centres it is common practice to withdraw the tube to the cords. If the upper end of the cuff impinges on the vocal cords however, pressure damage could result. On occasions part of the cuff may be positioned above the cords. This is most likely to occur when the cords cannot be seen at intubation and the tube is too short.

A number of alternative methods are available for checking the position of the tube in the trachea. The trachea can be palpated between the suprasternal notch and the cricoid cartilage and the distension of the trachea may be felt when the cuff is rapidly inflated [14]; alternatively, the filled pilot balloon can be lightly palpated and an increase in pressure should be detected in the balloon on applying pressure over the trachea at the site of the cuff [17]. A less desirable method of tube placement in adults is deliberately to intubate the right main branches and then to withdraw the tube 1–2 cm above the position at which bilateral air sounds are first heard [18]. An electromagnetic sensing device has also been described but this is not commercially available [19]. This allows detection of a foil marker band fixed into the tracheal tube at the level of the proximal cuff junction. The accuracy of the method was confirmed by comparing assumed placement with the method with the position of the tube assessed on a chest radiograph.

It is important to remember that the cuff and tip of a tube may move both in adults and children if the neck is flexed or extended [20]. Tracheal tube movement can therefore result in inadvertent endobronchial intubation on neck flexion and extubation on neck extension. With nasotracheal tubes in adults an average of 1.5 cm movement towards the carina occurred with neck flexion and 1.5 cm away from the carina with neck extension. The maximum movement observed away from the carina was 3.5 cm and towards the carina was 2.9 cm. Such movements of the cuff may also result in trauma to the tracheal epithelium. To minimize the risk both of extubation and accidental bronchial intubation associated with head movement it has been recommended that the cuff should be placed in the middle third of the trachea [20].

In normal practice for the adult the tube is cut to an appropriate length and the cuff is placed under direct vision 1–2 cm below the cords. If the tube is not seen passing through the cords other techniques may be required.

Cuff inflation

It is common clinical practice to inflate the cuff slowly until no leak is audible while applying positive pressure to the airway. It has been recommended that the pressure in large volume cuffs should be measured during inflation with an in line pressure gauge [41]. This should help to keep the cuff pressure within safe limits. However, it is not always possible with high volume cuffs to determine accurately the exact seal point. It has been suggested that it would be more practical to inflate large volume cuffs to a fixed pressure of 25–30 cm regardless of the cuff volume [105]. It is always essential to avoid overfilling the cuff. If the cuff is inflated by an impatient and unskilled assistant then it is common for the cuff to be inflated well past the seal point with resulting high pressures on the tracheal mucosa. Care and time should be taken during cuff inflation which should preferably be undertaken by the anaesthetist.

Tracheal wall pressures: method of measurement

Many methods have been described for measuring the lateral pressure exerted by the cuff on the tracheal wall. No single method is entirely satisfactory [26]. Indirect methods have been described for calculating the pressure exerted by tracheal cuffs on the tracheal wall [21, 22], although some of the assumptions made in the calculations have been questioned [23]. In an in vitro study Cross [24] stated that

$$P_{ic} = P_{tw} + P_{f(d,s)}$$

where P_{ic} = intracuff pressure,
P_{tw} = tracheal wall pressure
and $P_{f(d,s)}$ = a pressure which is a function of the cuff diameter (d) and the stiffness of the cuff material (s).

Therefore, if the cuff pressure is monitored the pressure on the tracheal wall will always be less than or equal to this easily measured value. If $P_{f(d,s)}$ is very low then pressure in the cuff approximates to the pressure on the tracheal wall.

Another in vitro method [28] involved inflating the cuff with a measured volume of air and measuring the cuff pressure (P_1); the cuff pressure was then measured in a model trachea when the cuff was inflated with the same volume of air (P_2). The pressure exerted on the model tracheal wall (P) was calculated from the formula:

$$P = P_2 - P_1$$

However, in a more detailed study of tracheal pressure in vitro with both high and low volume cuffs it was shown that this formula was not always correct [23]. There was a large difference between the measured tracheal wall pressure and the calculated tracheal wall pressure in some instances.

For direct measurement transducers have been implanted in a model trachea, in the tracheal wall in animals and in the excised human trachea [25–27]. Pressures on the trachea have also been measured in vivo with small balloons lying between the cuff of the tube and the tracheal wall [29, 30]. The mean pressure on the anterior tracheal wall at seal volume of the cuff (leak free ventilation) was 38 mmHg (range 24–68 mmHg) in 11 patients [29]. Latex armoured tracheal tubes were used. In another five patients the mean pressure was found to be 40.8 mmHg on the anterior tracheal wall and 27.2 mmHg on the posterior tracheal wall. Thus, in the normal head position the pressure on the anterior tracheal wall is greater than that on the posterior tracheal wall. This is because the membranous posterior tracheal wall is more distensible than the cartilaginous anterolateral portion. In the same study three patients were positioned with the head extended and the mean anterior and posterior wall pressures were 51 and 59 mmHg respectively; thus the difference in pressure was reduced and even reversed in some patients. In this position the vertebral column gives extra support to the posterior trachea. The pressures exerted on the tracheal wall became higher as patients recovered consciousness possibly due to increased muscle tone. The higher anterior

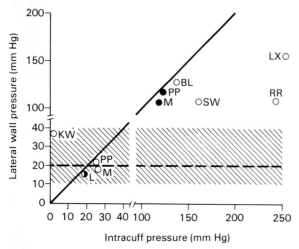

Fig. 4 Lateral wall pressure plotted against intracuff pressure during *in vitro* evaluation of tracheal tubes. Dashed line represents mean capillary pressure and shaded area theoretical limits of venous capillary pressure. ○ Tubes at seal-point pressure. ● Tubes inflated 5 ml beyond seal point. ◖ Lanz tubes at seal point and over inflated by 20 and 40 ml. BL = Portex blue line; PP = Portex profile; M = Mallinckrodt; L = Lanz; KW = Kamen-Wilkinson; RR = Red rubber; LX = Armoured latex; SW = Soft way. Modified from Leigh and Maynard [30], with kind permission of the authors and the *British Medical Journal*.

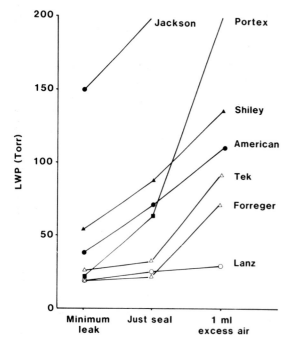

Fig. 5 Lateral tracheal wall pressure with different tracheostomy tubes and three different inflation points. From Wu et al [26], with kind permission of the authors and the publishers. © 1973 The Williams & Wilkins Co., Baltimore.

tracheal wall pressure explains why cuff related tracheal damage is most severe over the anterior trachea [31].

A number of authors have studied the pressure exerted on the tracheal wall with different tracheal tubes [23, 26, 27, 30]. A wide range of tracheal pressures have been reported with different tubes and slightly different experimental designs. Lateral tracheal pressures at airway seal varied with different tubes from 26 to 240 mmHg [26] in a model trachea, from 15 to 160 mmHg [30] in another model trachea (Fig. 4) and from 30 to 205 mmHg [27] in a dog. It is clear therefore that the design of the cuff is of paramount importance in limiting the pressure exerted on the tracheal wall. Cuff management is also important because inflation with as little as 1 ml of air after the seal point can result in potentially damaging increases in lateral wall pressure [26] (Fig. 5).

Intralaryngeal pressure exerted by tracheal tubes

Although major emphasis has been placed on tracheal trauma caused by the cuff the tube can exert considerable pressure on the larynx which can result in severe pathology [32]. Prolonged intubation can give rise to a varying amount of posterior glottic stenosis [33, 34]. Indeed the commonest cause of such stenosis is prolonged intubation [33]. The pressure exerted by tubes on the posterior glottis was quantified in dogs [32]. In three dogs pressures of 75–400 mmHg (often grossly in excess of capillary perfusion pressure) were exerted on the posterolateral portion of the larynx. Both the area of pressure and the extent of trauma is greater with a large diameter tube. It has therefore been recommended that the smallest tube compatible with acceptable ventilation should be used to minimize trauma to the posterolateral larynx [32, 35].

The conventional tube exerts forces on the airway due to its elastic recoil which can result in tracheal and laryngeal trauma [116] (Fig. 6). Such damage can be limited by the use of oral or nasal Lindholm tubes which conform to the lateral contours of the airway [106–110] (Fig. 7). Preliminary results with these tubes in a multicentre intensive care study indicate less severe lesions in the posterior subglottic and cuff areas during prolonged intubation [111].

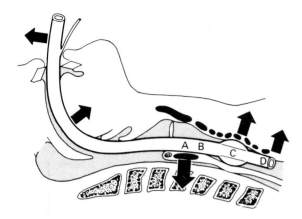

Fig. 6 Forces on airway. Arrows indicate forces acting to restore an elastic tracheal tube to its original shape when inserted into the patient's airway. A. Inner posterior part of larynx. B. Cricoid ring level which constitutes narrowest part of the airway. C. Cuff site. D. Tube tip. From Lindholm [116], with kind permission of the author and the editor of *Laekartidningen*.

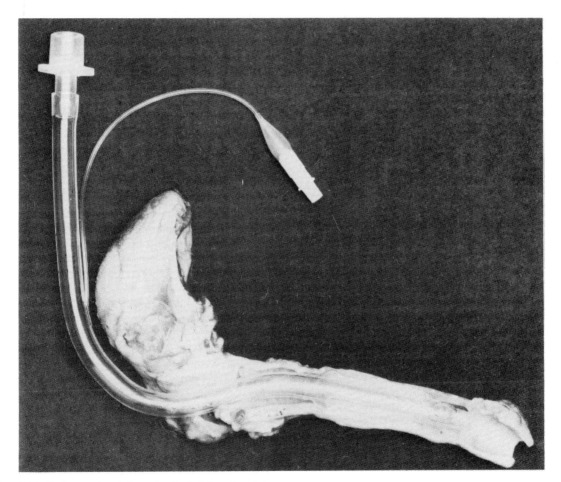

Fig. 7 Lindholm anatomical orotracheal tube placed in autopsy specimen of tongue–larynx–trachea from a young woman. From Lindholm and Grenvik [108], with kind permission of the authors and the publisher, Churchill Livingstone.

Control of tracheal wall pressure for long-term intubation

In two patients on artificial ventilation one with a Lanz tube and one with a red rubber tube both inflated to the seal point the pressures on the tracheal wall were 17 and 87 mmHg with intracuff pressures of 19 and 225 mmHg respectively [30]. A Lanz tube has a pressure regulating mechanism which prevents both excessive rise and fall in cuff and tracheal wall pressures (Figs 8a and b). This mechanism clearly must be used with a cuff capable of effecting a seal at the pressure fixed by the regulator. The pressures exerted on the tracheal wall by the cuffs were measured with a small balloon inserted between the cuff and the tracheal wall [30]. It was suggested that the use of the Lanz tube should be obligatory for all patients requiring long-term ventilation. Furthermore, although similar control of wall pressure was thought desirable during routine (short duration) anaesthesia financial constraints would clearly restrict the use of Lanz tubes on such a large scale. Measurements in vitro using eight different commonly used tubes showed that only three tubes (Lanz, Portex Profile and Mallinckrodt) were able to effect a seal with lateral wall pressures of less than 30 mmHg [30] (Fig. 4). In four of these types of tubes the lateral

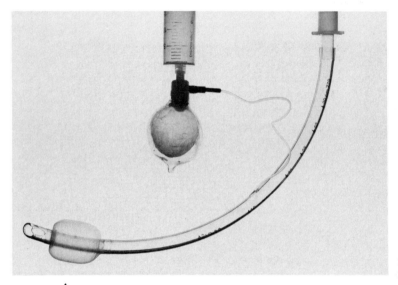

Fig. 8(a) Lanz tube with cuff and balloon inflated.

(a)

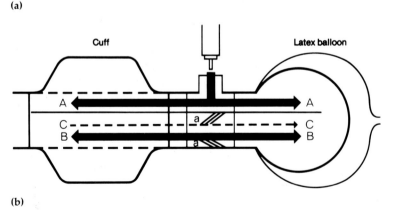

(b)

Fig. 8(b) The Lanz tube valve. A: A syringe is inserted into the Lanz valve and approximately 30 ml air is injected. The syringe is then removed. A cuff pressure not exceeding 25 mmHg is automatically provided. B: The valve system automatically keeps the cuff pressure below 25 mmHg for the duration of intubation. C: A special valve mechanism (a) regulates the speed of pressure release from the cuff to the latex balloon. The thin latex balloon expands and contracts within the operating range with no change in internal pressure. If the tracheal cuff pressure exceeds the balloon pressure the balloon expands and controls the cuff pressure. If the cuff pressure falls the balloon contracts forcing volume into the cuff maintaining a low pressure seal.

wall pressures at the seal point were greater than 100 mmHg including one in which the pressure was approximately 160 mmHg.

Long-term intubation practice in the United Kingdom

A postal questionnaire was used to determine the long-term intubation practice of members of the Intensive Care Society in the United Kingdom [112]. A mixture of tracheal cuffs had been in use; approximately 60% high volume, 25% intermediate volume and 10% low volume cuffs. The cuffs were generally inflated to no leak ventilation; cuff pressures were measured in only 17% of cases. The general policy of different units was to leave tubes in situ for periods ranging from less than 3 to more than 21 days before doing a tracheostomy. In 50% of cases a tracheostomy was done between 7 and 14 days. With proper control of cuff pressures and improved design of cuffs and tube shape the safety of long-term oral or nasotracheal intubation should be increased.

Ratio of cuff and tracheal diameters and tracheal wall pressure

An in vitro study was performed with a number of different makes of tubes and cuff sizes in an artificial trachea built with an elastic posterior wall to simulate the human trachea [36].

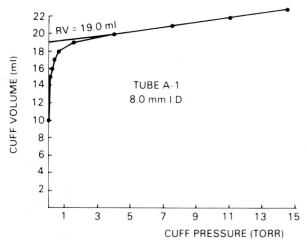

Fig. 9 Graphic extrapolation method for determining the residual volume of a cuff. From Tonnesen et al [36], with kind permission of the authors, the editor of *Anesthesiology*, and the publishers, J.B. Lippincott Co.

Residual volumes (RVs) were first obtained from cuff pressure volume graphs (Fig. 9). There were large differences between residual volumes of different makes of tubes and a trend towards an increase in volume with increased tube size. Residual volumes ranged from 1.8 to 27.3 ml. The seal volumes (SV = the volume preventing aspiration of water), the cuff pressures at SV, and the wall pressures were then measured in the model trachea. For tubes with a sealing volume/residual volume ratio (SV/RV) of 1 and over the ratio correlated with the wall pressures at seal point (Fig. 10). Thirty-seven

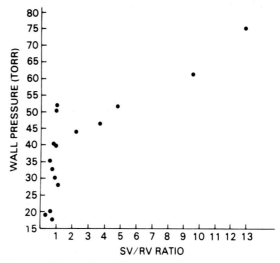

Fig. 10 Relationship between sealing volume/residual volume ratio and wall pressure at which a water tight seal was effected. Each point represents the mean value of nine or ten tubes for each brand and size. From Tonnesen et al [36], with kind permission of the authors, the editor of *Anesthesiology*, and the publishers, J.B. Lippincott Co.

per cent of tubes with an SV/RV ratio of one or less achieved a water tight seal at wall pressures of less than 35 mmHg. It is likely that the higher wall pressures (up to 52 mmHg) required to effect a seal in the other tubes with a SV/RV ratio less than one resulted from the extra pressure required to obliterate wrinkles formed in the large volume cuffs. In tubes with SV/RV ratio less than one, wall pressure and cuff pressure was very nearly identical (Fig. 11). In tubes with a SV/RV ratio greater than 1 however the cuff pressure was greater than the wall pressure. The wall pressure was greater with a small volume than a large volume cuff. It was concluded that the cuff should effect a seal

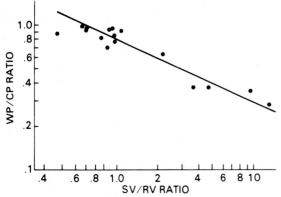

Fig. 11 Relationship (log vs log) between the seal volume/residual volume ratio and the wall pressure/cuff pressure ratio. The lower the SV/RV ratio the more closely the cuff pressure represents wall pressure. From Tonnesen et al [36], with kind permission of the authors, the editor of *Anesthesiology*, and the publishers, J.B. Lippincott Co.

before being filled to residual volume. A residual volume of more than 12 ml was required to effect a seal at low wall pressure in the model tested.

In clinical circumstances measurement of cuff pressure was considered valuable because cuff pressure always exceeded wall pressure. If a seal can be effected at a cuff pressure of 25 mmHg or less, then the risk of serious tracheal damage is minimized [40, 41]. Cuff and wall pressure difference increased as the residual volume of the cuff became smaller. The final pressure on the tracheal wall at the seal point was always higher with low rather than with high volume cuffs.

Cuff stiffness and tracheal wall pressure

Low pressure high volume cuffs have compliant walls and can adapt to the tracheal contour without deforming the shape of the trachea [37] (Fig. 12). In contrast stiff walled low volume cuffs deform the normal tracheal contours. In consequence such cuffs exert more pressure on the tracheal walls [27]. As the cuff is inflated it first touches the trachea at the narrowest point at that level. The areas in contact are subject to increasing pressure as the cuff is inflated. Cuff compliance is particularly important if the trachea constricts or becomes more rigid in vivo under autonomic control [38].

In 1969 when rigid cuffs were used routinely Geffin & Pontoppidan attempted to minimize tracheal distortion and damage by prestretching cuffs in a warm water bath with 20–30 ml air [39]. This effectively converted the early low volume into high volume cuffs. Following the introduction of the technique in the respiratory unit no patient developed respiratory obstruction following decannulation. Tracheal stenosis and respiratory obstruction were not uncommon however before introduction of the manoeuvre. With improvements in cuff design however, prestretching of cuffs is no longer required.

Pressure and tracheal blood flow

The blood flow in the mucosa of the rabbit's trachea has been investigated using isotope

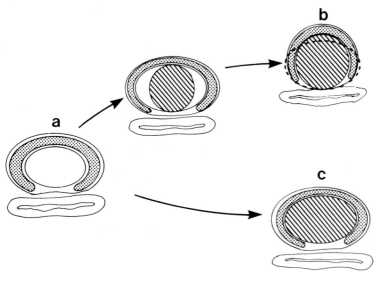

Fig. 12 The trachea and the cuff. (a) Normal trachea and oesophagus. (b) High pressure cuff distorts the trachea and makes the tracheal contour the same as the shape of the cuff. (c) Soft low pressure cuff conforms to the normal tracheal lumen. From Cooper and Grillo [37], with kind permission of the editor of *Chest*.

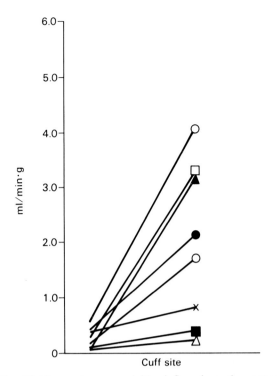

Fig. 13 Change in mucosal blood flow from the resting condition to the condition after insertion of the tracheal tube (with fixed cardiac output) but with no inflation of the cuff. (The symbols refer to individual animals.) From Nordin et al [40], with kind permission of the editor of *Acta Anaesthesiologica Scandinavica*.

labelled microspheres before and after insertion of a high volume cuffed tracheal tube [40]. The resting blood flow was 0.3 ml/min/g tissue which is about 60% of cerebral blood flow. Insertion of a tracheal tube with the cuff deflated surprisingly increased blood flow to approximately 10 times the control value (Fig. 13). This was thought to be due to release of histamine-like substances which decreased arteriolar tone. If the cuff of the tube was then inflated there was a linear decrease in blood flow so that there was virtually no flow at a cuff pressure of 80–120 mmHg (approximately arterial pressure). Nordin and his colleagues believed that pressure gradients exist and that initially as the cuff is inflated the flow to the mucosa over the cartilages is decreased and there is reactive hyperaemia between the cartilages [40]. The initial decrease in mucosal flow resulted from this phenomenon and there was a later flow reduction in the areas between the cartilages. With an ideal large diameter cuff the capillary perfusion decreases at pressures above 30 mmHg but does not cease until the tracheal pressure is much greater. A theoretical analysis indicated that a large volume cuff might exert pressure more evenly over the mucosa so minimizing the effect on the cartilage [40]. A rigid low volume cuff should exert pressure mainly over the cartilages with early reduction of blood flow. It was therefore recommended that the cuff should be inflated to a pressure not exceeding 30 cm H_2O.

Dobrin & Canfield investigated tracheal blood flow in the dog by measuring changes in tracheal temperature with a number of tracheal tubes with different characteristics and with varying cuff and wall pressures [27]. Cuff pressure was increased gradually resulting in a rise in measured wall pressure and a drop in tracheal temperature. When inflated to obtain a seal, compliant cuffs reduced the calculated blood flow to 98% of control while stiff cuffs reduced the flow to 20–40% of control. Stiff cuffs exerted a greater pressure on the mucosa than compliant cuffs. Further work showed that the blood flow was reduced more in the superficial mucosal layers rather than in the deeper tracheal structures.

In a later study Seegobin & van Hasselt used an endoscopic photographic technique to assess tracheal mucosal blood flow during intubation with large volume cuffed tubes [41]. The mucosa in contact with the cuff was examined for changes in colour which gave an indication of alteration in blood flow. At cuff pressures of 30 cm H_2O, impairment of mucosal flow could be observed over the anterior tracheal cartilages. Total obstruction of blood flow over the tracheal rings and over the stretched posterior muscular wall was observed at cuff pressures of 50 cm H_2O. It was recommended that the cuff should be inflated to a pressure not exceeding 30 cm H_2O. Mehta however pointed out that the intracuff pressures measured in the above experiments in large volume cuffs did not necessarily accurately reflect the pressure exerted on the tracheal wall [42]. The pressure exerted on the tracheal wall only equals the intracuff pressure with large volume, low pressure cuffs provided there is no tension in the wall of the cuff [43].

Tracheal pathology and cuff pressure

The effect of cuff pressures on the trachea was investigated in the rabbit by Nordin [117] who concluded that the severity of tracheal pathology was influenced by the product of the duration of intubation and the lateral wall pressure. However, pressure was more important in causing damage than time. At a wall pressure of 20 mmHg, superficial but non-progressive mucosal damage resulted within 15 min. At a higher pressure of 50 mmHg, changes were noted within 15 min with partial denuding of the basement membrane. At 100 mmHg after 4 h there was damage almost down to the cartilage accompanied by bacterial invasion. This study emphasized the importance of limiting the pressure exerted on the tracheal wall. If the lateral wall pressure is limited to 20 mmHg then the trachea can tolerate long-term intubation with a cuffed tube. Experiments in pigs demonstrated that intubation for 4.5 h caused variable damage to the ciliated epithelium which could result in obstruction to mucus transport [44]. It was not possible, however, to demonstrate a correlation between the extent of tracheal damage and the tendency to mucus arrest. In dogs following intubation for 2 h, ciliary regeneration could be seen 2 days after extubation and was nearly complete by 7 days [45].

Methods of decreasing tracheal trauma

Major complications were common following long-term ventilation with the rubber cuffs used prior to the introduction of plastics. Improvements in cuff design and management have

Table 1 Cuff management techniques and cuff design.

Management techniques	
Intermittent cuff deflation [46]	With modern high volume cuffs the tracheal wall pressure exerted does not restrict capillary blood flow thus rendering obsolete the practice of regular cuff deflation used with high pressure cuffs
Allowing small leaks around the cuff [47, 48]	Still frequently used during long-term ventilation. There is a risk of aspiration of pharyngeal contents with this method
Intermittent cuff inflation with equipment attached to the ventilator [49–53]	This equipment is cumbersome and the technique allows aspiration during expiration unless PEEP is applied. It was introduced to prevent complications developing with long-term tracheostomy tubes
Intermittent measurement of cuff pressures and adjustment of pressures as required	Simple but requires an appropriate measuring system. Should be routine clinical practice
Cuff with pressure control balloon which is used in place of the normal pilot balloon (the Lanz Tube) [22]	This mechanism prevents both rises and falls in cuff pressure. The final cuff pressure depends on the compliance of the large pilot balloon which is connected in series with the cuff
Fill cuff with gas of the same composition as that inspired during general anaesthesia	
Fill cuff with liquid to prevent diffusion of gas into the cuff	See 'Nitrous oxide' section, p. 61
Use of devices to prevent rises in cuff pressure above set value	
Design	
Self inflating cuffs [54–56]	These cuffs exerted a lateral tracheal wall pressure the same as airway pressure during inspiration. During expiration there is an increased risk of aspiration
Prestretching of cuffs [39]	This effectively converted early high pressure low volume cuffs into high volume low pressure cuffs with much lower intracuff pressures providing a seal
Kamen Wilkinson polyurethane foam cuff [57]	The pressure inside this self inflating cuff is equal to atmospheric pressure and the cuff exerts a very low pressure on the tracheal wall
High volume low pressure cuff [58]	The cuff and tracheal wall pressures should be identical if the cuff is carefully selected

been used to try to reduce the incidence of cuff related complications [22, 39, 46–59] (Table 1). These methods have been designed to limit the magnitude or the duration of the pressure applied to the tracheal mucosa. With a number of the early methods there was an increased risk of aspiration of pharyngeal contents and these are now rarely used.

The introduction of plastic tubes has enabled manufacturers to produce cuffs with improved characteristics which allow a seal to be achieved at cuff pressures which do not jeopardize capillary circulation in the tracheal wall. Thin walled, high volume, low pressure cuffs usually enable a tracheal seal to be obtained without any stretching of the cuff. The intracuff pressure will thus be equal to the pressure exerted on the tracheal mucosa. Careful monitoring and control of the cuff pressure is still indicated to prevent both increases and decreases in cuff pressure.

A system which automatically controls the cuff pressure, such as occurs with the Lanz tube, should be used. The introduction of the Lanz tube resulted in a tenfold decrease in the incidence of major tracheal complications and a significant decrease in deaths due to such sequelae during long-term ventilation [59]. These authors found that 25% of their intensive care patients required ventilation for more than 1 week and 10% required ventilation for more than 2 weeks [60]. A reliable system of control of cuff pressure is mandatory during such long-term ventilation.

Methods have also been described to limit the pressure increase due to diffusion of nitrous oxide into the cuff during general anaesthesia (see p. 61). This can result in a large increase in pressure but anaesthesia is usually of relatively short duration and this is therefore less important than the problems related to high cuff pressure in intensive care units.

Decrease in cuff pressure with time

In contrast to the numerous reports of increases in cuff pressure during general anaesthesia there is very little information available on decrease in cuff pressures during long-term ventilation. Jacobsen & Greenbaum, however, investigated the decrease in pressure in both high residual volume low pressure and low residual volume high pressure cuffs with time

Table 2 Decrease in cuff pressure and time. From Jacobsen & Greenbaum [61].

	Initial cuff pressure (mmHg)	Terminal cuff pressure (mmHg)	Time (h)
Low residual volume, high pressure cuffs	110	60	17
	95	75	6
	30	20	10
	65	25	30
	30	20	6
High residual volume, low pressure cuffs	23	15	6
	20	5	12
	20	5	9
	34	20	6
	15	5	10
	45	28	10
	20	20	6
	16	10	6

[61]. A wide range of initial cuff pressures occurred with high and low volume cuffs (Table 2). Cuff pressures decreased with time but no correlation was found between the magnitude of the decrease and time. The decrease in pressure was thought to result both from diffusion of gas and slow movement ('creeping') of the plastic in the cuff. The movement was speeded up by warm moist conditions in the trachea and transient increases in intracuff pressure [61]. The 'creeping' mimics the pre-stretching of cuffs advocated by Geffin & Pontoppidan [39]. It seems likely that the movement of the plastic occurs within the first few hours and after this the decrease in pressure is due to diffusion of gases through the cuff. The movement of the plastic results in an increase in cuff volume and a decrease in pressure [62]. Of course a leak from an improperly applied occluding device or leaking three-way taps will also reduce cuff pressure. A decrease in cuff pressure may result in aspiration of pharyngeal contents [63] or even inadequate ventilation.

Dynamic cuff pressure changes

The effect of ventilation on low and high pressure cuffs has been investigated both in vitro and in vivo [64]. The effect of ventilation on cuff pressure is less important in high (Fig. 14) than low pressure cuffs (Figs 15 and 16). Small changes in pressure in a high volume cuff

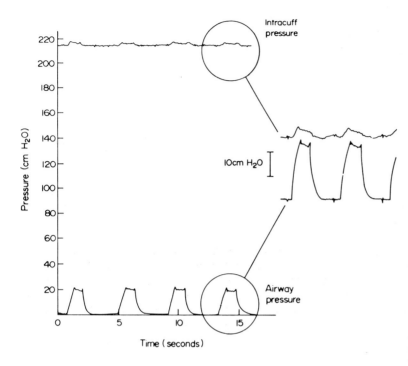

Fig. 14 Variation of intracuff and airway pressure for the low volume cuff in a patient. From Crawley & Cross [64], with kind permission of the authors and Academic Press, publishers of *Anaesthesia*.

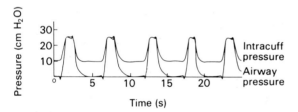

Fig. 15 Variation of intracuff and airway pressure for the high volume cuff in a model trachea. After Crawley and Cross [64], with kind permission of the authors and Academic Press, publishers of *Anaesthesia*.

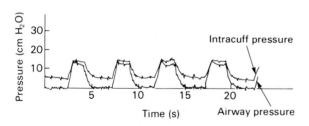

Fig. 16 Variation of intracuff and airway pressure for a high volume cuff in a patient. The small superimposed changes in pressure are due to cardiac displacement. After Crawley and Cross [64], with kind permission of the authors and Academic Press, publishers of *Anaesthesia*.

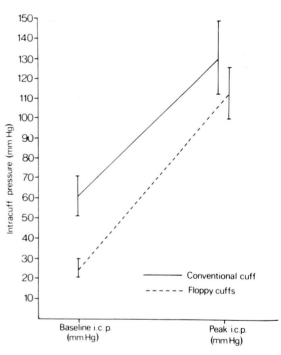

Fig. 17 Comparison of the increase in cuff pressure with coughing. (Bars represent s.e. mean.) From Jacobsen & Greenbaum [61].

seen on the trace (Fig. 16) are due to cardiac displacement; the intratracheal inflation pressure is transmitted to the cuff during inspiration. These dynamic changes show that it is not necessary for the cuff pressure to be above the inflation pressure to maintain a seal. In a spontaneously breathing patient the cuff pressure changed in a negative direction on inspiration and in a positive direction on expiration.

Transient large increases in cuff pressure were measured during coughing [61] (Fig. 17). These frequently occurred following the stimulus of tracheal suction. The open tube prevents a large increase in intrathoracic pressure thus precluding this as the causative mechanism. It was suggested that during a cough the trachea changes in shape and constricts the cuff of the tube. Cuff pressure with low pressure cuffs increased from 24 to 110 mmHg during coughing and with high pressure cuffs from 61 to 129 mmHg. There was no relationship between the cough force and peak cuff pressure. Such high pressures could theoretically at least cause collapse of the tube or cuff herniation.

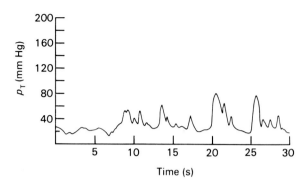

Fig. 20 The effect of 'fighting the ventilator' on tracheal wall pressure. After MacKenzie et al [65].

The pressure on the tracheal wall exerted by the cuff has also been shown to rise temporarily during vibration and 'bagging' physiotherapy [65] (Figs 18 and 19). It also rises when a patient 'fights the ventilator' (Fig 20). Therefore if this is prolonged, potential damage to the mucosa could result.

Nitrous oxide diffusion into cuffs

It was shown as early as 1965 that gas filled spaces in the body will expand during general anaesthesia when nitrous oxide is inspired [66]. When a 75% nitrous oxide concentration was inspired intestinal gas volumes increased 100–200% in 4 h and the volumes of a pneumothorax increased by 200–300% in 2 h. The increase was influenced by the blood gas solubility and blood flow.

In 1974 it was first demonstrated in vitro that nitrous oxide diffused into the cuffs of tracheal tubes with consequent increase in cuff volumes [67, 68]. In 1975 it was shown that both pressure and volume increase occurred in vivo [69]. The rise in pressure varied with different makes of tubes. The increase ranged from 1.35 to 5 times the initial pressure. It was suggested that these pressure changes could be limited by increasing the thickness of the cuff and that diffusion occurred less rapidly through latex rubber than through polyvinyl chloride. Cuff volumes increased by 42–89% over a test period of approximately 2 h. Analysis of cuff contents showed that 76–88% of the volume changes were due to nitrous oxide diffusion and 2–10% due to diffusion of oxygen. Less than 5% of the pressure increase in vivo occurred as a result of

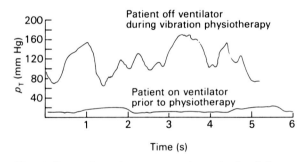

Fig. 18 Comparison of pressures on the tracheal wall during IPPV and vibration physiotherapy. After MacKenzie et al [65].

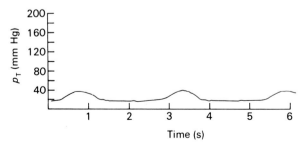

Fig. 19 The effect of 'bagging' on tracheal wall pressure. After MacKenzie et al [65].

warming the air in the cuff from room to body temperature. It was suggested that these changes would be less in vivo than in vitro because only the cuff area below the tracheal wall would be exposed for diffusion. Thin walled, high volume, low pressure cuffs have a large portion of the cuff in contact with the tracheal wall, which also acts as an area for diffusion, and this area is about 10 times that of the cuff not in contact with the trachea [70].

Cuff pressure and volume changes can be almost eliminated by filling the cuff with the same gas as that inspired [71]. When low pressure cuffs were filled with room air, however, pressures increased by approximately two times the control when breathing either 60% nitrous oxide in oxygen or 98% oxygen and 2% ethrane. Volume and pressure changes following nitrous oxide anaesthesia were similar with both low and high pressure cuffs. It was recommended that cuffs should routinely be filled with gas of the same composition as that of the inspired mixture. It is interesting that these increases can not be prevented by breathing oxygen.

A linear increase in pressure occurred over the first 3 h in air filled high-volume low-pressure and small-volume cuffs during nitrous oxide anaesthesia [72]. This effectively converts a low pressure to a high pressure cuff. These changes were prevented by filling the cuff with gas of the same composition as that inspired or saline (Fig. 21). It was recommended that the

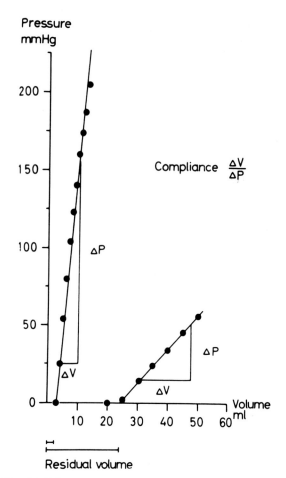

Fig. 22 Volume-pressure relations in one small and one large volume cuff tested in vitro. From Revenas & Lindholm [72], with kind permission of the editor of *Acta Anaesthesiologica Scandinavica*.

cuff pressure should be measured even when the cuff is filled with the same gas as the inspired mixture. If the cuff residual volume is low the filling volume at which the cuff pressure remains low is limited. The volume pressure relationships of one large and one small cuff were demonstrated in vitro by Revenas & Lindholm (Fig. 22) [72].

A number of different tubes were investigated both for cuff volume changes with time after being exposed to nitrous oxide in vitro and also for the physical characteristics of the cuffs [73]. The rate of nitrous oxide transfer varied inversely with cuff thickness and directly with the partial pressure of nitrous oxide. Cuff thickness ranged from 0.033 to 0.55 mm. Diffusion rates also varied with cuffs of the same

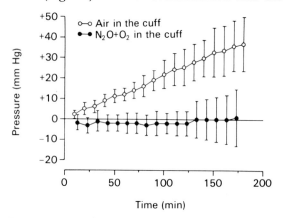

Fig. 21 Pressure changes as a function of time using the large volume cuff during nitrous oxide-oxygen anaesthesia (70–30%). The cuff was filled with air or the nitrous oxide/oxygen mixture. Mean and 95% confidence interval. After Revenas & Lindholm [72], with kind permission of the editor of *Acta Anaesthesiologica Scandinavica*.

composition but different densities, as well as with cuffs of different compositions. Most cuffs were made of polyvinyl chloride. The factors influencing the volume of gas diffusing into a cuff were defined in the following equation by Mehta [74]:

$$V = \frac{KAT\,(P_1 - P_2)}{X}$$

where V = volume of gas diffusing into the cuff, A = area available for diffusion, T = time available, X = thickness of the membranes, $P_1 - P_2$ = difference in pressure of the gas on the two sides of the membrane

and K is a constant which depends on diffusion and solubility characteristics.

Permeability is also affected by the nature of the permeating gas and the physical characteristics of the cuff material.

The use of large diameter, thin walled cuffs was recommended by Bernhard and his colleagues [73]. However, a thin cuff wall facilitates nitrous oxide transfer and cuff pressures during anaesthesia should therefore be adjusted at 30 min intervals [73] or be used with pressure regulating devices [75, 76, 77, 113].

A later simple cuff pressure regulator working on the principle of a tube immersed in water was also shown to be effective in clinical

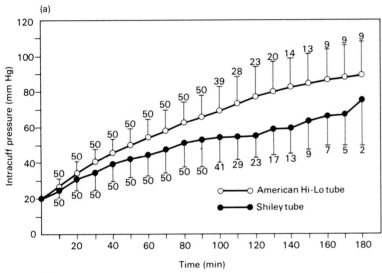

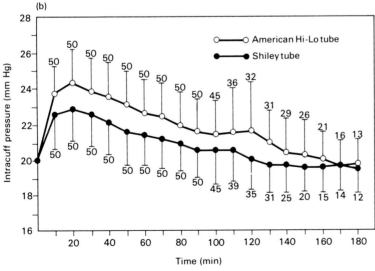

Fig. 23 Intraoperative changes in intracuff pressure of two types of tracheal tubes when the intracuff pressure was not controlled (a) and when it was controlled (b) by the 'Tracheal tube cuff pressure stabilizer'. Intracuff pressure started at 20 mmHg in all tubes. Vertical bars indicate standard deviation of the mean. Number of tubes is shown at the end of each vertical bar. After Kim [77], with kind permission of the International Anesthesia Research Society.

practice [77]. In a group of patients with high volume, low pressure cuffs a large increase in cuff pressure due to nitrous oxide diffusion was demonstrated during anaesthesia (Fig. 23). Any significant rise in pressure was prevented by the use of the 'Tracheal Tube Cuff Pressure Stabilizer'. An electropneumatic device, 'the Cardiff Cuff Controller', will prevent both rises and falls in cuff pressure [113]. Major changes in cuff pressure due to diffusion of nitrous oxide have also been demonstrated during cardiopulmonary bypass [78].

In conclusion, the increases in cuff pressures and volumes due to diffusion of nitrous oxide are well documented. Clear recommendations have been made that cuff pressures should be measured during clinical anaesthesia and appropriate measures taken to prevent an undue rise (Table 3).

Table 3 Techniques to reduce the effect, or limit the diffusion, of nitrous oxide into the cuff.

Fill the cuff with the same mixture as that inspired	Easily done but mixture needs to be changed if inspired mixture changed [71]
Fill the cuff with saline	Easily done and no further adjustments required [72]
Fill the cuff with air	Measure cuff pressure regularly and adjust as required
Fill cuff with air and use devices which limit rises in cuff pressure	1 Use pressure release valve [76] 2 Use 'Tracheal Tube Cuff Pressure Stabilizer' [77] 3 Lanz tube with pressure limiting balloon [75] 4 Use of an electropneumatic control system [113]
Kamen Wilkinson Tube with foam cuff	This cuff is self inflating and the cuff can be left open to the atmosphere

However, it is also clear that most clinicians ignore these recommendations and make no effort to prevent rises in cuff pressure during general anaesthesia. It is particularly important to control cuff pressures during long-term anaesthesia to decrease the risk of developing pressure related complications.

Aspiration

'Silent' regurgitation of stomach contents into the pharynx during tracheal anaesthesia has been reported in 22 out of 152 patients (14.5%) [79] and 58 of 472 patients (12.3%) [80]. Upper abdominal surgery, the prone position or artificial ventilation were all associated with an increased incidence of regurgitation. Therefore the risk of aspiration is decreased by frequent oropharyngeal suction to prevent the accumulation of fluid in the pharynx [81]. Pharyngeal contents can accumulate in the trachea above the cuff of an endotracheal tube. To minimize the volume collecting in the trachea it has been recommended that the cuff should be placed just beyond the vocal cords and after cuff inflation the tube should be withdrawn until resistance is met [16]. At extubation patients should be placed in a 10° head down and lateral position and suction applied to the tube.

Speaking tracheostomy tubes (Vocalaid tubes from Portex) have a channel just above the cuff. This channel is normally used for insufflation of oxygen to enable the patient to phonate but can be used for aspiration of secretions which collect above the cuff. We have noted sometimes when these tubes are used in the intensive care unit that quite large volumes of fluid can be aspirated through the oxygen channel. In patients with such large volumes of pharyngeal secretions aspiration will certainly occur if the cuff is not properly inflated. It has been shown that aspiration past the cuff of tracheostomy tubes can result in fever and pulmonary complications [87]. Aspiration of these secretions through the oxygen channel can result in daily volumes as high as 600 ml being collected with rapid improvement in pulmonary complications. Thus a cuff protects against massive aspiration but not necessarily against repeated small volumes in patients with laryngeal dysfunction.

Aspiration past tracheal tubes has been studied in vivo with dye placed in the mouth [82, 83]. Aspiration of dye occurred in 56% of intensive care patients with low volume, high pressure cuffs and 20% of patients with high volume, low pressure cuffs [83]. However, there was no data on cuff pressures. In patients with a tracheostomy using a high volume, low pressure cuff aspiration occurred in about 16% of patients [84]. Unrecognized aspiration has been suggested as one of the causes of postoperative pulmonary complications; 16% of 300 unselected patients undergoing anaesthesia had evidence of dye aspiration postoperatively [85].

Table 4 Tube and cuff types, intracuff pressures and incidences of aspiration. From Bernhard et al [82], with kind permission of the authors, the editor of *Anesthesiology*, and the publishers, J.B. Lippincott Co.

Tube	Cuff size	Intracuff pressure (cm H$_2$O)	Tracheal aspiration of dye (% of cases)
Lanz	Large	20	38.5
American/NCC Hi-Lo	Large	20	38.5
Lanz	Large	25	0
American/NCC Hi-Lo	Large	25	0
Lanz	Large	27–34	0
American/NCC Hi-Lo	Large	Minimal occluding volume (25–27)	0
Portex Blue Line	Large	Minimal occluding volume (25–27)	35.3
Rusch Red Rubber	Small	Minimal occluding volume (approx 250)	0

Table 5 Cuff physical characteristics, intracuff pressures and incidences of aspiration. From Bernhard et al [82], with kind permission of the authors, the editor of *Anesthesiology*, and the publishers, J.B. Lippincott Co.

Tube	Cuff diameter (mm)±s.d.	Cuff thickness (mm)±s.d.	Intracuff pressure (cm H$_2$O)	Aspiration
American Hi-Lo	33.28±0.76	0.044±.005	25	No
Lanz	30.07±0.63	0.104±.007	27–34	No
Portex Blue Line	28.75±1.63	0.25±.029	Minimal occluding volume (25–27)	Yes
Rusch	14.52±0.44	0.537±.029	Minimal occluding volume (±250)	No

A prospective investigation has been made to determine the cuff pressure required to prevent aspiration with different cuffs in vivo [82]. Evans Blue dye was placed in the pharynx and afterwards the respiratory tract was inspected for evidence of soiling. Aspiration occurred when cuff pressures were kept at 20 cm H$_2$O but not at 25 cm H$_2$O or above with both Lanz and Hi-Lo cuffs. Aspiration however did occur even at a cuff pressure of 25–27 cm H$_2$O with the thicker walled Portex tubes (Tables 4 and 5).

Folds or wrinkles (Fig. 24) can occur in high volume cuffs when the circumference of the cuff is greater than that of the trachea [86]. The magnitude of aspiration of liquid past the wrinkles depends on three main factors [115]. These are the viscosity of the liquid, the hydrostatic pressure of the liquid above the cuff and the number and size of the folds or wrinkles. With stiff thick walled cuffs the wrinkles become collapsed less easily than with thin walled cuffs. Higher cuff pressures are therefore required to prevent leaks with such high volume cuffs particularly where the cuff wall is thicker and less pliable. Aspiration has been reported in two spontaneously breathing patients [86, 90] past properly inflated large volume cuffs and one of the patients soon died from hypoxia [90]. In the other patient aspiration was controlled by inserting a low volume high pressure cuffed tube. The extent of aspiration may be accentuated in a spontaneously breathing patient if a subatmospheric pressure is generated distal to the cuff. A thin walled, high volume cuff is required that will fit the tracheal contours at a low inflation pressure without forming wrinkles. Such a cuff would have a diameter when just inflated which is approximately the same as that of the trachea.

In vitro tests with three different types of tubes showed that in all instances irrespective of wrinkle formation leaks could be eliminated by increasing intracuff pressures to high levels

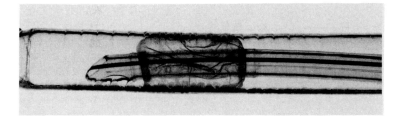

Fig. 24 Large volume cuff inflated in a model trachea to demonstrate the formation of wrinkles in the cuff.

Table 6 Mean cuff diameters (in 10 cuffs) and aspiration in two types of tubes with the same cuff thickness. Tubes were tested in a model trachea connected to a model lung. From Mehta [89], with kind permission of the editor of *Annals of the Royal College of Surgeons of England*.

Tube	Wall thickness (mm)	Circumference and (diameter) at residual volume (mm)	Residual volume (ml)	Cuff diameter / Tracheal diameter	Mean cuff pressure to produce leak free ventilation (kPa)*	Mean cuff pressure at which aspiration started to occur (kPa)*
Portex Profile	0.125	93.6 (29.8)	13.05	1.49	4.16	2.93 (with two tubes aspiration occurred at 5.98)
Searle Sensiv	0.125	69.9 (22.2)	6.9	1.11	1.06 (in no case higher than 1.47)	0.54 (in no case higher than 1.08)

*1 kPa = 10.2 cmH$_2$O

[86]. However, aspiration should be prevented with low cuff and tracheal wall pressures so as to decrease the risk of tracheal trauma. Leaks could be minimized when the cuff diameter was approximately the same as the tracheal diameter and wrinkles were not formed [86]. However, in the short term and in high risk situations such as in spontaneously breathing patients the cuff can be temporarily overinflated to decrease the risk of aspiration [88]. Tests with two types of tubes showed that the cuff pressures required to produce leak free ventilation were greater than that at which aspiration occurred in a model trachea with 2 cm H$_2$O above the cuff [89] (Table 6). The peak airway pressure was fixed at 1.96 kPa. The two tubes had the same cuff thickness but the circumference and stiffness of the Portex cuff was greater than that of the Searle cuff.

The incidence of minor aspiration of pharyngeal contents in clinical practice is not easy to determine and will be influenced by the volume of pharyngeal contents, posture and cuff pressure and design characteristics of the cuff. There may be a difference between the viscosity of aqueous dye and pharyngeal secretions. Thus the clinical incidence of aspiration past the cuff at a given pressure may not correlate with the expected incidence from in vitro tests.

In conclusion, aspiration can be prevented by overinflating the cuff. The cuff is often overinflated during short-term intubation for surgery and serious complications are not normally evident. For the longer term it is important to control cuff pressures accurately.

The cuff and other factors and postoperative sore throat

A sore throat after intubation usually lasts for only a few days and is considered a minor unavoidable complication of general anaesthesia [91]. Severe pain elsewhere following major surgery often ensures that the less severe pain in the throat is largely ignored. After minor surgery however, a sore throat may be the main cause of postoperative discomfort. This complication occurs more commonly in women than men [98].

The incidence of sore throat after general anaesthesia administered by mask varies from 15% [97] to 22% [94, 96] and is generally short lasting and of minor severity (Table 7) [92–101, 104]. These studies have tried to isolate and study individual contributing causes. In some areas, however, such as the effect of local anaesthetics on the cuff, the evidence is conflicting. The cause of sore throats associated with mask anaesthesia has been attributed to inspiring unhumidified gas with consequent drying of the mucous membranes of the pharynx and trachea. A bolus of succinylcholine administered during mask anaesthesia however resulted in 68.2% incidence of sore throat [102]. The incidence in a control group not receiving succinylcholine was 9.5%. The severity of sore throat correlated with the degree of postoperative myalgia. Atropine, oropharyngeal airway, laryngoscopy and pharyngeal suction were avoided in that study.

Table 7 The cuff and postoperative sore throat

Authors and reference	Year	Tube	Design of study (all relatively short term intubations)	Study variables	Incidence of sore throat (%)	Severity of sore throat	Method and time of investigation of sore throat	Comment
Lund & Daos [92]	1965	Not stated	Double blind investigations of effect of *local anaesthetic* and *lubricant* on sore throat incidence	No lubricant on tube Heavy viscous lubricant Heavy lubricant with 5% lignocaine Light lubricant	22.8 20.8 6.6 21.2	No	Direct questioning	A reduction in incidence was noted with the heavy viscous lubricant containing local anaesthetic
Stock & Downs [101]	1982	7.0–9.0 mm int. diam High vol. low pressure cuffs	Effect of different *lubricants* on incidence of sore throat	Mask Dry tube Normal saline Water soluble jelly Lignocaine jelly Lignocaine ointment	21 45 42 45 41 50	Yes (scale 0–3)* 0.3 1.1 0.8 0.8 0.9 0.9	Interview 20–30 h after extubation	Same incidence of sore throat and hoarseness with lubricated and unlubricated tubes. Lignocaine in jelly or ointment did not influence the incidence. Intubation was mechanically easier with lubricated tubes
Stanley [93]	1975	Not stated	To study the changes in cuff volume and pressure with diffusion of *nitrous oxide* into air filled cuffs when used *in vivo*	5 different low pressure cuffs and 3 different high pressure cuffs	Not measured	No	Not measured	Similar increase in cuff volume and pressure occurred with both types of cuffs. It was inferred that cuff expansion might cause tracheal trauma and sore throat
Saarni-vaara & Grahne [98]	1981	Shiley high vol. low pressure cuff	Investigation of diffusion of *nitrous oxide* into air filled cuff on cuff pressures and postoperative sore throat and hoarseness. The tubes were lubricated with 10% lignocaine ointment	*Group I* Adjusting the cuff pressure and keeping the pressure from rising above 25 mmHg *Group II* Allowing the cuff pressure to rise freely	Time (min) post extubation I II 30 0 13 60 0 13 120 4 6 180 9 7 240 0 0	No	Studied for 240 min after extubation	No significant difference in incidence of hoarseness in the 2 groups. The incidence ranged from 12 to 28%. The incidence of sore throat ranged from 0 to 13%. The incidence of side-effects was greater in women than in men

(continued over pp. 68–70)

Table 7 (continued)

Authors and reference	Year	Tube	Design of study (all relatively short term intubations)	Study variables	Incidence of sore throat (%)	Severity of sore throat	Method and time of investigation of sore throat	Comment
Jensen et al [100]	1982	7.5–9.0 mm int. diam.	Further investigations of effect of *high or low pressure cuffs* on incidence of sore throat. Intracuff pressures were adjusted to just seal point every 15 min in groups. The tubes were lubricated with jelly without local anaesthetic, cuffs were filled with room air	Group —mask —Rusch red rubber 'low' pressure 'high' pressure —Portex blue line —Shiley low pressure	18 45 52 63 65	Yes (scale 0–3)* 0.32 0.58 0.86 1.08 1.03	Direct questioning at 24–30 h postoperatively	Lower incidence and severity of sore throat with low volume high pressure cuffs than high volume low pressure cuffs *provided* that cuff pressures were maintained at the just seal point. The incidence of sore throat was higher in women than men
Loeser et al [94]	1976	7.0–8.5 mm int. diam. tubes	Investigation of *cuff design* on incidence of sore throat. Patients with nasogastric tubes, difficulty with intubation or coughing during intubation or extubation were excluded. All tubes were lubricated with 5% lignocaine ointment and all patients were ventilated.	No tube (mask) *Low pressure cuffs* 1 Foregger 2 American 3 Extra Corporeal 4 Portex *High pressure cuffs* 1 Harlake 2 Rusch 3 American 4 Shiley	22 48 58 58 54 24 38 24 25	Yes (scale 0–3)* 0.26 0.64 0.78 0.82 0.68 0.24 0.40 0.26 0.25	Direct questioning at 20–30 h postoperatively	Cuff tracheal surface contact area may be directly related to the extent of mucosal damage. Bulky cuffs may also produce damage both on intubation and extubation. Wrinkling of high pressure cuffs may produce areas of high pressure on the trachea. The high incidence after Rusch tubes was attributed to residual cidex after re-sterilization (all other tubes were disposable). A low cuff tracheal contact area is desirable

Table 7 (continued)

Authors and reference	Year	Tube	Design of study (all relatively short term intubations)	Study variables		Cuff length (mm)	Intra-cuff seal pressure (mmHg)	Incidence of sore throat (%)	Severity of sore throat	Method and time of investigation of sore throat	Comment
Loeser et al [96]	1980	7.5, 8.0 or 8.5 mm int. diam. tubes	Investigation of cuff tracheal contact area on influence of sore throat. Same design features as above study. All the tubes were lubricated with 5% lignocaine	National catheter cuffs	Standard	25	133	24	Yes (scale 0–3)*	Direct questioning at 20–30 h postoperatively	Sore throat incidence is highly correlated with the length of cuff used. It is not related to intubation time, age of patient, type of operation or intracuff pressure. Tubes with narrow cuffs cause a low incidence and severity of sore throats (half that of mask anaesthesia). This may be because the dry gas dehydrates upper airway mucosa with mask anaesthesia
					Hilo	37	18	58	0.74		
					Medium	30	17	47	0.6		
					Narrow	22	17	10	0.1		
				Portex cuffs	Taper	29	15	38	0.5		
					Large volume	39	17	54	0.68		
				Mask				22	0.26		
Stenqvist & Nilsson [99]	1982	8.0 mm int. diam. I Portex Blue Line II Mallinckrodt Hilo	Investigation of I low, II high volume cuffs. The cuff tracheal contact area was calculated as 11 cm² in group I and 20 cm² in group II	Cuffs were inflated with the inspired mixture. No stylets or lubricants were used. The inspired mixture was humidified				I 55 II 44	No	Direct questioning on first day postoperatively	No difference between the 2 groups. In long-term intubation the cuff causes more damage than the intubation procedure. In short-term intubation the influence of the intubation procedure relative to the cuff is great
Loeser et al [97]	1980	7.5–8.5 mm int. diam. Portex tubes	To determine incidence of sore throat with uncuffed and cuffed tubes of two designs. To determine the influence of local anaesthetic or saline on the tubes on the incidence of sore throat. The cuffs were filled with the inspired mixture. Patients breathed humidified heated humidified gas spontaneously for orthopaedic procedures	Tube	Lubricant				Yes (scale 0–3)*	Not stated	The use of 4% lignocaine jelly on uncuffed tubes is disadvantageous (an irritant to the mucosa). It was postulated that unhumidified air is entrained during spontaneous ventilation with uncuffed tubes causing airway damage. Tube causing lowest incidence of sore throat was one with unlubricated low volume cuffs
				Uncuffed	lignocaine jelly (4%)			90	2.1		
				Uncuffed	lignocaine solution (4%)			40	0.45		
				Uncuffed	saline			40	0.4		
				Large volume cuff	none			46	0.49		
				Low volume cuff	none			25	0.31		
				Mask	none			15	0.2		

(continued on p. 70)

Table 7 (continued)

Authors and reference	Year	Tube	Design of study (all relatively short term intubations)	Study variables	Incidence of sore throat (%)	Severity of sore throat	Method and time of investigation of sore throat	Comment
Loeser et al [95]	1978	7.0–8.5 mm int. diam tubes	Investigation of tracheal *tube conformity* to the pharyngeal contour and *cuff design* on incidence of sore throat. Same design features as above study	*Low volume, high pressure cuffs* 1. Standard tube 2. Pharyngeal moulded tube *High volume, low pressure cuffs* Standard tube Pharyngeal moulded tube Foam-filled cuff (Kamen-Wilkinson)	24 44 58 54 65	Yes (scale 0–3)* 0.26 0.54 0.74 0.75 0.9	Direct questioning 20–30 h postoperatively	Pharyngeal moulded tubes have a higher incidence of sore throat for short-term use rather than standard tubes. Possibly this is due to a greater tube mucous membrane contact area. Cuff surface area in contact with the trachea thought to be more important than increase in pressure by nitrous oxide diffusion in influencing incidence of sore throat
Alexopoulos & Lindholm [104]	1983	Standard or Lindholm design. Both with high vol. low pressure cuffs	To investigate the effect of specially *designed tubes* shaped to conform to the shape of the airway on the incidence of sore throat	1. Standard PVC tube 2. Preformed PVC tube (with asymmetric double curve in sagittal plane)	1a 26 b 55 2a 14 b 21	No	1. Spontaneous complaint within 2 days. 2. Direct questioning at 4 days	Higher risk of sore throat with standard tubes. Also at laryngoscopy higher incidence of mucosal lesions at cricoid plate and at posterior laryngeal commissure

*0 = no sore throat; 3 = severe sore throat.

The incidence of sore throat after short-term tracheal intubation varies from 6.6% [92] to 90% [97] (Table 7). A figure widely quoted in the literature is 60% [103]. This is, however, higher than the average values of 30–40% (Table 7). It is not always possible to determine whether a sore throat results from the presence of a tube in the trachea or from the trauma of the intubation [99]. The incidence of sore throat is higher in patients intubated with uncuffed tubes compared to those intubated with cuffed tubes [97].

Table 8 Factors which may influence the incidence of post operative sore throat

Trauma at intubation to:
  tonsillar pillars
  pharynx
  tongue
  larynx
  trachea

Use of stylet

Ryle's tube

Coughing on intubation or extubation

Blind pharyngeal suction

Use of pharyngeal pack

Cuff not deflated at extubation

Tube characteristics
  Pharyngeal contour tubes [107]
  Cuff:
    material
    cuff to tracheal contact area
    wrinkles on the cuff
    cuff to tracheal wall pressure

Method of investigation
  Direct questioning
  Indirect questioning

The use of cuffs with low tracheal contact areas [94, 96, 97, 100] reduces the incidence of sore throat. It also seems sensible to adjust cuff pressures intermittently to avoid major pressure rises due to diffusion of nitrous oxide into the cuff [98, 100]. Lubricants are applied routinely to tubes in most centres as an aid to easy and atraumatic intubation. There is conflicting evidence, however, on the use of local anaesthetic lubricants on the incidence of sore throat [91, 96, 100]. Recent evidence [100] suggests that lubrication of the tube with water soluble jelly, lignocaine ointment or lignocaine jelly does not influence the incidence of sore throat [100].

It is clear that the cuff related causes only partly influence the incidence of postoperative sore throat (Table 8). However reducing cuff contact area, intracuff pressure control and improved tube design [104] should all decrease the incidence of this annoying complication.

Cuff design recommendations

Different recommendations have been made regarding the optimal size of large volume cuffs relative to the tracheal size. Lomholt recommended that the cuff diameter should be at least one and a half times the tracheal diameter [105]. It is well recognized, however, that wrinkles can form with large volume cuffs. The number and size of these are influenced by the cuff – tracheal circumference ratio, cuff thickness, cuff composition and by the intracuff pressure. Other recommendations are that the cuff circumference and diameter at residual volume should be close to those of the trachea [89, 106]. This should minimize wrinkle formation. At the same time the intracuff pressure should approximate to the tracheal wall pressure. Small volume, high pressure cuffs are undesirable as they produce high minimum sealing pressures and increase the potential for tracheal trauma.

The cuff material should be strong and tear resistant but thin, soft, pliable and flexible. This should ensure a low pressure seal and minimize the size of any wrinkles formed. It should be biologically compatible and not allow diffusion of anaesthetic gases [89]. Early low volume cuffs had large tracheal contact areas; a later recommendation is that a smaller cuff tracheal contact area should be used. Pear shaped or tapered cuffs were thought to be preferable to cylindrical cuffs [89].

Summary

Improvements in cuff design and management can confidently be expected in the future. This should enable long-term intubation to be accomplished with increased safety.

REFERENCES

1 Waters R M, Rovenstine E A & Guedel A E (1933) Endotracheal anaesthesia and its historical development. *Anesth Analg* 12:196.

2 Trendelenburg F (1871) Beitrage zur den operationen au den Luftwegen Tamponade der Trachea. *Arch J Klin Chir* 12:121.

3 Macewen W (1880) Clinical observations on the introduction of tracheal tubes by the mouth instead of performing tracheotomy or laryngotomy. *Br Med J* 2:122,163.

4 Eisenmenger V (1893) Zur Tamponade des Larynx nach Prof Maydl. *Wien Med Wochenschr* 43:199.

5 Rowbotham E S & Magill I W (1921) Anaesthetics in plastic surgery of the face and jaws. *Proc R Soc Med* 14:17.

6 Magill I W (1930) Technique in endotracheal anaesthesia. *Br Med J* 2:817.

7 Guedel A E & Waters R M (1928) A new intratracheal catheter. *Anesth Analg* 7:238.

8 Dorrance G M (1910) On the treatment of traumatic injuries of the lungs and pleurae: with the presentation of a new intratracheal tube for use in artificial respiration. *Surg Gynecol Obstet* 2:160.

9 Macintosh R R (1943) Self-inflating cuff for endotracheal tubes. *Br Med J* 2:234.

10 Ibsen B (1952) The anaesthetist's viewpoint on the treatment of respiratory complications in poliomyelitis during the epidemic in Copenhagen. *Proc R Soc Med* 47:72.

11 Lassen H C A (1953) A preliminary report on the 1952 epidemic of poliomyelitis in Copenhagen. With special reference to the treatment of acute respiratory insufficiency. *Lancet* i:37.

12 Zwillich C W, Pierson D J, Creagh C E et al. (1974) Complications of assisted ventilation. *Am J Med* 57:161.

13 Whitehouse A C & Klock L E (1975) Evaluation of endotracheal tube position with the fibreoptic intubation laryngoscope. *Chest* 68:848.

14 Chander S & Feldman E (1979) Correct placement of endotracheal tubes. *N Y State J Med* 79:1843.

15 Hamilton W K & Stevens W C (1966) Malpositioning of endotracheal catheters. *JAMA* 198:1113.

16 Mehta S (1972) The risk of aspiration in the presence of cuffed endotracheal tubes. *Br J Anaesth* 44:601.

17 Triner L (1982) A simple maneuver to verify proper positioning of an endotracheal tube. *Anesthesiology* 57:548.

18 Wallace C T & Cooke J E (1976) A new method for positioning endotracheal tubes. *Anesthesiology* 44:272.

19 Cullen D J, Newbower R S & Gemer R (1975) A new method for positioning endotracheal tubes. *Anesthesiology* 43:596.

20 Conrady P A, Goodman L R, Lainge F & Singer MM (1973) Nasotracheal tube mobility with flexion and hyperextension of the neck. *Crit Care Med* 1:117.

21 Dobrin P B, Goldberg E M & Canfield T R (1974) The endotracheal cuff. A comparative study. *Anesth Analg* 53:456.

22 McGinnis G E, Shively J G, Patterson R L & Magovern G J (1971) An engineering analysis of intratracheal tube cuffs. *Anesth Analg* 50:557.

23 Black A M S & Seegobin R D (1981) Pressure on endotracheal tube cuffs. *Anesthesia* 36:498.

24 Cross E D (1973) Recent developments in tracheal cuffs. *Resuscitation* 2:77.

25 Carrol R, Hedden M & Safar P (1969) Intratracheal cuffs. Performance characteristics. *Anesthesiology* 31:275.

26 Wu W-H, Lim I-T, Simpson F A & Turndorf H (1973) Pressure dynamics of endotracheal and tracheostomy cuffs. Use of a tracheal model to evaluate performance. *Crit Care Med* 1:197.

27 Dobrin P & Canfield T (1977) Cuffed endotracheal tubes: mucosal pressures and tracheal wall blood flow. *Am J Surg* 133:562.

28 MacKenzie C F, Klose S & Browne D R G (1976) A study of inflatable cuffs on endotracheal tubes. Pressures exerted on the trachea. *Br J Anaesth* 48:105.

29 Knowlson G T G & Bassett H F M (1970) The pressures exerted on the trachea by endotracheal inflatable cuffs. *Br J Anaesth* 42:834.

30 Leigh J M & Maynard J P (1979) Pressure on the tracheal mucosa from cuffed tubes. *Br Med J* 1:1173.

31 Cooper J D & Grillo H C (1969) Experimental production and prevention of injury due to cuffed tracheal tubes. *Surg Gynecol Obstet* 129:1235.

32 Weymuller E A, Bishop M J, Fink B R, Hibbard A W & Spelman F A (1983) Quantification of intralaryngeal pressure exerted by endotracheal tubes. *Ann Otol Rhinol Laryngol* 92:444.

33 Olson N R & Bogdasarian R S (1980) Posterior glottic laryngeal stenosis. *Otolaryngol Head Neck Surg* 88:765.

34 Keane W M, Denneny J C, Rowe L D & Atkins JP (1983) Complications of intubation. *Ann Otol Rhinol Laryngol* 91:584.

35 Stenqvist O, Sonander H & Nilsson K (1979) Small endotracheal tubes. Ventilator and intratracheal pressures during controlled ventilation. *Br J Anaesth* 51:375.

36 Tonnesen A S, Vereen L & Arens J F (1981) Endotracheal tube cuff residual volume and lateral wall pressure in a model trachea. *Anesthesiology* 55:680.

37 Cooper J D & Grillo H C (1972) Analysis of problems related to cuffs on intratracheal tubes. *Chest* 62:21S.

38 Palombini B & Coburn R F (1972) Control of the compressibility of the canine trachea. *Respir Physiol* 15:365.

39 Geffin B & Pontoppidan H (1969) Reduction of tracheal damage by the prestretching of inflatable cuffs. *Anesthesiology* 31:462.

40 Nordin U, Lindholm C-E & Wolgast M (1977) Blood flow in the rabbit tracheal mucosa under normal conditions and under the influence of tracheal intubation. *Acta Anaesthesiol Scand* 21:81.

41 Seegobin R D & Van Hasselt G L (1984) Endotracheal cuff pressure and tracheal mucosal blood flow: endoscopic study of effects of four large volume cuffs. *Br Med J* 288:965.

42 Mehta S (1984) Endotracheal cuff pressure. *Br Med J* 288:1763.

43 Carroll R G, McGinniss G E & Grenvik A (1974) Performance characteristics of tracheal cuffs. *Int Anaesthesiol Clin* 12:111.

44 Alexopoulos B, Jannson B & Lindholm C-E (1984) Mucus transport and surface damage after endotracheal intubation and tracheostomy. An experimental study in pigs. *Acta Anaesthesiol Scand* 28:68.

45 Klainer A S, Turndorf H, Wu W-H, Maewal H & Allender P (1975) Surface alterations due to endotracheal intubation. *Am J Med* 58:674.

46 Andrews M J & Pearson F G (1971) Incidence and pathogenesis of tracheal injury following cuffed tube tracheostomy with assisted ventilation. *Ann Surg* 173:249.

47 Hardy K L, Fettel B E & Shiley D P (1970) New tracheostomy tube. *Ann Thorac Surg* 10:58.

48 Gibson P (1967) Aetiology and repair of tracheal stenosis following tracheostomy and intermittent positive pressure respiration. *Thorax* 22:1.

49 Crosby W M (1964) Automatic intermittent inflation of tracheostomy-tube cuff. *Lancet* ii:509.

50 Kirby R R, Robison E J & Schulz J (1970) Intermittent cuff inflation during prolonged positive pressure ventilation. *Anesthesiology* 32:364.

51 Rainer W G & Sanchez M (1970) Tracheal cuff inflation: synchronous timed with inspiration. *Ann Thorac Surg* 9:384.

52 Arens J F, Ochsner J L & Gee G (1969) Volume limited intermittent cuff inflation for long term respiratory assistance. *J Thorac Cardiovasc Surg* 58:837.

53 Nordin U & Lyttkens L (1976) New self-adjusting cuff for tracheal tubes. *Acta Otolaryngol (Stockh)* 82:455.

54 Benveniste D (1967) Endotracheal and tracheostomy tubes with self-inflating cuff. *Acta Anaesthesiol Scand* 11:85.

55 Abouav J & Finley T N (1976) Self-inflating parachute cuff. A new tracheostomy and endotracheal cuff. *Am J Surg* 125:657.

56 Jackson R R & Rokowski W J (1967) A disposable endotracheal tube with self inflating cuff. *Arch Surg* 94:160.

57 Kamen J M & Wilkinson C J (1971) A new low-pressure cuff for endotracheal tubes. *Anesthesiology* 34:482.

58 Lomholt N (1967) A new tracheostomy tube. *Acta Anaesthesiol Scand* 11:311.

59 Lewis F R, Schlobohm R M & Thomas A N (1978) Prevention of complications from prolonged tracheal intubation. *Am J Surg* 135:452.

60 Lewis F R, Blaisdell F W & Schlobohm R M (1977) Incidence and outcome of posttraumatic respiratory failure. *Arch Surg* 112:436.

61 Jacobsen L & Greenbaum R (1981) A study of intracuff pressure measurements, trends and behaviour in patients during prolonged periods of tracheal intubation. *Br J Anaesth* 53:97.

62 Hill D W (1976) Physics Applied to Anaesthesia, 3rd edn, p. 226. Butterworths, London.

63 Bernhard W N, Cottrell J E, Sivakumaran C, Patel K, Yost L & Turndorf H (1979) Adjustment of intracuff pressure to prevent aspiration. *Anesthesiology* 50:363.

64 Crawley B E & Cross D E (1975) Tracheal cuffs. A review and dynamic pressure study. *Anaesthesia* 30:4.

65 MacKenzie C F, Klose S & Browne D R G (1976) A study of inflatable cuffs on endotracheal tubes. *Br J Anaesth* 48:105.

66 Eger E I & Saidman L J (1965) Hazards of nitrous oxide anesthesia in bowel obstruction and pneumothorax. *Anesthesiology* 26:61.

67 Stanley T H (1974) Effects of anesthetic gases on endotracheal tube cuff gas volumes. *Anesth Analg* 53:480.

68 Stanley T H, Kawamura R & Graves C (1974) Effects of nitrous oxide on volume and pressure of endotracheal tube cuffs. *Anesthesiology* 41:256.

69 Stanley T H (1975) Nitrous oxide and pressures and volumes of high and low-pressure endotracheal tube cuffs in intubated patients. *Anesthesiology* 42:637.

70 Brandt L (1982) Nitrous oxide in oxygen and tracheal tube cuff volumes. *Br J Anaesth* 54:1238.

71 Stanley T H & Liu W-S (1975) Tracheostomy and endotracheal tube cuff volume and pressure changes during thoracic operations. *Ann Thorac Surg* 20:144.

72 Revenas B & Lindholm C-E (1976) Pressure and volume changes in tracheal tube cuffs during anaesthesia. *Acta Anaesthesiol Scand* 20:321.

73 Bernhard W N, Yost L, Turndorf H, Cottrell J E & Paegle R D (1978) Physical characteristics of and rates of nitrous oxide diffusion into tracheal tube cuffs. *Anesthesiology* 48:413..

74 Mehta S (1981) Effects of nitrous oxide and oxygen on tracheal tube cuff gas volumes. *Br J Anaesth* 53:1227.

75 Magovern G J, Shiveley J G, Fecht D & Thevoz F (1972) The clinical and experimental evaluation of a controlled pressure intratracheal cuff. *J Thorac Cardiovasc Surg* 64:747.

76 Stanley T H, Foote J L & Liu W-S (1975) A simple pressure relief valve to prevent increases in endotracheal tube cuff pressure and volume in intubated patients. *Anesthesiology* 43:478.

77 Kim J-M (1980) The tracheal tube cuff pressure stabilizer and its clinical evaluation. *Anesth Analg* 59:291.

78 Ikeda S & Schweiss J F (1980) Tracheal tube cuff volume changes during extracorporeal circulation. *Can Anaesth Soc J* 27:453.

79 Turndorf H, Rodis I D & Clark T S (1974) 'Silent' regurgitation during general anesthesia. *Anesth Analg* 53:700.

80 Blitt C D, Gutman H L, Cohen D D, Weisman H & Dillon J B (1970) 'Silent' regurgitation and aspiration during general anaesthesia. *Anesth Analg* 49:707.

81 Macrae W & Wallace P (1981) Aspiration around high-volume low-pressure endotracheal cuff. *Br Med J* 283:1220.

82 Bernhard W N, Cottrell J E, Sivakumaran C, Patel K, Yost L & Turndorf H (1979) Adjustment of intracuff pressure to prevent aspiration. *Anesthesiology* 50:363.

83 Spray S B, Zuidema G D & Cameron J L (1976) Aspiration pneumonia. Incidence of aspiration with endotracheal tubes. *Am J Surg* 131:701.

84 Bone D K, Davis J L, Zuidema G D & Cameron J L (1974) Aspiration pneumonia. Prevention of aspiration in patients with tracheostomies. *Ann Thorac Surg* 18:30.

85 Cameron J L & Zuidema G D (1972) Aspiration pneumonia. Magnitude and frequency of the problem. *JAMA* 219:1194.

86 Pavlin E G, Van Nimwegan D & Hornbein T F (1975) Failure of a high-compliance low-pressure cuff to prevent aspiration. *Anesthesiology* 42:216.

87 Shahvari M B G, Kigin C M & Zimmerman J E (1977) Speaking tracheostomy tube modified for swallowing dysfunction and chronic aspiration. *Anesthesiology* 44:290.

88 Egatinski J (1975) Overinflating low-pressure cuffs to prevent aspiration. *Anesthesiology* 42:114.

89 Mehta S (1982) Performance of low-pressure cuffs. An experimental evaluation. *Ann R Coll Surg Engl* 64:54.

90 Routh G, Hanning C D & McLedingham I (1979) Pressure on the tracheal mucosa from cuffed tubes. *Br Med J* 1:1425.

91 Riding J E (1975) Minor complications of general anaesthesia. *Br J Anaesth* 47:91.

92 Lund L O & Daos F G (1965) Effects on postoperative sore throats of two analgesic agents and lubricants used with endotracheal tubes. *Anesthesiology* 26:681.

93 Stanley T H (1965) Nitrous oxide and pressures and volume of high- and low-pressure endotracheal tube cuffs in intubated patients. *Anesthesiology* 42:637.

94 Loeser E A, Orr D L, Bennett G M & Stanley T H (1976) Endotracheal tube cuff design and post operative sore throat. *Anesthesiology* 45:684.

95 Loeser E A, Machin R, Colley J, Orr D, Bennett G M & Stanley T H (1978) Postoperative sore throat — importance of endotracheal tube conformity versus cuff design. *Anesthesiology* 49:430.

96 Loeser E A, Bennett G M, Orr D L & Stanley T H (1980) Reduction of postoperative sore throat with new endotracheal tube cuffs. *Anesthesiology* 52:257.

97 Loeser E A, Stanley T L, Jordan W & Machin R (1980) Postoperative sore throat: influence of tracheal cuff lubrication versus cuff design. *Can Anaesth Soc J* 27:156.

98 Saarnivaara L & Grahne B (1981) Clinical study on an endotracheal tube with a high-residual volume, low pressure cuff. *Acta Anaesthesiol Scand* 25:89.

99 Stenqvist O & Nilsson K (1982) Postoperative sore throat related to tracheal tube cuff design. *Can Anaesth Soc J* 29:384.

100 Jensen P J, Hommelgaard P, Sondergaard P & Eriksen S (1982) Sore throat after operation: influence of tracheal intubation, intracuff pressure and type of cuff. *Br J Anaesth* 54:453.

101 Stock C & Downs J B (1982) Lubrication of tracheal tubes to prevent sore throat from intubation. *Anesthesiology* 57:418.

102 Capan L M, Bruce D L, Patel K P & Turndorf H (1983) Succinylcholine induced postoperative sore throat. *Anesth Analg* 62:245.

103 Wylie W D & Churchill-Davidson H C (1972) Examination of the respiratory tract and tracheal intubation. In: *A Practice of Anaesthesia*, 3rd edn, pp. 368–371. Year Book Medical Publishers, Chicago.

104 Alexopoulos C & Lindholm C E (1983) Airway complaints and laryngeal pathology after intubation with an anatomically shaped tube. *Acta Anaesthesiol Scand* 27:339.

105 Mehta S (1984) Endotracheal cuff pressure. *Br Med J* 288:1763.

106 Lindholm C E & Carroll RG (1975) Evaluation of tube deformation pressure *in vitro*. *Crit Care Med* 2:196.

107 Lindholm C E (1973) Experience with a new oro-tracheal tube. *Acta Otolaryngol (Stockh)* 75:389.

108 Lindholm C E & Grenvik A (1977) Flexible fibreoptic bronchoscopy and intubation in intensive care. In: McLedingham I (ed) *Recent Advances in Intensive Therapy*, p. 55. Churchill Livingstone, Edinburgh.

109 Alexopoulos C, Larsson S G & Lindholm C E (1983) Anatomical shape of the airway. *Acta Anaesthesiol Scand* 27:185.

110 Alexopoulos C, Larsson S G & Lindholm C E (1983) The anatomical shape of the airway after orotracheal intubation. *Acta Anaesthesiol Scand* 27:331.

111 Lindholm C E & Grenvik A (1982) Tracheal tube and cuff problems. *Int Anesthesiol Clin* 20:103.

112 Pippin L K, Short D H & Bowes J B (1983) Long-term tracheal intubation practice in the United Kingdom. *Anaesthesia* 38:791.

113 Morris G & Latto I P (1985) An electropneumatic instrument for measuring and controlling the pressures in the cuffs of tracheal tubes: 'The Cardiff Cuff Controller'. *J Med Eng Technol* (in press).

114 Browning D H & Graves S A (1983) Incidence of aspiration with endotracheal tubes in children. *J Pediatr* 102:582.

115 Mehta S (1984) Safe lateral wall cuff pressure to prevent aspiration. *Ann R Coll Surg Engl* 66:426.

116 Lindholm C E (1977) Den iatrogent fororsakade trakealstenosens etiologi. *Lakartidningen* 74:2344.

117 Nordin U (1976) The trachea and cuff induced tracheal injury. An experimental study on causative factors and prevention. *Acta Otolaryngol* 345:1.

CHAPTER 5 Intubation procedure and causes of difficult intubation

INTRODUCTION

Difficulty with intubation may not be anticipated preoperatively. However, anticipation of such a possibility can decrease morbidity and mortality, especially in an emergency situation.

It is therefore essential to be prepared for impending difficulty at all times which will enable the operator calmly to make and follow a rational plan of action with the correct equipment immediately available as described in Chapter 7. Preoperative examination is an important step in the preparation. Intubation difficulty can arise either from inability to visualize the larynx or from obstruction to the passage of the tracheal tube, or from a combination of these.

INTUBATION PROCEDURE

Difficulty in passing a tracheal tube may be encountered because of errors in technique or choice of equipment.

Patient position

Chevalier Jackson (1913) stressed the importance of anterior flexion of the lower cervical

spine in addition to the more obvious extension of the atlanto-occipital joint [1]. Bannister & MacBeth (1944) described the axial alignment of mouth, pharynx and larynx with this position, commonly referred to as 'sniffing the morning air' [2]. The axial planes can be seen in Figs 1a, b and c.

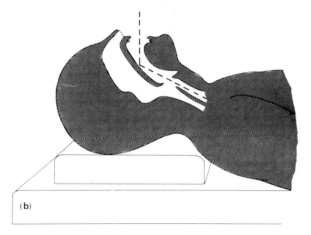

(b)

Fig. 1 (b) Supine position with flexion of the lower portion of the cervical spine produced by a pillow placed under the occiput, thus producing alignment of the pharynx and trachea.

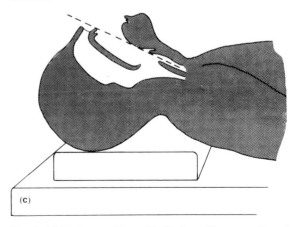

(c)

Fig. 1 (c) Supine position with flexion of lower portion of cervical spine and extension of the atlanto-occipital joint. Mouth, pharynx and trachea are in perfect alignment.

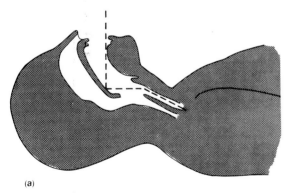

(a)

Fig. 1 (a) Supine position demonstrating the axial planes of mouth, pharynx and trachea.

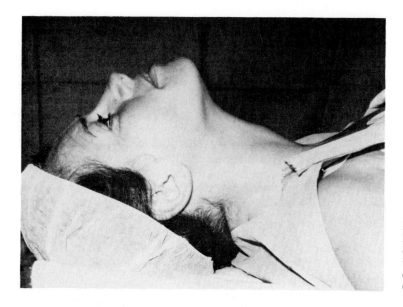

Fig. 2 Perfect position for intubation. Flexion of the lower portion of the cervical spine produced by a pillow under the head. Axial alignment completed by extension of the atlanto-occipital joint (voluntary).

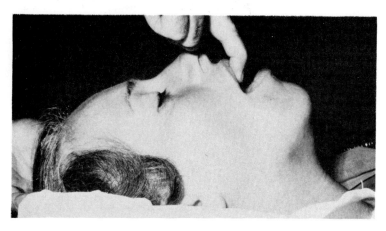

Fig. 3 Intubation position in the unconscious patient. Note the pillow under the head producing flexion of the lower portion of the cervical spine. Extension of the atlanto-occipital joint is initially produced by caudad pressure from the left hand on the top of the head and upward traction from the index finger of the right hand on the upper teeth or gum.

In practice, the lower portion of the cervical spine is maintained in a position of flexion by means of a pillow under the head (Fig. 2). Extension of the atlanto-occipital joint is achieved by traction on the upper teeth or gum with the left index finger, whilst the middle finger of that hand depresses the mandible, thus opening the mouth. In addition to depressing the mandible, the middle finger also ensures the lips are not trapped between the teeth and the blade (Figs 3 and 5).

The relative increase in the anteroposterior plane in the head of a child usually makes the use of a pillow unnecessary to flex lower cervical vertebrae.

Instruments and technique

Laryngoscope blades are straight or curved. The tip of the curved laryngoscope blade (Fig. 4), is inserted into the right corner of the mouth and advanced at the side of the tongue towards the right tonsillar fossa, so that the tongue lies in the recess on the left side of the laryngoscope blade. The tip of the blade is moved into the midline when the right tonsillar fossa is visualized. During these manoeuvres, it is important to ensure that the lips and tongue are not trapped between the teeth and the blade (Fig. 5). The blade is then cautiously advanced behind the base of the tongue, elevating it, until

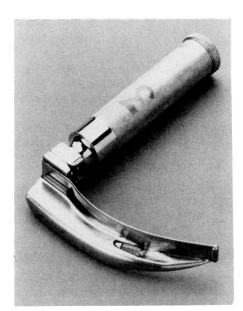

Fig. 4 Macintosh laryngoscope.

the epiglottis is visualized. The tip of the blade is advanced into the vallecula, anterior to the base of the epiglottis, which is lifted forwards to expose the vocal cords (Fig. 6).

Modifications are required when using a straight blade. The straight blade is inserted into the midline, thus depressing the tongue, to expose the epiglottis. The tip of the blade is then placed immediately posterior to the epiglottis, directly lifting the structure forwards to expose the underlying glottic aperture (Fig. 7).

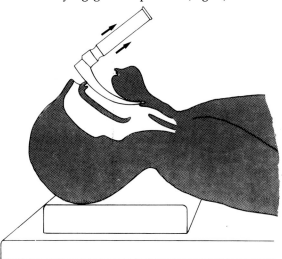

Fig. 6 Diagram to show final position of the curved laryngoscope blade. N.B. The arrows denote the direction of traction on the handle.

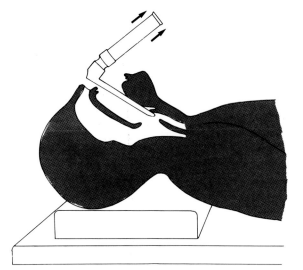

Fig. 7 Diagram to show final position of the straight laryngoscope blade. N.B. The arrows denote the direction of traction on the handle.

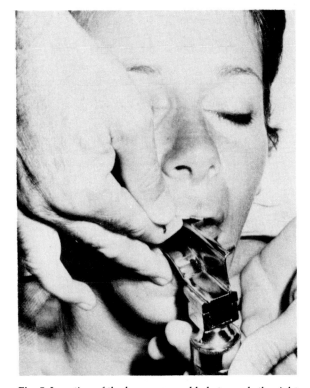

Fig. 5 Insertion of the laryngoscope blade towards the right tonsillar fossa. Maintenance of intubation position with index finger of the right hand. Middle finger of right hand depresses the mandible to open the mouth and also clears the lip from the laryngoscope blade and lower dentition or gum.

With both types of laryngoscope blade, traction is applied along the handle, at right angles to the blade to expose the glottis. This should not be achieved by leverage on the upper teeth or alveolar margins.

These guidelines are intended for a right handed anaesthetist. Laryngoscope blades are also manufactured for left handed operators which should be used with a similar technique applied to the opposite side.

The tip of a blade may pass inadvertently into the oesophagus, although this is unlikely if the procedure is carried out slowly and methodically. The operator should be alerted by failure to visualize the larynx at the appropriate level and recognition of oesophageal mucosa. Passage of the 'tracheal' tube without visualizing the larynx may result in oesophageal intubation and possible disaster. Unrecognized, it inevitably leads to hypoxia and eventual death. If there is delay in recognition it may have caused gastric distension and regurgitation.

Children

Older children can usually be intubated in the same way as adults since the anatomy is virtually identical. However in younger children, infants and neonates certain differences exist.

The larynx is situated at a higher level in relation to the cervical spine and therefore in relation to the mandible and base of the tongue. The result is that the larynx is placed more anteriorly. To obtain adequate exposure, it may be necessary to apply external pressure on the thyroid cartilage. In the neonate, this can be achieved by using the little finger of the left hand; the remaining fingers hold the handle of the laryngoscope blade (Fig. 8).

The glottis is flaccid and leaf-like at this age, protruding into the pharynx and obscuring the glottic aperture. It has the shape of an elongated 'U'. Access into the mouth and adequate exposure of the larynx in the neonate and infant is facilitated by the use of a small, straight laryngoscope blade, such as the Seward (Fig. 9)

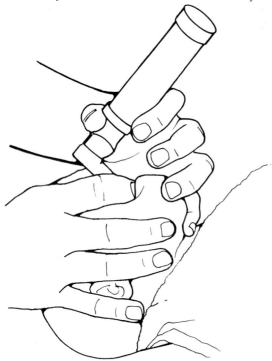

Fig. 8 Intubation of the neonate.

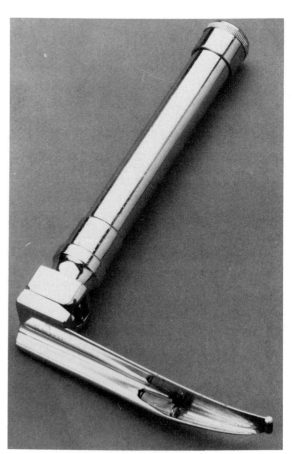

Fig. 9 Seward laryngoscope.

combined with a narrow handle. Some clinicians purposely pass the blade into the oesophagus, distal to the glottic aperture and expose the latter by slow withdrawal. The tip of the blade then slips posteriorly to the epiglottis. The straight blade can also be inserted into the vallecula (anterior to the epiglottis) and used in the same manner as a curved blade.

The narrowest portion of the larynx at this age is the cricoid ring. To reduce laryngeal trauma, it is important that loose-fitting, non-cuffed tracheal tubes are employed, which allow a slight leakage of gases during inflation of the lungs.

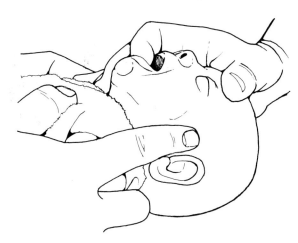

Fig. 10 Skilled assistance for the intubation of the small child.

Intubation in the neonate is facilitated by experienced assistance. It may be necessary to elevate the shoulder to overcome the increased anteroposterior depth of the skull; movement of the head from side to side is also prevented by the assistant's index fingers (Fig. 10). Awake intubation can be successful in the neonate without any form of anaesthesia but trauma should be avoided. If initial attempts prove difficult despite adequate skilled assistance, it is safer to anaesthetize the child.

Muscle relaxants are commonly utilized for intubation in children. If venous access is difficult, intramuscular suxamethonium may be useful (2–3 mg/kg); the onset of relaxation is slower than intravenous administration and recovery is prolonged.

Muscle relaxation

Adequate muscle relaxation should be present prior to intubation. A common cause of difficulty is an attempt to intubate before a short-acting relaxant has worked or after the effect has worn off if the attempt is prolonged. Muscle relaxants may not be indicated if there is pre-existing respiratory obstruction, or obvious anatomical deformities complicating intubation, or during certain emergency procedures. Mouth opening may be limited despite adequate muscle relaxation. Occasionally, muscle spasm can be produced by certain drugs such as fentanyl but it can be antagonized by muscle relaxants [3]. Droperidol may also present a similar picture [4]. Malignant hyperpyrexia is often preceded by abnormal muscle spasm, frequently triggered by the use of suxamethonium or halothane. Myotonia congenita is characterized by abnormal muscle contracture – greatly augmented by the injudicious use of suxamethonium.

ANATOMICAL ABNORMALITIES

Physiological

Certain anatomical configurations which are compatible with a normal existence can give rise to concern during intubation. The most common problem is inability to visualize the larynx which may be encountered in association with the following features:

1 short muscular neck (bull neck);
2 receding mandible;
3 prominent upper incisors;
4 'narrow' mouth with high arched palate;
5 limited movement of mandible;
6 large breasts.

X-ray measurements in patients with laryngoscopy problems were initially discussed by Cass et al (1956) (Fig. 11). The distances mentioned as being relevant were [5]:

1 incisor tooth to posterior border of ramus;
2 alveolar margin to lower border of the mandible;
3 angle of mandible.

Malocclusion was also identified as a contributory factor. Absolute measurements were not given by the authors.

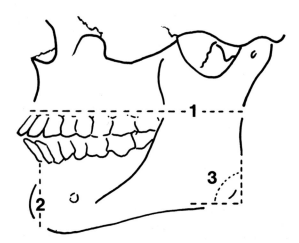

Fig. 11 X-ray measurements. From Cass et al [5], with kind permission of the authors and the *British Medical Journal*.

White & Kander [6] compared radiological measurements in normal patients and those in whom direct laryngoscopy had proved difficult. The radiograph predictors of difficult laryngoscopy were:

1 Increased posterior depth of the mandible (measurement 6, Fig. 12) in relation to the effective mandibular length (measurement 5, Fig. 12). It was found that if the ratio of effective mandibular length to the posterior depth of the mandible was greater than 3.6 difficult intubation was unlikely.
2 Increased depth of the mandible (measurement 7, Fig. 12).
3 Reduction in the distance between the occiput and the spinous process of C_1 (atlanto-occipital distance), and to the lesser extent C_1–C_2 interspinous gap (measurement 10, Fig. 12).
4 Reduced mobility of the mandible.

Nichol & Zuck [7] stressed the importance of the atlanto-occipital distance as a determinant of the ability to extent the head during laryngoscopy. Evans & Cormack (1984) produced a computer-generated equation linking this distance with the posterior depth of the mandible [8]:

$$Y = 27.1 - 12.2\,X_1 + 1.3\,X_2$$

where

X_1 = measurement 6, posterior depth of the mandible (cm);
X_2 = measurement 10, atlanto-occipital distance (cm).
If Y is negative then difficulty with laryngoscopy and intubation may occur.

Maxillary protrusion

A study of Nigerian patients [9] demonstrated maxillary protrusion in 20% of patients in the surgical population as determined by measurement of distance between the upper incisors and vocal cords. There was a statistically significant correlation between 'upper incisor to vocal cords' and 'tragus of ear to the nasal septum' measurements; thus the latter measurement could be utilized to predict maxillary protrusion. It must be emphasized that malocclusion is usually obvious in these patients and difficulty with laryngoscopy can be anticipated.

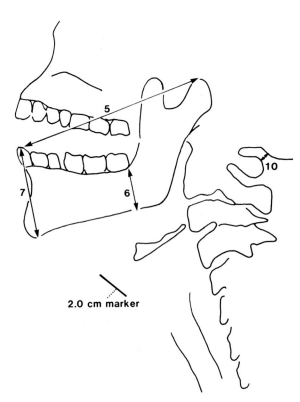

2.0 cm marker

Fig. 12 X-ray measurements. From White & Kander [6].

Mandibular coronoid hyperplasia

An infrequent disorder of the mandible is hyperplasia of the coronoid process which if bilateral will present as inability to open the mouth, in the absence of obvious pathology. Bilateral mandibular hyperplasia usually occurs in males.

Cervical rigidity

Physiological reduction in the mobility of the cervical spine occurs with advancing age. The normal range of flexion–extension movements is 90–160° but the movement in any individual will be reduced by 20% by the seventh decade of life, without an obvious disease state [10]. Although this could theoretically hinder laryngoscopy, this does not seem to be a problem in practice. Nichol & Zuck (1983) [7] discuss an unexpected difficult intubation in a 9-year-old child.

Congenital

Failure of normal embryological development may produce defects in the respiratory passage which can prevent the successful passage of a tracheal tube.

Absence of the nose

This rare condition is often associated with a high arched palate. Surgery may be required because of accompanying feeding difficulties.

Choanal atresia

This soft tissue or bony obstruction at the posterior border of the hard palate can be a cause of neonatal mortality if not recognized at birth by the passage of a small soft catheter through the nares. Atresia exists if the catheter is halted in the nasopharynx at a distance less than 32 mm. A strong familial tendency exists and a sibling with this condition should increase the degree of expectation in the newborn. It is often accompanied by congenital heart defects. In undiagnosed cases attempts at feeding can result in aspiration and secondary pneumonitis. Episodes of respiratory obstruction and cyanosis also occur.

An effective emergency treatment is the insertion of a rubber 'dummy' with ventilation holes, and attachments which can be strapped around the ears. After a few days the child learns to coordinate alternate breathing and swallowing. Surgery is then performed at the age of 1 year. Alternatively a surgical sound can be used to perforate the obstruction and definitive surgery is performed at the age of 2 weeks. An awake intubation or an inhalational induction with oral intubation is then required.

Encephalocoele

This is a protrusion of meningeal-covered brain substance in the nasofrontal region, which although rare, could produce difficulty in visualizing the cords and subsequent passage of the endotracheal tube.

Congenital fusion of the jaws

This rare abnormality has been reported in association with a cleft palate [11]. Other associations are aglossia, facial hemiatrophy and retrognathia.

Radiographs of the temporomandibular joints may be normal; the fusion of the joints is due to fibroepithelial and fibrocartilaginous material. Intubation may be impossible and elective tracheostomy is preferable to the inadvertent trauma produced by blind probing with a tracheal tube.

Macroglossia

This condition may be idiopathic, or it may be due to lymphangioma or haemangioma. In the Beckwith–Wiedemann Syndrome [12] macroglossia is accompanied by hypoglycaemia and an omphalocoele. An enlarged tongue will sometimes obstruct direct vision of the vocal cords.

Maxillofacial cleft

This condition may affect the lip or palate or both. There is an incidence of 1 in 700 in the newborn. In 1973 Zawistowska et al classified this type of abnormality in 787 patients according to increasing difficulties met by the anaesthetist during intubation [13]. These may be seen in Table 1. The main problem is lack of

Table 1 Classification of the congenital defects of the maxillofacial cleft. From Zawistowska et al [13].

Defect	Grade of difficulty
Isolated cleft lip	0
R-sided cleft of lip and alveolar process / R-sided cleft of lip, alveolar process and palate	1
L-sided cleft of the lip and alveolar process / Bilateral cleft of lip and alveolar process / L-sided cleft of the lip, alveolar process and palate	2
Bilateral cleft of lip, alveolar process and palate	3

support for the laryngoscope blade and these authors suggest three solutions:

1 the use of a tongue depressor as a support;

2 the insertion of the laryngoscope at the extreme right hand side of the mouth;

3 extension of the head by the assistant to open the mouth and conventional approach with a curved laryngoscope blade. The forward thrust of the laryngoscope handle compensates for the lack of support by the alveolar margins.

Treacher-Collins syndrome (mandibulofacial dysostosis)

This condition results from an embryological disturbance in the formation of the first branchial arch. It produces a hypoplastic mandible, a receding chin, macroglossia, glossoptosis, maxillary protrusion and trismus related to temporomandibular joint abnormalities. The palate is high and the teeth abnormally placed. In addition to the problems with intubation, it is difficult to maintain an airway even with the insertion of an artificial airway [14]. This syndrome should be recognized prior to induction of anaesthesia.

Features which aid the preoperative recognition of this syndrome include abnormalities of:

1 Ears – there is deformity of the pinna frequently accompanied by atresia of the external auditory meatus. Partial or complete deafness may be present.

2 Eyes – there is an oblique palpebral fissure with droop of canthus and often a notch in the lower eyelid at the junction between the medial two-thirds and the outer one-third. Meibomian glands are absent and there is no intermarginal strip. The eyelashes in the medial two-thirds are absent. The eyes lie on an oblique axis.

3 Miscellaneous features:

    (a) normal mentality;

    (b) familial incidence;

    (c) relationship with hare-lip and cleft palate;

    (d) long second metatarsal – a constant feature.

The Pierre Robin disorder and hemi-facial microsomia also present with mandibular hypoplasia which displace the tongue backwards producing an apparent 'anterior larynx'.

Craniofacial dystosis (Crouzon's syndrome)

These patients may present for correction of exophthalmus. Other characteristics are hypertelorism, parrot-beaked nose, high arched palate, nasal obstruction and obliteration of the paranasal sinuses. Breckner (1968) described a patient suffering additionally with the Pickwickian syndrome. A fascinating feature of that case was the presence of a calcified and enlarged anterior longitudinal ligament extending anteriorly down the bodies of the cervical vertebrae and bulging into the pharynx, which produced airway obstruction [15].

Klippel-Feil syndrome

The neck is shortened. Cervical movement is limited due to a reduction in number, fusion or abnormal shape of the cervical vertebrae.

Engelmann's disease (osteopathia hyperostotica scleroticans multiplex infantilis)

This rare disease of the skeleton causes intubation difficulties with limited opening of the mouth and an immobile neck. Retrograde catheterization techniques have been used to facilitate intubation [16].

Achondroplasia (chondodystrophia fetalis)

This inherited condition produces a dwarf-like appearance due to abnormality of cartilage development [17]. Difficulties are due to an angular kyphosis between C_2 and C_3. Full extension of the head results in the axis of

C_1–C_2 making a forward angle of inclination of 25° with respect to C_2–C_3, thus producing an anteriorly placed larynx.

Fetal alcohol syndrome

This occurs in offspring of alcoholics. Deformities relevant to the anaesthetist include maxillary and mandibular hypoplasia [18]. Children with this syndrome have been intubated using bougie techniques [19].

Subglottic cysts

These cysts present at birth or appearing shortly afterwards are a remnant from the thyroglossal duct. They arise from the epiglottis and aryepiglottic folds and may be lined with respiratory or squamous epithelium. Healing of a mucosal lesion after intubation produces a subglottic cystic lesion, although stenosis is the more common event. Intubation may be impossible, and a tracheostomy may be required.

Cystic hygroma

This is due to a congenital defect in the formation of lymphatic channels. The lymphangioma may be unilateral or bilateral and extend into the mediastinum or axilla. Some cysts are small, whilst others are large involving many structures in the neck. They present as multiple cavernous cysts containing serous fluid, serosanguinous fluid, or frank blood.

The lesion may be present at birth but usually occurs during the first year of life. Involvement of the upper airway may include tongue, lips, floor of the mouth, styloid process, larynx, epiglottis and aryepiglottic folds.

Upper respiratory tract obstruction can occur, necessitating tracheostomy. Intubation of these children can be hazardous [20].

Aspiration of the cysts may be carried out as an emergency procedure but the fluid soon tends to reaccumulate.

Vascular compression of trachea

The trachea may be compressed by enlarged great vessels, the most common being the innominate artery, although occasionally it may be due to double aortic arch. The condition may

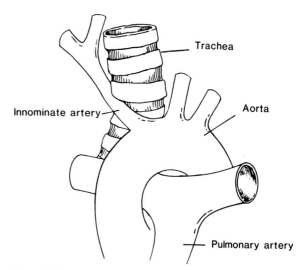

Fig. 13 Compression of the trachea by the innominate artery.

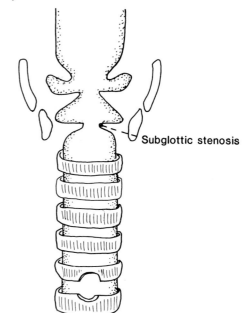

Fig. 14 Schematic representation of subglottic stenosis.

remain symptomless until accompanied by intercurrent respiratory tract infection (Fig. 13).

Subglottic stenosis

Recurrent croup or persistent stridor may occasionally present with subglottic stenosis which prevents the passage of the correct size tube. More commonly, this condition can arise after prolonged intubation (Fig. 14).

Mucopolysaccharide disease

Clinical features of this group include:
1 skeletal changes;
2 coarse facies;
3 corneal clouding;
4 mental retardation.

(1) Hurler's syndrome (gargoylism). This disease may be inherited as an autosomal recessive trait or a sex-limited recessive trait affecting males. No physical abnormalities are seen at birth but these develop slowly after 6 months and are apparent in the second year. A grotesque, coarse facial appearance develops and of importance to the anaesthetist, a large tongue with a short neck and limited extension. These children are prone to respiratory failure and may suffer intimal thickening of the coronary arteries and valves.

(2) Hunter's syndrome. These children are similar to those with Hurler's syndrome but have a longer lifespan.

(3) Morquio's syndrome. Intubation may be hazardous because of a flattened face and degenerate odontoid peg with the possibility of spinal cord damage [21]. Associated factors include kyphosis, pigeon chest, poor vision and deafness.

Laryngeal web

This rare abnormality may be congenital or acquired and can create a variable degree of obstruction. The congenital variety can occur at the glottic, supraglottic or subglottic levels [22].

Inflammatory

Bacterial

Difficult intubation can occur in any inflammatory process producing oedema, contracture or abscess formation in the upper respiratory tract. The following have been described.

Quinsy and retropharyngeal abscess. Infection in the pharyngeal area can produce pathological enlargement either by oedema, exudate or frank abscess. Inability to open the mouth (trismus) may occur, but this sometimes improves once anaesthesia is established. Swelling may obscure visualization of the larynx and hinder the subsequent passage of the tracheal tube.

Epiglottitis. This is caused by a rapidly progressive bacterial infection involving supraglottic structures, distal spread being prevented by tightly adherent mucosa on the vocal cords. The causative organism is usually *Haemophilus influenzae* (type B), occasionally *Staphylococcus, Streptococcus, Neisseria catarrhalis*, pneumococci or virus. It commonly affects children aged from 1 month to 3½ years. For the first 3 months of life passive immunity is acquired from the mother; natural immunity is usually acquired after entry into school.

Respiratory arrest can occur quite suddenly in these children. Once the diagnosis has been confirmed the child should be intubated. This should always be performed by experienced personnel with the appropriate facilities and equipment. Conservative management may be indicated in isolated cases but it is dangerous since results are unpredictable. Cantrell et al (1976) reviewed 749 patients with a mortality rate of 6.1% with a conservative approach [23].

Increasing awareness has reduced mortality. The incidence of epiglottitis has been reported to be 0.1% of paediatric admissions, 8% of which present with respiratory distress [24]. Most anaesthetists are asked at some time to deal with this disease, especially in endemic areas. There are other causes of epiglottitis – inhalation of steam, ingestion of corrosives and diphtheria, and it may arise without obvious cause in the adult.

Diagnosis is made by the history and then confirmed with a lateral cervical X-ray – if time permits. Examination of the pharynx should be carried out in theatre under anaesthesia, as sudden excitement can precipitate acute complete respiratory obstruction. Tracheal intubation may be carried out following an inhalational induction using a tracheal tube a size smaller than anticipated. Experience has shown that continued intubation (up to 4 days) is preferable to tracheostomy [25–27]. Extubation is usually possible after 48 h thus avoiding the complication of laryngeal granulomata.

Leprosy. This is a rare cause of obstructive granulation tissue in the upper respiratory tract.

Diphtheria. This membrane-producing disease is now virtually extinct in the Western hemisphere.

Viral

Infectious mononucleosis. In the glandular variety, infection is due to the Epstein–Barr virus (EBV), lymphadenopathy being the predominant feature. Proliferation of tonsillar and adenoidal lymphoid tissue can produce severe pharyngeal obstruction.

Croup. This is an oedematous viral infection which occurs below the vocal cords, the majority of cases responding to medical management. A small number require intubation with a smaller tracheal tube than calculated.

Non-infective inflammation

Rheumatoid arthritis

Juvenile chronic arthritis and rheumatoid arthritis are clinically and biochemically distinct entities, which occur under and over the age of 16 respectively [28]. However, difficulties in intubation can occur in both cases, and distinction between the types of arthritides is less important to the anaesthetist.

Rheumatoid arthritis can be associated with the following.

Instability of the cervical spine. Approximately 3% of patients with biochemical evidence of rheumatoid arthritis will also have cervical instability. This usually occurs at the atlanto-axial joint but may occur at lower levels. Subluxation is present in 30% of hospital inpatients with rheumatoid arthritis. Spinal cord compression or transection occasionally occurs, especially with forced flexion.

Preoperatively instability of the cervical spine should be suspected from the following:
1 vertebral artery insufficiency producing vestibular symptoms and diplopia;
2 abnormal neurological signs in the limbs;
3 obvious inability to maintain extension of head and neck with loss of angle between the occiput and cervical spine;
4 neck pain radiating into the occiput (neck pain itself is a frequent concomitant of rheumatoid arthritis);

5 abnormal protrusion of the axial arch felt by a finger in the pharynx;
6 abnormal radiological appearances:
    (a) abnormal vertebral movement on flexion;
    (b) erosion of the dens;
    (c) narrowing of the space between skull and C_1, C_1 and C_2, with or without the presence of bony erosion;
    (d) increased distance between the anterior surface of the odontoid peg and the anterior surface of C_1. The normal variation in distance is from 2 to 4 mm. Any increase in the distance between the odontoid process and the anterior arch of the atlas in the lateral X-ray of the flexed cervical spine, as compared with the same view in extension, is abnormal.

Cervical fixation. This commonly affects the lower cervical vertebrae, producing a fixed flexion deformity, which prevents adequate extension of the head and difficulty introducing

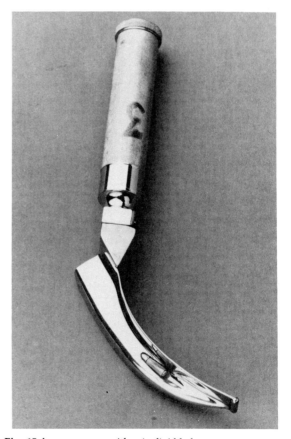

Fig. 15 laryngoscope with a 'polio' blade.

the laryngoscope blade. If it is the only problem it can be circumvented by using a polio blade – a blade which makes an obtuse angle with the handle (Fig. 15).

Temporomandibular disease. Cervical fixation is often accompanied by temporomandibular joint disease, producing major difficulties with intubation due to an inability to open the mouth.

Cricoarytenoid disorders. Disease affecting these joints can impede the passage of the tracheal tube due to glottic stenosis. Jenkins & McGraw [29] recommend a preoperative tracheostomy if this condition exists. It should be suspected if, preoperatively, the rheumatoid patient presents with hoarseness, dyspnoea on exertion, stridor, dysphagia or fullness in the throat. The diagnosis is confirmed by indirect laryngoscopy which shows decreased cricoarytenoid movement, or bowing of the cords during inspiration.

Hypoplastic mandible. This may be associated with rheumatoid arthritis. A comprehensive review of anaesthetic problems associated with rheumatoid arthritis is presented by Jenkins & McGraw (1963) [29]. The disorders of the airway which occur with rheumatoid arthritis and their relevance to the anaesthetist have been described by D'Arcy et al (1976) [30] (Table 2).

Table 2 A classification of the difficulties in airway management with rheumatoid arthritis. From D'Arcy et al [30], with kind permission of the authors and Academic Press, publishers of *Anaesthesia*.

	Usual clinical characteristics	Quality of airway	Conventional intubation
Group I	Good movement of neck and jaw	Good	Good
Group II	Stiff cervical spine but good jaw movement	Satisfactory	Very difficult
Group III	Stiff neck and restricted jaw movements	May obstruct at any time	Impossible
Group IV	Stiff neck and jaw with skeletal stunting	Obstructs with sedation	Impossible

Ankylosing spondylitis

This inflammatory arthropathy has been reviewed by Sinclair & Mason (1984) [31]. Upper airway management can be severely compromised by rigidity of the cervical spine, usually in a position of flexion. This is sometimes accompanied by a tendency to cervical fracture at the C_5–C_7 level [32], and as a result, the possibility of cord damage. A small proportion of these patients (10–40%) have limited mouth opening due to temporomandibular disease [33].

Neoplasm

Benign or malignant tumours extending into the airway can obscure the operator's view and obstruct the passage of a tracheal tube.

Laryngeal papillomatosis

This is an uncommon, but well recognized, cause of stridor in childhood which can progress to respiratory failure and death. Most tumours in children are benign; despite certain characteristics of viral infection, electron microscopy has failed to demonstrate characteristic inclusion bodies or viruses. Laryngeal papillomata are seen in the newborn but can occur at any age, and regression may be seen at puberty. Harper et al (1973) described a patient with persistent laryngeal obstruction and respiratory failure, dependent on hypoxaemia as a stimulant for respiration; relief of hypoxaemia resulted in episodes of apnoea [34]. The history from the parents may suggest the possibility of laryngeal papillomata; huskiness prior to dyspnoea is the vital clue.

Calcification of the stylohyoid ligament

Several reports in the literature have cited calcification of the stylohyoid ligament producing difficulty with intubation [35, 36], which arises due to an inability to elevate the soft tissue around the vallecula and hyoid bone. There is shortening and immobility of the stylohyoid ligament and associated muscles.

It had been previously suggested that these patients could be identified preoperatively by a prominent skin crease over the hyoid bone [35], but this was absent in two cases reported by Akinyemi & Elegbe [36]. The common feature seen on laryngoscopy is a difficulty in lifting the epiglottis away from the posterior laryngeal wall with a curved laryngoscope.

If this condition is suspected preoperatively, it may be confirmed by preliminary X-rays. Coincidental finding on X-ray should alert the anaesthetist to a difficult intubation.

Endocrine

Obesity

Obesity produces difficulty in insertion of the laryngoscope blade through the mouth. It may be corrected by the use of the 'polio' blade in place of the usual right angled blade. Thus, the handle of the blade is no longer deflected by protuberant breast tissue. This problem may be accentuated in the pregnant patient.

Acromegaly

This disease, which results from hyperactivity of the pituitary gland, in addition to other features, may produce abnormalities in the upper airway. The relevant features are:
1 macroglossia;
2 thickening of pharyngeal tissues;
3 thickening of laryngeal soft tissues and vocal cords;
4 recurrent laryngeal nerve palsy;
5 decrease in the width of the cricoid arch;
6 fixation of the vocal cords;
7 prognathism;
8 hypertrophy of the aryepiglottic and ventricular folds.

It may be difficult to ventilate an apnoeic acromegalic patient with a mask because of the large nose, hypertrophied nasal cartilages and spreading teeth.

In addition, it may also be difficult to intubate because of difficulty in visualizing the larynx. Indeed, the above changes can be so severe as to cause respiratory obstruction and death unrelated to anaesthesia or surgery [37].

Thyroid goitre

In the author's experience, visualization of the cords has not been difficult, even in the presence of extremely large goitres. Deviation of the trachea, which occurs more commonly than

compression, tends to obstruct the subsequent passage of too rigid a tracheal tube but a latex armoured tube is suitable as it is flexible but will not collapse from compression. However this may necessitate using a tracheal tube with a smaller diameter than anticipated.

Trauma

Trauma to the face and neck can compromise the airway and produce problems with intubation due to haemorrhage, haematoma, oedema and accompanying distortion of the tissues.

Intubation may be difficult due to an inability to visualize the larynx and there may be obstruction to the passage of a tracheal tube.

Facial injuries

Mandibular fractures. Fractures of the mandible are frequently bilateral and often indirect. Problems associated with intubation are:
1 hypermobility of tongue, resulting in pharyngeal obstruction;
2 distortion of the normal dental configuration which can obstruct the passage of a tracheal tube as well as obscuring the larynx from vision. The author was presented with a patient whose dentures were firmly embedded in the lower posterior pharyngeal wall following facial trauma;
3 haemorrhage and oedema involving tissues within the tongue which present a major obstruction to oral intubation;
4 trismus prevents adequate opening of the mouth in the conscious state and may be due to deformity or pain. Until the patient is anaesthetized it is difficult to be sure which is the cause. Under the effect of general anaesthesia, trismus due to pain rapidly diminishes, allowing normal mouth opening and uncomplicated tracheal intubation. However, trismus due to anatomical deformity will prevent the operator from passing the laryngoscope and a very dangerous situation may be present;
5 risk of vomiting or regurgitation of stomach contents which may include large clots of blood in addition to recently ingested food;
6 concomitant cervical injuries which could jeopardize the spinal cord during intubation.

It must be stressed that definitive surgery for mandibular fractures can be delayed for 24 h during which time conditions for intubation could become far more favourable – but many of these injuries are compound and undue delay could lead to osteomyelitis. Nasal intubation must be achieved for surgical access. If inspection of the mouth and pharynx suggests no obvious difficulty with intubation, then pre-oxygenation, paralysis with suxamethonium and cricoid pressure is the method of choice. Tracheostomy prior to surgery is rarely indicated; the fractured mandible is mobile when the patient is unconscious and intubation is rarely a problem to the trained anaesthetist.

Maxillary fractures (middle third fractures). Injury to this region may necessitate early oral intubation even prior to projected surgery to provide the airway. Laryngoscopy and intubation may be impeded by the presence of haemorrhage and anatomical distortion. When the nasal fractures have been surgically corrected the oral tube can be replaced by a nasal tube to improve surgical access.

Laryngeal and tracheal trauma

Injuries to the trachea, larynx and pharynx can be divided into open and closed. The open injuries can be further subdivided into incisional and contused (macerated).

1. Open injuries

Incisional injuries. Intubation may be difficult for several reasons:
1 A tendency for the tongue and epiglottis, which are freed from their attachments, to obscure or obstruct the laryngeal opening, when the incision occurs above the hyoid bone.
2 Haemorrhage into the respiratory tract will obscure vision as well as asphyxiate the patient. The greatest danger occurs with incisions at tracheal level, when they may lacerate common carotid or inferior thyroid arteries.
3 Recurrent laryngeal nerve damage may occur with a low incision.
4 Infection with cellulitis and oedema will occur if treatment is delayed.

Contusional injuries. In addition to the lacerations, widespread damage to the underlying structures may occur producing maceration, oedema and damage to the more rigid structures in the throat. The hyoid bone and laryngeal cartilages may be damaged producing considerable distortion.

2. Closed injuries

Life-threatening events may follow massive closed neck injuries. The most common cause of these injuries is sudden deceleration as seen in a car crash.

Rupture of the trachea and larynx are often accompanied by surgical emphysema [38]. Although symptoms such as pain on swallowing, dyspnoea, and haemoptysis may be present this is not always the case, and injury to the larynx and trachea may only become apparent during intubation.

Concomitant cervical spine injuries may prevent the patient being placed in the traditional 'sniffing the morning air' position. In the conscious patient, neurological examination and cervical radiology should be carried out to exclude cord damage before attempting intubation.

Muscle relaxants should not be used prior to intubation in these patients. Inflation will increase the surgical emphysema, and effective ventilation of the lungs may be difficult. Local anaesthesia is impracticable because of the injuries and may even be dangerous in the presence of vomiting from a full stomach. An inhalational induction would therefore seem to be the best choice.

Direct trauma to the neck can produce traumatic dislocation of the arytenoid cartilages [39] so that the arytenoid falls anteromedially causing respiratory obstruction which is augmented by relaxation of the corresponding vocal cord. However, provided that oedema is minimal, this should not obstruct the subsequent passage of the tracheal tube.

Tracheal rupture, as a result of closed injury or laceration, may produce a difficulty with intubation. The former has been rectified by rapid surgical exploration of the cervical tissues and subsequent manipulation of the tube past the injured segment [38]. Occasionally with massive cervical injury, the trachea can be intubated directly through the injured area.

REFERENCES

1 Jackson C (1913) The technique of insertion of intra-tracheal insufflation tubes. *Surg Gynecol Obstet* 17:507.
2 Bannister F & MacBeth R G (1944) Direct laryngoscopy and tracheal intubation. *Lancet* ii: 651.
3 Askgaard B, Nilson T, Ibler M et al (1977) Muscle tone under fentanyl-nitrous oxide anaesthesia measured with a transducer apparatus in cholecystectomy incisions. *Acta Anaesthesiol Scand* 21:1.
4 Patton C M (1975) Rapid induction of acute dyskinesia by droperidol. *Anaesthesiology* 43:126.
5 Cass N M, James N R & Lines V (1956) Difficult direct laryngoscopy complicating intubation for anaesthesia. *Br Med J* 1:488.
6 White A & Kander P L (1975) Anatomical factors in difficult direct laryngoscopy. *Br J Anaesth* 47:468.
7 Nichol H C & Zuck D (1983) Difficult laryngoscopy – the 'anterior' larynx and the atlanto-occipital gap. *Br J Anaesth* 55:141.
8 Evans R & Cormack R S (1984) Correspondence – Difficult intubation. *Points West* 17:79.
9 Magbagbeola J A O & Ayeni O (1972) Some aspects of endotracheal anaesthesia in Nigerians. *West Afr Med J* 21:161.
10 Kattle F J & Mundale M O (1959) Range of mobility of the cervical spine. *Arch Phys Med* 40:379.
11 Seraj M A, Yousif M & Channa A B (1984) Anaesthetic management of congenital fusion of the jaws in a neonate. *Anaesthesia* 39:695.
12 Filippi G & McKusick V A (1970) The Beckwith–Weidemann Syndrome – report of two cases and review of the literature. *Medicine* 49:270.
13 Zawistowska J, Menzel M & Wytyczak M (1973) Difficulties and modifications of intubation technique in infants with labial, alveolar and palatal clefts. *Anaesth Resus Intensive Therap* 1:211.
14 Ross E D T (1963) Treacher Collins Syndrome. An anaesthetic hazard. *Anaesthesia* 18:350.
15 Brechner V L (1968) Unusual problems in the management of airways: flexion-extension mobility of the cervical vertebrae. *Anaesth Analg* 47:362.
16 Mason J & Slee I (1968) Anaesthesia and Engelmann's disease. *Anaesthesia* 23:250.
17 Mather J S (1966) Impossible direct laryngoscopy in achondroplasia. *Anaesthesia* 21:244.
18 Clarren S K & Smith D W (1978) The fetal alcohol syndrome. *N Engl J Med* 298:1063.
19 Finucane B T (1980) Difficult intubation associated with the foetal alcohol syndrome. *Can Anaesth Soc J* 27:574.
20 Weller R M (1974) Anaesthesia for cystic hygroma in a neonate. *Anaesthesia* 29:588.
21 Birkinshaw K J (1975) Anaesthesia in a patient with an unstable neck. *Anaesthesia* 30:46.
22 Capistrano-Baruh E, Wenig B, Steinberg L, Stegnajajic A & Baruh S (1982) Laryngeal web: a cause of difficult endotracheal intubation. *Anesthesiology* 57:123.
23 Cantrell R W, Bell R A & Morioka W T (1976) Acute epiglottitis. *Trans Pac Coast Otoophthalmol Soc Annu Meet* 57:75.
24 Vetto R R (1960) Epiglottitis. *JAMA* 173:990.
25 Oh T H & Motoyama E K (1977) Comparison of nasotracheal intubation and tracheostomy in the management of acute epiglottitis. *Anesthesiology* 46:214.
26 Tos M (1973) Nasotracheal intubation in acute epiglottitidis. *Arch Otolaryngol* 97:373.
27 Milko D A, Marshak G & Striker T W (1974) Nasotracheal intubation in the treatment of acute epiglottitis. *Pediatrics* 53:674.
28 Huskisson E C & Hart F D (1978) Joint Disease: All the Arthropathies, 3rd edn. John Wright, Bristol.
29 Jenkins L C & McGraw W R (1969) Anaesthetic management of the patient with rheumatoid arthritis. *Can Anaesth Soc J* 16:407.
30 D'Arcy E J, Fell R H, Ansell B M & Arden G P (1976) Ketamine and juvenile chronic polyarthritis (Still's disease). *Anaesthesia* 31:624.
31 Sinclair J R & Mason R A (1984) Ankylosing spondylitis. The case for awake intubation. *Anaesthesia* 39:3.
32 Murray G C & Persellin R H (1981) Cervical fracture complicating ankylosing spondylitis. *Am J Med* 70:1033.
33 Resnick D (1974) Temporo-mandibular joint involvement in ankylosing spondylitis. *Radiology* 112:587.
34 Harper J R, Thomas K & Wirk H (1973) A complicated case of juvenile laryngeal papillomatosis. *Anaesthesia* 28:71.
35 Sharwood-Smith G H (1976) Difficulty in intubation. Calcified stylohyoid ligament. *Anaesthesia* 31:508.
36 Akinyemi O O & Elegbe E O (1981) Difficult laryngoscopy and tracheal intubation due to calcified stylohyoid ligaments. *Can Anaesth Soc J* 28:80.
37 Chappel W F (1896) A case of acromegaly with laryngeal and pharyngeal symptoms. *J Laryngol Otol* 10:142.
38 Sirker D & Clark M M (1973) Rupture of the cervical trachea following road traffic accident. *Anaesthesia* 45:909.
39 Seed R F (1971) Traumatic injury to the larynx and trachea. *Anaesthesia* 26:55

CHAPTER 6 Awake intubation

INTRODUCTION

General anaesthesia is not essential for the performance of tracheal intubation. Indeed, in certain circumstances, consciousness is best maintained. In a patient who is awake and breathing spontaneously, it is of little importance if time is taken to complete the intubation process. There need be no sense of urgency, since hypoxia is unlikely to occur. With the use of local anaesthetic agents, the pharyngeal and laryngeal reflexes are obtunded but when vomiting or regurgitation occurs the patient can usually respond to the threat to his airway; the head and thorax are voluntarily turned to the side and the pharynx is cleared by coughing, retching or repeatedly swallowing.

The main disadvantage of 'awake intubation' is the patient's reaction. Closing the mouth, swallowing, gagging, or adducting the vocal cords can make intubation more difficult. Contraction of the pharyngeal muscles can be prevented by a blockade of the glossopharyngeal nerve.

The degree of psychological and physical disturbance to the patient is related to the experience of the operator and his gentleness. It is important that teaching programmes should be arranged using techniques of awake intubation on suitable elective patients with adequate psychological preparation and advice to the patient.

INDICATIONS

Upper airway obstruction

It is axiomatic in anaesthetic practice that patients with airway obstruction are not given muscle relaxants until it is clear that artificial ventilation can be carried out. Avoiding the use of muscle relaxants but attempting intubation under deep general anaesthesia may also be hazardous. In these circumstances, awake intubation is an attractive and safe method and avoids the risk of upper airway obstruction which can occur with general anaesthesia. This may not be acceptable or practical, however, with children or very nervous patients.

Difficult intubation

It is highly desirable to maintain spontaneous respiration in cases of difficult intubation. In a patient with a previous history of difficult or failed intubation a local anaesthetic may be employed. Awake intubation appears more popular in the USA than in the UK perhaps because in a litigious atmosphere it seems safer and easier to justify.

Respiratory failure

These patients are often in extremis. Pharmacological intervention with central nervous system depressants is ill advised. Cardiovascular instability is often a problem and the abrupt commencement of intermittent positive pressure ventilation can produce devastating results with an abrupt reduction in venous return and arterial carbon dioxide tension. Cessation of respiration prior to intubation may be critical in patients with a low arterial oxygen tension, and thus it may be inadvisable to produce sudden muscle relaxation prior to intubation.

Drug overdose

Intubation may be required to treat ensuing respiratory failure or protect the airway to allow safe conduct of gastric lavage following the ingestion of sedative drugs in excess of quantities recommended by the relevant manufacturers. In the latter circumstance the use of central nervous system depressants or muscle relaxants may complicate the monitoring of vital signs.

Moribundity

The use of general anaesthesia is fraught with hazard in the moribund patient. Indeed intubation can often easily be carried out without general anaesthesia, muscle relaxation or topical anaesthesia. Benefit may accrue from the temporary increase in cardiac output, apart from the improvement in oxygen delivery [1].

Full stomach

Awake intubation may be performed on patients with a full stomach in an attempt to prevent aspiration. Patient comfort is sacrificed to avoid subsequent aspiration. Walts (1965) [2] and DeHollander (1974) [3] recommended that local anaesthesia be limited to the supraglottic structures and sedation be minimal. Kopriva et al (1974) [4] demonstrated that topical anaesthesia was slightly safer in this respect than sedation with fentanyl. Libman (1976) [5] expressed the extreme view that topical anaesthesia should be limited to the lower lip and the outer half of the tongue, whilst Thomas (1969) [6] advocated sparing of the subglottic regions by omission of the transtracheal injection.

FIBREOPTIC INTUBATION

The use of a fibreoptic bronchoscope or laryngoscope as a guide to the subsequent passage of a tracheal tube in cases of difficult intubation is discussed elsewhere. This method may also have advantages where it is mandatory to avoid hypertension and tachycardia [7].

The following description of local anaesthetic techniques and sedation used in conjunction with 'awake intubation' apply to both fibreoptic and rigid laryngoscopy, although the suction port of the fibreoptic bronchoscope can be used for a 'spray-as-you-go' technique.

SEDATION

It is desirable that intubation of the conscious patient is performed with the aid of sedation provided that patient safety is not compromised. Agents commonly used for this purpose belong mainly to the benzodiazepine group of drugs (diazepam, midazolam) or the neurolept group (droperidol) often in combination with a short acting opiate (fentanyl or alfentanil).

Diazepam

The intravenous use of diazepam is accompanied by an unacceptable incidence of superficial vein thrombosis. This problem is virtually eliminated by the addition of lipid as solvent to form the preparation Diazemuls. There is often a variation in response [8] and there may be prolonged action with second peak effect [9, 10]. The dose ranges from 5 to 20 mg for a 70 kg patient.

Midazolam

This has a shorter duration of action compared to diazepam [11] and is more suitable for brief procedures such as intubation when this is not followed by general anaesthesia. Water soluble midazolam is virtually devoid of thrombophlebitic problems [12]. The dose range for a 70 kg patient is 2–7.5 mg intravenously.

Fentanyl

This opioid drug is commonly used with droperidol, to produce neuroleptanalgesia. The cough and gag reflex are depressed and the patient often accepts a tracheal tube whilst still capable of obeying a command. The dose range for a 70 kg patient is 50–150 µg intravenously.

Phenoperidine

Phenoperidine is used where a more prolonged analgesia is required following intubation. The dose range for a 70 kg patient is 0.5–1.0 mg.

ANTISIALOGOGUE ADMINISTRATION

Whenever possible, it is helpful and indeed advisable to premedicate with an antisialogogue such as atropine (0.3–0.6 mg, i.v. or i.m.) hyoscine (0.3–0.4 mg, i.v. or i.m.) or glycopyrrolate (0.3 mg, i.v. or i.m.). The resultant reduction in secretions not only reduces the desire by the patient to swallow repeatedly, but also increases the effectiveness of the topical local anaesthetic agent.

LOCAL ANAESTHETIC TECHNIQUES
Topical anaesthesia

During the following discussion on topical anaesthesia, reference will be made to surface-active local anaesthetic agents which will not be specifically named but which include:

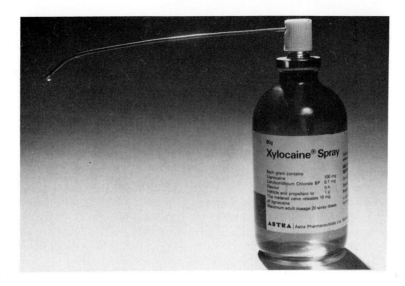

Fig. 1 Metered-dose spray.

cocaine 4–10% (spray or paste)
lignocaine 4–10% (spray or viscous gel)
amethocaine 60 mg (lozenge)

Lignocaine, because of its wider safety margin, is the most commonly used agent for this purpose.

Surface anaesthesia of the nasal mucosa

The nose is packed with ribbon gauze soaked in a local anaesthetic solution. Cocaine, with its intrinsic vasoconstrictive properties, is most commonly used for this purpose but excess solution must be removed prior to insertion to avoid systemic toxicity. Alternatively, the nasal mucosa may be sprayed with lignocaine or cocaine immediately prior to intubation.

Surface anaesthesia of the oropharyngeal-laryngeal regions

'Spray-as-you-go'. Surface anaesthesia may be produced by a 'spray-as-you-go' technique, commencing at the nose or mouth and slowly advancing towards the glottis and infraglottic areas. Despite the advantage of the metered dose with the modern cannister sprays (Fig. 1), older models such as the Swerdlow (Fig. 2) spray have the advantage of a long blunt-ended nozzle which enables safe entry into the glottis and trachea. Toxicity can be avoided by first placing a calculated safe dose for each patient in the reservoir chamber (Table 1).

Lozenges. Anaesthesia of the mouth and upper pharynx can be achieved by the administration

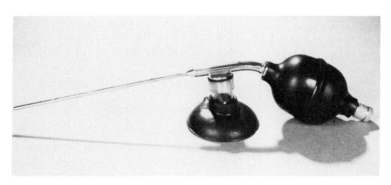

Fig. 2 Swerdlow spray.

Table 1 Maximum safe dose of local anaesthetic agents (topical application)

Lignocaine	3 mg/kg
Cocaine	1.5 mg/kg
Amethocaine	0.8 mg/kg

of an amethocaine lozenge (60 mg) 30 min prior to intubation.

Gargle. An alternative to the lozenge is for the patient to gargle a 4% lignocaine gel which is bitter but can be flavoured to improve patient acceptance.

Ultrasonic nebulizer. An ultrasonic nebulizer containing 10 ml of 4% plain lignocaine (400 mg) inhaled through a mask for 10 min was effective in 95% of 1000 patients, being prepared for bronchoscopy [13]. Serum levels of lignocaine were below the toxic limit of 5 µg/ml.

Labat's syringe. The glottis and infraglottic areas can be anaesthetized using Labat's syringe (Fig. 3) or a similar curved applicator. The patient is placed in the sitting position facing the operator. The tongue is extended and held with a gauze swab by the operator or the patient. In the latter situation the operator is able to utilize an indirect laryngoscope with a warmed mirror for accurate droplet placement. Indirect laryngoscopy is not essential for good results in experienced hands.

The curved applicator of the syringe is introduced over the dorsum of the tongue, which is held extended with a gauze swab, keeping strictly to the midline. The patient is requested to take shallow breaths and to avoid coughing. The local anaesthetic solution is then allowed to fall in droplets onto and then through the laryngeal inlet. Fry [14] recommended additional application to the pyriform fossae with the aid of the indirect laryngeal mirror, thus anaesthetizing the superior laryngeal nerves.

Cricothyroid puncture. The infraglottic mucosa can be anaesthetized by cricothyroid or transtracheal puncture. The most widely accepted term for this procedure is translaryngeal anaesthesia, although transcricothyroid membrane analgesia would be the least confusing [15].

With the head held in a position of maximum extension, the superior notch of the thyroid cartilage is readily palpable in the midline at the junction of the floor of the mouth and the anterior aspect of the neck.

The ring-shaped cartilage below the thyroid cartilage is the cricoid cartilage; the gap between these structures which is bridged by the cricothyroid membrane is easily recognized in the majority of patients (Fig. 4). A cross is marked on the skin midway between these structures in the midline thus denoting the point of needle entry.

Following sterilization of the skin, a bleb is raised using lignocaine at the designated point of entry. A needle is then introduced at right angles to the skin to penetrate the cricothyroid membrane and enter the lumen of the upper trachea. The use of a needle and syringe connected by a short length of flexible tubing, e.g. 21 SWG 'Butterfly' needle will reduce the possibility of needle breakage or trauma to the larynx. Following aspiration of air to confirm that the needle tip is in the trachea, 2 ml of local anaesthetic agent are injected. This often produced violent coughing. If performed at the end of inspiration, the local anaesthetic is rapidly coughed in expiration towards the glottic region, thus anaesthetizing the infraglottic mucosa and the lower surface of the vocal cords. If the patient is placed in a reverse Trendelenburg position and a second injection performed on expiration, the anaesthesia will extend to distal regions of the respiratory tract thus preparing the patient for subsequent bronchoscopy. Violent coughing occurs when the local anaesthetic solution reaches the carina, which also serves to reinforce anaesthesia above the level of injection.

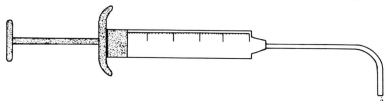

Fig. 3 Labat's syringe.

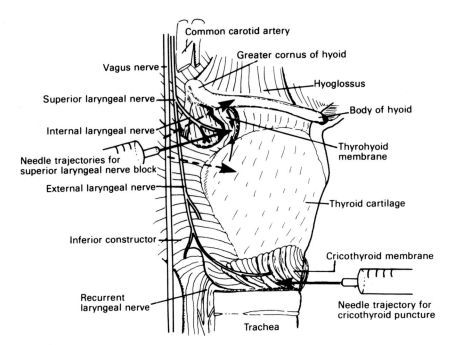

Fig. 4 Anatomical relationships of hyoid bone, thyroid and cricoid cartilages, showing needle trajectories for cricothyroid puncture and superior laryngeal nerve block. Modified from Zuck, with kind permission of the author and the editor of *Anaesthesia*.

REGIONAL BLOCKS

Regional nerve blocks can produce profound analgesia using small quantities of local anaesthetic solution.

Maxillary nerve block

This block is reported [16] to produce profound surface analgesia of most of the nasal cavity, thus aiding nasal intubation.

Anatomy

Sensory fibres from the second division of the trigeminal nerve pass through the pterygopalatine (sphenopalatine) ganglion to supply the hard and soft palate, septal and lateral walls of the nasal cavity and the nasopharynx (see Chapter 1, Figs 2 and 3).

Method

A 4 cm needle is angled to 45° at the hub, care being taken to prevent fracture and is introduced into the greater palatine canal through the greater palatine foramen (Fig. 5) in the posterolateral aspect of the palate. The needle is then passed into the pterygopalatine (sphenopalatine) fossa as shown in Figs 6 and 7.

An additional benefit may be gained if a local anaesthetic agent with a vasoconstrictor, or inherent vasoconstrictor properties such as

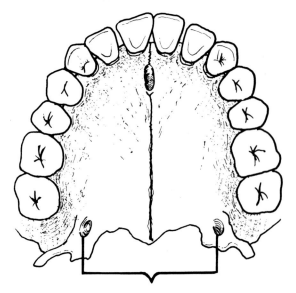

Fig. 5 Hard palate with the greater palatine foraminae. From Baddour et al [16], with kind permission of the editor of *Anesthesia Progress*.

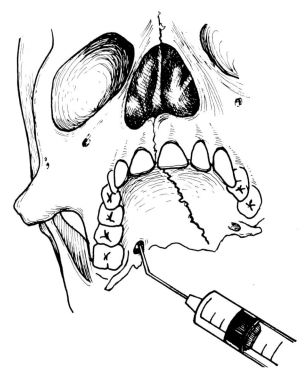

Fig. 6 Injection into the greater palatine canal. From Baddour et al [16], with kind permission of the editor of *Anesthesia Progress*.

cocaine, is used. The blood supply to the nasal mucosa is reduced by constriction of the sphenopalatine artery as it transverses the pterygopalatine fissure.

Glossopharyngeal nerve block

Bilateral glossopharyngeal nerve block produces anaesthesia at the posterior third of the tongue, tonsillar region, and oropharynx. There is a loss of sensation to pressure in these areas which does not occur with surface analgesia, and the gag reflex is also completely suppressed. A major disadvantage is paralysis of the pharyngeal muscles and relaxation of the base of the tongue which may produce sudden respiratory obstruction requiring immediate treatment.

Note

A glossopharyngeal nerve block is an additional block in patients with an active gag reflex who fail to relax. Therefore, it may follow one of the methods of oral laryngeal topical analgesia or superior laryngeal nerve block. It is important that the superior laryngeal nerve block should always be carried out first to avoid respiratory obstruction.

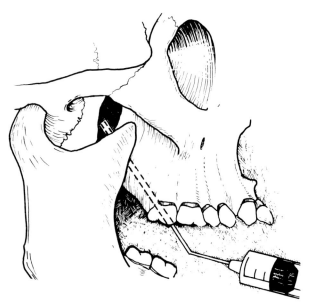

Fig. 7 Lateral view of the skull showing the path of the needle *into* the pterygopalatine fossa. From Baddour et al [16], with kind permission of the editor of *Anesthesia Progress*.

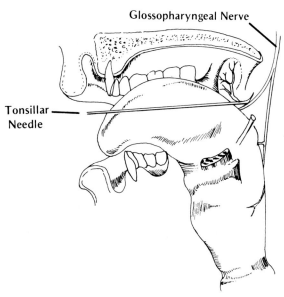

Fig. 8 Glossopharyngeal nerve block. From DeMeester et al [24].

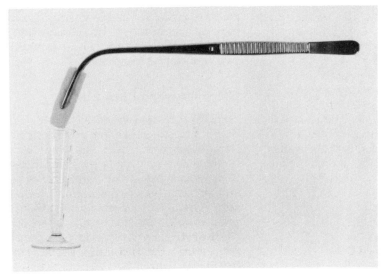

Fig. 9 Krause's forceps.

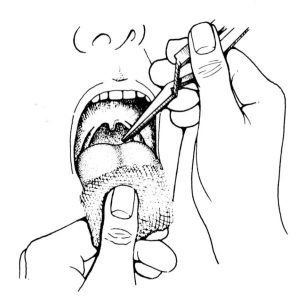

Fig. 10 Insertion of Krause's forceps. Left hand of operator holding the tongue with a gauze swab. From Macintosh & Ostlere [23], with kind permission of the authors and the publisher, E.S. Livingstone.

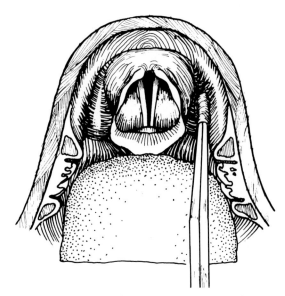

Fig. 11 Superior view of larynx – final position of Krause's forceps in the pyriform fossa. From Macintosh & Ostlere [23], with kind permission of the authors and the publisher, E.S. Livingstone.

Method

After applying surface analgesia to the dorsal aspect of the tongue, the latter is then depressed and the posterior tonsillar pillar placed under tension. An angled tonsillar needle is inserted behind the posterior tonsillar pillar at its mid point, to a depth of 1 cm (Fig. 8). Following aspiration, 3 ml of local anaesthetic are injected and procedure repeated on the other side.

Superior laryngeal nerve block

Transmucosal block (Krause's forceps)

The superior laryngeal nerve can be blocked by the oral route along the floor of the pyriform fossa, using Krause's forceps (Figs 9–11).

Method. Following oropharyngeal anaesthesia the patient is placed in the sitting position facing the operator and asked to stick out the tongue fully. The tongue is then held in this position with the aid of a gauze swab. Krause's forceps, firmly holding a dental pledget soaked in local anaesthetic solution, is passed into each pyriform fossa following the downward continuation of the tonsillar fossa, close to the lateral pharyngeal wall. The position may be checked by palpating the neck lateral to the superior aspect of the thyroid cartilage. The pledget is held in position for about 1 min to allow the solution to diffuse to the superior laryngeal nerve.

Percutaneous block

Method. The cornua of the hyoid bone and the superior cornua of the thyroid cartilage are palpated and the positions marked with a skin pencil. This block can be accomplished either by starting from the hyoid landmark or from the thyroid cartilage as shown in Fig. 4.

A point is marked on the skin 1 cm medial to the superior cornua of the hyoid bone. A skin weal is raised and a 3 cm, 23 SWG needle is inserted to contact the hyoid bone. The needle is then walked off the bone in a caudad direction to pierce the thyrohyoid membrane. In an alternative method, the needle is inserted, after local infiltration, onto the superior cornua of the thyroid cartilage and walked off the cartilage piercing the thyrohyoid membrane as in Fig. 4. In both cases an injection of 2 ml of local anaesthetic solution is made following careful aspiration. Aspiration of air indicates that the nedle has entered the larynx and must be withdrawn prior to injection. The block is repeated on the other side.

Warning. It is important that the thyroid cartilage is not pierced since deposition of local anaesthetic solution can lead to oedema of the vocal cords.

SYSTEMIC TOXICITY

Absorption of local anaesthetic agents from the mucous membrane in the upper respiratory tract is extremely rapid, and attention must be paid to safe limits shown in Table 1. Foldes [17] noted objective signs of lignocaine toxicity at venous levels of 5.29 μg/ml. These were tachy-cardia, moderate hypertension, T-wave flattening and S–T segment depression in the ECG, accompanied by slow activity in the EEG. The most common complication, however, is cerebral excitation which can present as a frank convulsion. This may be preceded by a prodromal period during which the patient describes a perioral tingling sensation and isolated twitching movements. It is important that techniques involving the administration of large doses of local anaesthetic agents should always be performed by skilled personnel with adequate resuscitation equipment, an indwelling venous cannula, and intravenous anticonvulsant agents such as diazepam and thiopentone.

Absorption of local anaesthetic agents from topical anaesthesia prior to intubation has been studied and the following points emerge.

1 There is a faster absorption of local anaesthetic agents in children. Differences also exist in children of different age groups [18].

2 Peak levels of serum lignocaine following topical application in adults [19] occur between 15 and 60 min. This emphasizes the need for careful supervision in the recovery phase.

3 Peak levels of active metabolites of lignocaine may occur 3–4 h following administration.

4 Estimations of serum lignocaine have been reported as well below the toxic limits despite the administration of amounts which exceeded the manufacturers' recommended values by 25–30%. Indeed, even in some patients where levels were greater than those reported to have caused toxicity, adverse reactions were not observed [20].

5 Absorption is greater in the lower respiratory tract than in the pharynx and larynx [20].

CARDIOVASCULAR CONSEQUENCES

In adults the pressor response to laryngoscopy and tracheal intubation is attenuated by awake intubation and local anaesthesia but by no means abolished [21]. Bradycardia, which may be of reflex origin, has been reported in children after laryngeal spraying [22]. This effect may be augmented by concurrent administration of suxamethonium or general anaesthetic agents. Peak levels of lignocaine occur too late to be of value in preventing arrhythmias during intubation.

The pressor response and increase in heart rate are minimized using fibreoptic nasotracheal intubation combined with thorough topical analgesia [7].

CONCLUSION

A combination of cricothyroid injection and preoperative amethocaine lozenge in the presence of sedation and antisialogogue administration seem the simplest combination of techniques in less experienced hands. The techniques should be carried out only where immediate facilities are available for resuscitation. However, there is a reasonable evidence to suggest that limits set by manufacturers for the use of local anaesthetic agents in this context are unnecessarily low. Even in children, where absorption is greatest, it would seem a dose of 4 mg/kg of lignocaine is safe [18].

REFERENCES

1 Tomori Z & Widdicombe J G (1969) Muscular bronchomotor and cardiovascular reflexes elicited by mechanical stimulation of the respiratory tract. *J Physiol* 200:25.

2 Walts L F (1965) Anaesthesia of the larynx in the patient with a full stomach. *JAMA* 192:705.

3 D'Hollander A A, Monteny E, Dewachter B, Sanders M & Dubois-Primo J (1974) Intubation under topical supraglottic analgesia in unpremedicated and non-fasting patients: amnesic effects of sub-hypnotic doses of diazepam and innovar. *Can Anaesth Soc J* 21:467.

4 Kopriva C J, Eltringham R J & Siebert M Q (1974) A comparison of the effects of intravenous Innovar and topical spray on the laryngeal closure reflex. *Anesthesiology* 40:596.

5 Libman R H (1976) Topical anaesthesia and intubation. *JAMA* 236:2393.

6 Thomas J L (1969) Awake intubation. Indications, techniques and a review of 25 patients. *Anaesthesia* 24:28.

7 Ovassapian A, Yelich S J, Dykes M H M & Brunner E E (1983) Blood pressure and heart rate changes during awake fibreoptic nasotracheal intubation. *Anesth Analg* 62:951.

8 Dundee J W & Haslett W H K (1970) The benzodiazepines. A review of their actions and uses relative to anaesthetic practice. *Br J Anaesth* 42:217.

9 Baird E A & Hailey D M (1972) Delayed recovery from a sedative: correlation of plasma levels of diazepam with clinical effects after oral and intravenous administration. *Br J Anaesth* 44:803.

10 Kaplan S A, Jack M L, Alexander K & Weinfeld R E (1973) Pharmacokinetic profile of diazepam in man following single intravenous and oral and chronic oral administration. *J Pharm Sci* 62:1789.

11 Brown C R, Sanquist F H, Canup C A & Pedley T A (1979) Clinical electroencephalographic and pharmacokinetic studies of a water-soluble benzodiazepine, midazolam maleate. *Anesthesiology* 50:467.

12 Shou Olesen A & Huttel M S (1980) Local reactions to I.V. diazepam in three different formulations. *Br J Anaesth* 52:609.

13 Palva T, Jokinen K, Saloheimo M & Karvonen P (1975) Ultrasonic nebuliser in local anaesthesia for bronchoscopy. *J Oto-Rhino-Laryngol* 37:306.

14 Fry W A (1978) Techniques of topical anaesthesia for bronchoscopy. *Chest* 73:694.

15 Allen H L (1983) Letter: Rediscovering the larynx. *Anesth Analg* 62:855.

16 Baddour H M, Hubbard A M & Tilson H B (1979) Maxillary nerve block used prior to awake nasal intubation. *Anesth Prog* 26:43.

17 Foldes F F, Malloy R, McNall P G & Koukal L R (1960) Comparison of toxicity of intravenously given local anaesthetic agents in man. *JAMA* 172:1493.

18 Eyres R L, Bishop W, Oppenheim R C & Brown T C K (1983) Plasma lignocaine concentrations following topical laryngeal application. *Anaesth Intensive Care* 11:23.

19 Jones D A, McBurney A, Stanley P J, Tovey C & Ward J W (1982) Plasma concentrations of lignocaine and its metabolites during fibreoptic bronchoscopy. *Br J Anaesth* 54:853.

20 Curran J, Hamilton C & Taylor T (1975) Topical analgesia before tracheal intubation. *Anaesthesia* 30:765.

21 Kautto U-M & Heinonen J (1982) Attenuation of circulatory response to laryngoscopy and tracheal intubation; a comparison of two methods of topical anaesthesia. *Acta Anaesthesiol Scand* 26:599.

22 Mirakhur R K (1982) Bradycardia with laryngeal spraying in children. *Acta Anaesthesiol Scand* 26:130.

23 Macintosh R R & Ostlere G (1955) *Local Analgesia. Head and Neck*, p. 10. E.S. Livingstone, Edinburgh

24 De Meester T R, Skinner D B, Evans R H & Benson D W (1977) Local nerve block anesthesia for peroral endoscopy. *Annals of Thoracic Surgery* 24:278.

CHAPTER 7 Management of difficult intubation

INCIDENCE

Difficult intubation can occur unexpectedly in clinical practice. However, some cases of difficulty can be foreseen. It is important, therefore, always to carry out a careful preoperative clinical examination, and also, if possible, to check previous anaesthetic records and if judged necessary to obtain skull, cervical spine and mandibular radiographs. Sia & Edens estimated that 90% of cases of difficult intubation should be anticipated and in only 10% should there be an unexpected problem [1]. In a prospective study of 1200 patients from Cardiff however, 22 of 43 difficult intubations (51%) were anticipated and 21 (49%) were not [156]. Difficult intubation was anticipated in 84 patients; however, only 22 were actually difficult. It is clear therefore that unexpected cases of difficulty occur commonly in clinical practice and that some cases of anticipated difficulty may be simple to manage. The incidence of very difficult cases requiring awake intubation often with a complex technique is rare, probably about 1–5% of difficult cases. Awake intubation was required in only one of the above 43 patients (2.3%).

An incidence of 2.3% of difficult intubation was reported from a general hospital [2]. The Cardiff Anaesthetic Record System between 1972 and 1977 recorded an incidence of 1%, in which 65% of 109 000 patients had tracheal intubation. However, a smaller unpublished prospective study of intubation problems revealed a 3.6% incidence of difficult intubations in 1200 cases [156]. About half of these intubations were performed by staff in training and the true incidence is probably lower. Of course, the number of cases which present a problem with tracheal intubation depends upon the experience of the reporting clinician and the type of patient and surgery involved. Aro and his colleagues found that 85% of difficult intubations could be managed by experienced clinicians with the use of an introducer [2]. In 15% of difficult intubations (0.3% of all intubations) a more complicated approach was necessary.

There are many possible definitions of 'difficult' intubation. A grading can also be made according to the view obtained at laryngoscopy [154].

Grade 1 Most of the glottis is visible and there should be no difficulty.

Grade 2 Only the posterior extremity of the glottis is visible. This may give rise to slight difficulty. Pressure on the neck may improve the exposure of the larynx.

Grade 3 No part of the glottis is visible. The epiglottis can be seen. This can result in severe difficulty.

Grade 4 Not even the epiglottis can be seen. Intubation with complex methods may be required. This occurs with obvious pathology but is very rare if the anatomy is normal.

Some authors classify difficult intubation arbitrarily (including Cardiff data). Others classify according to whether the individual anaesthetist needs to use an intubation aid. Still others categorize according to the type of aid required to intubate successfully. Experienced clinicians may be able to intubate a patient whose cords are not visible. Although they may have no difficulty the record is marked as difficult to warn a trainee who might subsequently intubate the patient. Others who have some difficulty through forgetfulness, or pride, omit to mark the form so statistics may not be reliable. A precise definition of difficult intubation is essential before undertaking a prospective evaluation of incidence.

CLINICAL MANAGEMENT

The practical management of a difficult intubation depends on the availability of specialized skills and apparatus, the urgency of the surgery

Table 1 Plan for failed intubation [3].

Maintain cricoid pressure ↓	
Position patient head down and on left side ↓	
Oxygenate by positive pressure ventilation, use airway and aspirate pharynx if required ↓	
If ventilation and oxygenation are easy ventilate with nitrous oxide and oxygen and either methoxyflurane or ether until spontaneous ventilation occurs and the patient is surgically anaesthetized	→ If oxygenation by positive pressure ventilation is difficult with patient on side try releasing cricoid pressure
↓	↓
Pass wide bore stomach tube and aspirate stomach. Instil 15 ml magnesium trisilate into the stomach	If oxygenation is still difficult allow effect of relaxant to wear off and patient to wake up. Then empty stomach and undertake an inhalation induction followed by inhalation anaesthesia with a face mask
↓	
Remove stomach tube aspirate pharynx, level the table and use lateral tilt ↓	
Proceed with surgery using inhalation anaesthesia and face mask ↓	
Consider the alternatives of regional or local analgesia	Repeated and prolonged attempts at intubation resulting in hypoxia should be avoided

Table 2 Apparatus in Cardiff difficult intubation box.

Clock for timing duration of the procedure

Nasal airways

Large Macintosh laryngoscope blade

Left handed Macintosh laryngoscope blade

Straight laryngoscope blade

Polio blade

Plastic tooth bridge

Gum elastic catheter

Stylet

Equipment for retrograde techniques:
 Tuohy needle
 Epidural catheter
 Seldinger wire
 Hook to deliver epidural catheter from mouth

Equipment for transtracheal ventilation:
 Needle and cannula
 Connections from cannula to the anaesthetic machine

and the type of surgery planned. It is mandatory to ensure that oxygenation is maintained with resumed artificial ventilation at intervals during attempts to pass a tracheal tube. The risk of aspiration of gastric contents should be minimized. When the situation occurs unexpectedly, particularly in obstetric anaesthesia, the patient always has a potentially full stomach and it is important to have a rational and safe plan of action for a failed intubation such as that described by Tunstall [3] (Table 1) or that described in chapter 9.

It is a matter of individual judgement as to how long the clinician should persevere in attempted intubation even if there is adequate oxygenation. A decision will be influenced both by the urgency of the surgery and whether trauma results from the attempts. Desperate and prolonged attempts at intubation resulting in intermittent hypoxia should be avoided. It is essential to avoid trauma and certainly to reduce this to a minimum. Sufficient sets of simple apparatus which might be urgently required should be kept readily available in the theatre suite in a special 'difficult intubation box' [4], and the contents of the Cardiff box are shown in Table 2. In addition it is valuable, and it may soon be considered essential, to have fibreoptic equipment available together with personnel trained in its use. There have, as yet, been no prospective clinical trials comparing different methods of intubation, and therefore it is not possible to make firm recommendations on choice of a primary method for any individual patient. Each situation has to be carefully evaluated by the clinician and only then can the exact choice of technique be determined.

Choice of technique: retrospective survey

A survey of methods chosen by British anaesthetists to facilitate tracheal intubation and expertise with the methods was conducted at a Symposium on Intubation in October 1982 [5]. Questionnaires were completed by 163 clinicians. Simple methods were used intially and are shown in order of preference in Fig. 1.

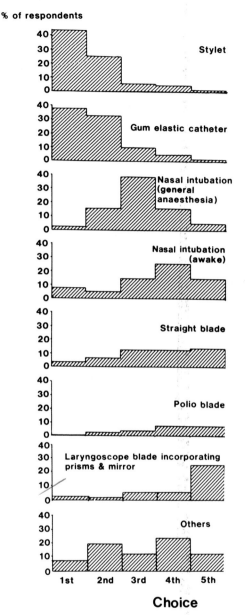

% of respondents

Stylet

Gum elastic catheter

Nasal intubation (general anaesthesia)

Nasal intubation (awake)

Straight blade

Polio blade

Laryngoscope blade incorporating prisms & mirror

Others

1st 2nd 3rd 4th 5th

Choice

Fig. 1 Retrospective survey. Choice of simple techniques. From James & Latto [5], with kind permission of the authors.

One-third of respondents used these methods exclusively and had no experience with any of the complex methods. It is clear that the most popular first and second choices are the gum elastic catheter or bougie and the stylet. The use of more complex methods is shown in Table 3. These are only required rarely in clinical practice

so that many clinicians have not developed competence with them. Formalized training programmes are necessary for clinicians who lack the requisite skills. Two-thirds of clinicians who had used the retrograde technique at least once considered themselves competent with that method, which may be required for a very difficult and urgent intubation. This may commonly occur since fibreoptic equipment and expertise is not yet widely available. The first choice of complex methods for difficult cases presenting both expectedly and unexpectedly is presented in Table 4.

Choice of technique: prospective survey

An unpublished prospective analysis of techniques used in 43 cases of difficult intubation [156] is shown in Fig. 2, which should be compared with Fig. 1.

IDENTIFYING THE PRACTICAL PROBLEM

There are many causes of difficult intubation which are discussed in chapter 5. On a practical level however, in any particular case of difficulty during induction of a general anaesthetic a specific problem may be identified (Table 5). For cases of both expected and unexpected difficulty clinicians initially use simple familiar techniques and mainly succeed. A plan for difficult intubation is essential. A suggested plan for elective cases is shown in Table 6.

Expected difficulty

In cases where a moderately difficult intubation is anticipated induction of general anaesthesia with an attempt at intubation precedes any other more complex approach. Such patients should be preoxygenated for at least 3 min before induction of anaesthesia and it is essential to ensure that ventilation and oxygenation can be maintained before using muscle relaxants. Should failure to intubate result it is common for a trainee to call for the assistance of a more experienced clinician. Most trainees do not gain sufficient expertise with complex techniques. If the experienced clinician fails with a simple technique then fibreoptic endoscopy or retrograde techniques may be required.

Table 3 Expertise of the 64% (105 out of 163) of anaesthetists who had used complex methods of intubation [5].

	Anaesthetists using the method				Mean number of cases per anaesthetist				Ratio of total number of patients subjected to procedure non-difficult/difficult difficult intubations	Anaesthetists who considered themselves competent: number (%) of total using method
	Number (% of 163 total)	% using for difficult cases only	% using for difficult and non-difficult cases	% using for non-difficult cases only	Difficult only	Difficult and non-difficult		Non-difficult only		
						Difficult	Non-difficult			
Retrograde	27(16.5)	81	11	7	2.6	5.3	2.7	1.5	1/6.6	18(66.7)
Fibreoptic bronchoscope	60(36.8)	17	28	55	2.8	3.8	21.7	8.4	7/1	23(38.3)
Fibreoptic laryngoscope	75(46)	8	29	63	4	6.4	18.8	7.6	4.7/1	29(38.7)
Light wand	19(11.6)	16	26	58	8	4.6	13.2	3.7	2.3/1	7(36.8)

Table 4 First choice of a complex method of intubation from retrospective survey [5].

Method	% of respondents first choice of complex method	
	Expected difficulty	Unexpected difficulty
Fibreoptic bronchoscope	26.9	21.5
Fibreoptic laryngoscope	17.2	19.6
Retrograde method	21.4	22.1
Light wand	1.8	7.3
None	17.2	17.7
Total (%)	94.5*	87.9*

*Data excluded from respondents who did not give a single first choice.

Table 5 Some problem orientated solutions to difficult intubation.

Inability to open mouth	1 Inadequate relaxation. Give more relaxant or wait for relaxant already given to become effective 2 If trismus is present intubate under local or assess the effect of inhalation anaesthesia in relaxing jaw muscles 3 Awake intubation in patients with jaws that are permanently closed
Mouth open but difficulty in inserting laryngoscope blade	1 Detach blade from handle and insert separately 2 Use polio blade
Laryngoscope deflected by irregular teeth	Use plastic tooth bridge
Mouth open but tube deflected by irregular teeth	Use rigid introducer to facilitate positioning the tube
Cords partially visible Cords not visible	Initially use either a gum elastic catheter, stylet or other simple technique
Epiglottis partly or wholly concealed	Complex methods will probably be required

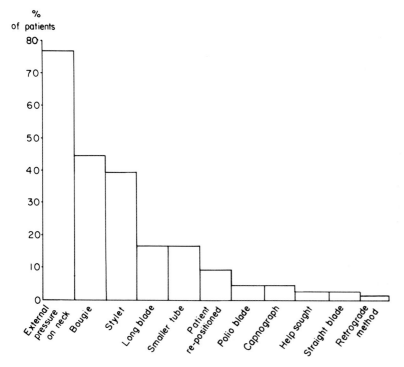

Fig. 2 Prospective survey. Simple methods used in 43 cases of difficult oral intubation (3.6% of total of 1200 cases). From Eastley et al [156], with kind permission of the authors.

Table 6 Commonly adopted plans for difficult intubation in
elective cases using general anaesthesia (assumes minimal
risk of gastric reflux).

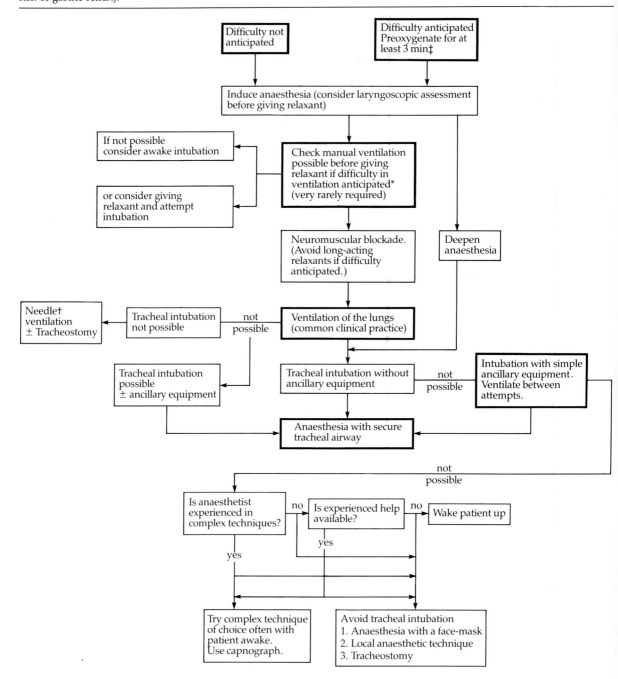

*The 16 stone, bull-necked, heavy drinking individual may be managed with a rapid sequence
induction technique after lengthy preoxygenation. Spontaneous ventilation should be resumed
within 3 min if intubation or effective ventilation are not possible. Awake intubation may then be considered.

†Life threatening situation without prompt management.

‡The tyro should call for assistance before induction if difficulty is anticipated.

Table 7 Cardiff plan for anticipated very difficult intubation. Incidence not known but it is less than 5% of difficult intubations.

Attempt oral or nasal intubation		Avoid oral and nasal intubation			
Fibreoptic technique under local anaesthesia	Retrograde technique under local anaesthesia	Tracheostomy under local anaesthesia	Consider doing operation under local block	Needle ventilation [131]	Consider cardiopulmonary bypass in cases of distal main airway obstruction [157, 158]

Obtain expert assistance if required
Obtain capnograph to confirm tube placement

When a case of very difficult intubation is identified preoperatively and there is doubt about the ability to ventilate, a different management plan should be adopted. Awake intubation under local anaesthesia is the safer approach (Table 7). Under no circumstances should intubation be attempted under general anaesthesia. For a clinician who has not gained expertise with fibreoptic or retrograde techniques, blind nasal intubation may seem appropriate; it is essential to avoid trauma to the airway and bleeding with its potentially fatal results [6]. Retrograde or fibreoptic techniques are usually preferable. Fibreoptic techniques should not be attempted for the first time by the inexperienced clinician in a difficult intubation. A retrograde technique can be tried in an emergency since it is easy to perform and should not result in major complications. A clinician with no expertise in either fibreoptic or retrograde techniques might wisely decide to recommend a tracheostomy under local anaesthesia to ensure a secure airway. Occasionally even this option may not be available in a patient with a fixed flexion neck deformity.

For very short procedures clinicians may choose to avoid intubation and manage the patient with a facemask breathing spontaneously. It is important to be aware of the potential danger of difficulty in maintaining the airway under these circumstances [7]. The patient with mucopolysaccharide disease has a short neck, a high epiglottis and infiltration of nasopharyngeal tissues. In these patients an oral airway can push the epiglottis back which can then occlude the larynx. However, a nasopharyngeal airway keeps the epiglottis forward and helps to maintain a clear airway should it be lost. Rapid intubation may often not be possible; and there may be fatal consequences. This approach should therefore be used with caution. Alternatively, it may be possible to perform the operation under local anaesthesia and avoid intubation. There are real risks to this too. If a local block is insufficient or wears off during surgery then it may be necessary to induce general anaesthesia under emergency conditions. If a complication such as a total spinal occurs it would be difficult to manage since rapid intubation would not be possible.

These cases represent a considerable challenge to even the most experienced anaesthetist and difficulties in management should not be underestimated. It is important to consider and adopt a plan which minimizes risks to the patient.

CONFIRMATION OF CORRECT PLACEMENT OF TRACHEAL TUBE

There have been detailed reports of seven cases [8–11] in which tests commonly used by the anaesthetist to confirm correct tube placement were misleading (Table 8). However, it should be stressed that the usual tests are misleading in only a tiny minority of patients. Pollard & Junius [8] reported four cases, two of whom suffered irreversible brain damage. On occasions chest movement is poor due to low lung or chest wall compliance or breath sounds may be abnormal due to obstructive airway disease even when the tube is in the trachea. On the other hand breath sounds, chest movement and the 'feel' of the reservoir bag can all be apparently normal even when the tube is in the oesophagus [8]. With experience, problems are only likely to occur when the cords cannot be seen during intubation. An inexperienced clinician, however, may be confused by the anatomy and mistake the view of the tube passing into the oesophagus with that of the tube passing through the vocal cords. A cadaver study with a tracheal tube in the oesophagus showed that oesophageal ventilation could result in both chest and epigastric movements [8]. The stomach was intermittently inflated and then deflated into the oesophagus. The feel of the inflation bag was normal. When the lower part of the oesophagus was occluded chest movement still occurred as the oesophagus became distended and lifted the heart and upper mediastinum forwards thus elevating the sternum and ribs. The compliance however was reduced.

An analysis of anaesthetic misadventures reported to the Medical Defence Union revealed 37 deaths and 13 cases of cerebral damage from unrecognized oesophageal intubation over the 8 year period from 1970 to 1977 [17]. Twenty-six per cent of operating room deaths or brain damage due mainly to error resulted from inadvertent oesophageal intubation or mismanaged tracheal intubation [17].

Many tests have been described to confirm correct tube placement [8–10, 12–15] (Table 9),

Table 8 Description of cases where tests commonly used to confirm correct placement of tracheal tube were misleading.

Reference	Clinician	Clinical comments	Cords visualized	Observed chest movement with ventilation	Auscultation	Bag compression and release	Cyanosis	Results
Pollard & Junius (1980) [8]	4th year	Lengthy preoxygenation and anticipated difficult intubation	No	Normal	Normal	Normal	Surgical incision made 15 min after induction and blood was seen to be dark	Tube removed; patient became pink on mask. Second attempt at intubation successful
	Trainee with student	Unexpectedly difficult in a patient with cardiac disease	No	Normal	Normal	Normal	Yes	Cardiac arrest with irreversible brain damage
	Specialist	Preoxygenation and intubation without difficulty	Not stated	Normal	Normal	Normal	Blood dark on skin incision but no clinical cyanosis	Cardiac arrest at time tube misplacement diagnosed. Irreversible brain damage
	Resident with specialist	Gas heard entering stomach on auscultation of epigastrium	Not stated	Normal	Normal	Normal	Yes	Tracheal tube removed and replaced
Howells & Riethmuller (1980) [9]	Not stated	Initial bradycardia then tachycardia	No	Normal	Sounds compatible with air entry plus scattered rhonchi	Normal	Yes	Tracheal tube removed and oxygen given by mask
Cundy (1981) [10]	Trainee with consultant	'Death rattle' of fluid was heard in the tracheal tube	Not stated	Normal	Normal	Normal	Yes	Tracheal tube removed and replaced
Stirt (1982) [11]	Probably trainee with consultant	Blind nasal intubation under local anaesthesia. Tube initially in pharynx then in oesophagus	No	Tube connected to circle system (4 litres/min oxygen) reservoir bag emptied and filled approximately 150/200 ml with each breath. Air came from tracheal tube with each breath. Positive pressure ventilation produced chest expansion and breath sounds	Faint breath sounds in both mid and axillary lines		No	Tube pulled back from oesophagus and then readvanced blindly into the trachea

Table 9 Tests for confirming correct tube placement

Reference	Methods to confirm the placement of tubes in the trachea		Reliability	Comment
Pollard & Junius (1980)	*Commonly used methods*			
	1	Seeing the tube pass through the vocal cords	Reliable	Reliable for experienced clinician only. Inexperienced clinician may confuse the anatomy and think the tube is in the trachea when it is in the oesophagus
[8]	2	Hearing breath sounds over the lung fields	Unreliable	
	3	Bilateral chest movement with ventilation	Unreliable	
	4	Characteristics feel of inflation bag during manual ventilation	Unreliable	
	5	Sound of gas escaping round the tube in the oesophagus	Unreliable	
	6	Deterioration of colour and cardiovascular changes associated with hypoxia	Probably reliable	Not positive sign but should be taken as indicating tube misplacement unless positively disproved
	Less commonly used methods			
	7	Listening to stomach for air entry if tube is in oesophagus	Probably reliable	*No reported instance of this being misleading. We use this test routinely in all cases of doubt*
	8	Inspection of epigastrium to detect distension	Unreliable	
	9	Listen over open end of tube when pressing on sternum	May be unreliable	
	10	Listen over trachea for air entry	Reliable	
	11	Feel over trachea for cuff movement as tube is moved	Reliable	
Cundy (1981) [10]	12	Sound of fluid in the tracheal tube Signs 2, 3 (see above)	Reliable Unreliable	Case report of oesophageal tube placement
Howells & Riethmuller (1980) [9]		Signs 2, 3 (see above)	Unreliable	Breath sounds unless *normal* are an unreliable sign of tracheal tube placement
Chander & Feldman (1979) [12]	13	Rapid inflation of cuff with air. The cuff can then be palpated in the suprasternal notch. Used for placement of the cuff of the tube	Unreliable	Difficult in obese short necked individuals
Warden (1980) [13]				Preoxygenation delays the development of hypoxia and therefore may delay the onset of cyanosis and diagnosis of tube misplacement
Ionescu (1981) [14]	14	End tidal carbon dioxide monitor trace disappears if tube is placed in the oesophagus	Reliable	Claimed to be the only rapid and reliable guide in difficult cases *Test with capnograph immediately when site of placement is in doubt*
Murray & Modell (1983) [15]		Sign 14 (see above)	Reliable	This technique is useful for confirming intubation when cords not visible. Also useful in patients where breath sounds are distant and access is difficult intraoperatively. Useful for confirming proper ventilation with double lumen tubes

but it is apparent that some can be unreliable. Visualization of the tube entering the larynx [8] provides a certain and simple confirmation of correct tube placement. Auscultation over the stomach was only performed in one of the seven failed cases [8–11] (Table 8) and the tube was then replaced in the trachea. No cases of misplacement have been reported in which auscultation was carried out over the epigastrium. We believe that this test should be used in all cases in addition to auscultating over the apices of the lungs and the trachea.

Monitoring of end tidal carbon dioxide concentration gives positive evidence that the tube is correctly placed [14–16] and a capnograph is valuable if difficult intubation is anticipated preoperatively. However elevated carbon dioxide values (maximum values of 4.4 and 4.9 vol % in two patients) were obtained even during oesophageal ventilation [16]. This occurred when there was gastric distension with exhaled air during initial mask ventilation. The carbon dioxide values, however, are only transient and decrease in less than a minute to zero (Fig. 3). These misleading carbon dioxide percentages can occur in conjunction with backflow of gases and apparently normal filling of the rebreathing bag. It has also been shown that oesophageal ventilation resulted in some pulmonary ventilation due to chest movement [16] (Fig. 4), which explains why faint breath sounds may be heard on auscultation.

Normally, with a tube in the oesophagus, ventilation results in zero percentage of 'expired' carbon dioxide [15] (Fig. 5). A positive carbon dioxide reading can occur when the tip of the tube is in the pharynx (Fig. 6). An important rule is to remove the tube and ventilate with a mask in all cases where there is doubt about the correct placement of the tube

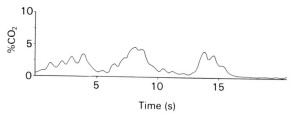

Fig. 4 Carbon dioxide recorded at the open end of a tracheal tube during simultaneous ventilation into the oesophagus. In 18 out of 20 patients ventilation into the oesophagus caused pulmonary ventilation with maximum peak carbon dioxide concentrations similar to those found during tracheal ventilation. After Linko et al [16], with kind permission of the editor of *Acta Anaesthesiologica Scandinavica*.

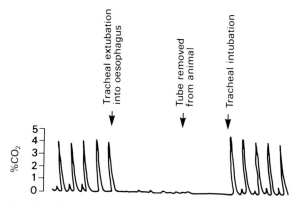

Fig. 5 Carbon dioxide tracing of tidal gas during tracheal extubation with the tip of the tube lodged in the oesophagus. After Murray & Modell [15], with kind permission of the authors, the editor of *Anesthesiology*, and the publishers, J.B. Lippincott Co.

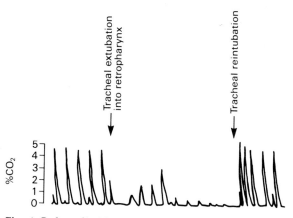

Fig. 6 Carbon dioxide tracing of tidal gas during tracheal extubation with retropharyngeal lodgement of the tip of the tube. After Murray & Modell [15], with kind permission of the authors, the editor of *Anesthesiology*, and the publishers, J.B. Lippincott Co.

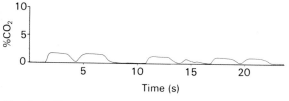

Fig. 3 Accidental oesophageal intubation. Gastric distension noted during mask ventilation. Capnography during oesophageal ventilation showed flat irregular carbon dioxide curves that gradually diminished. Back flow was felt in breathing bag. After Linko et al [16], with kind permission of the editor of *Acta Anaesthesiologica Scandinavica*.

associated with clinical deterioration – 'when in doubt take it out'. Delay in instituting effective ventilation and oxygenation has resulted in irreversible cerebral damage. Problems in recognizing oesophageal intubation should occur only when the tube is not seen going through the cords and a capnograph is not available. Under these circumstances, auscultation over the stomach during positive pressure ventilation should be conclusive.

A technique has been described to confirm correct placement of the tracheal tube [155]. When it is impossible to visualize the cords the laryngoscope is left in the mouth and the tracheal tube displaced posteriorly towards the hard palate. This brought the tube and cords into view in 21 cases where the larynx was obscured during intubation.

Muscle relaxants

If difficult intubation is suspected it is important to ensure that the airway can be maintained and positive pressure ventilation applied *before* giving a muscle relaxant. Most clinicians avoid the use of a non-depolarizing relaxant under these circumstances and would prefer a smaller dose of a short acting depolarizing relaxant. If failure to intubate or to ventilate occurs then most patients should start breathing spontaneously in 2–3 min.

SIMPLE TECHNIQUES

One or more of the following techniques may be required in cases of difficult intubation.

Head position and pressure on front of neck

A common difficulty is caused by failure to position the patient properly. The optimum position is flexion of the cervical spine and extension of the head at the atlanto-occipital joint [18]. Simple repositioning may enable the anatomy to become visible and intubation to be successfully accomplished. In addition pressure directed posteriorly on the cricoid or thyroid cartilage on the front of the neck may render the larynx more easily visible. This is particularly helpful when the larynx is anteriorly placed and therefore difficult to see.

Cricoid pressure can result in difficult intubation

Cricoid pressure was described to avoid aspiration during induction by Sellick in 1961 [19]. Backward pressure on the front of the cricoid cartilage obstructs the upper oesphagus, which prevents regurgitation and aspiration prior to intubation (Fig. 7). It also prevents gastric distension during positive pressure ventilation with a face mask. In the original description the head and neck were fully extended and cricoid pressure was applied before induction of anaesthesia. However, in modern clinical practice the patient is often positioned with the neck flexed and head extended to ensure ease of tracheal

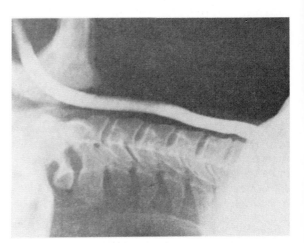

Fig. 7 (a) Lateral X-ray of neck showing lumen of upper oesophagus filled by latex tube containing contrast medium.

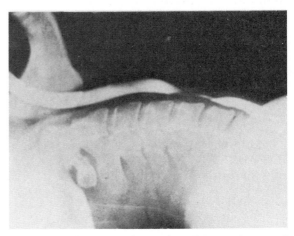

Fig. 7 (b) Obliteration of oesophageal lumen by cricoid pressure at level of 5th cervical vertebrae. From Sellick [19], with kind permission of the editor of *Lancet*.

intubation. Sellick later recommended that firm cricoid pressure, the onset of unconsciousness and the achievement of full muscular relaxation should be achieved simultaneously [20]. With these precautions he believed that the risk of oesophageal rupture from vomiting (not regurgitation) was negligible. The technique was designed to be an alternative to induction in the sitting position.

Anatomical distortion can occasionally result from pressure on the neck rendering intubation more difficult [21, 22]. Crawford described a 'contra cricoid' cuboid support applied to the back of the neck before induction of anaesthesia which minimized this distortion thus reducing the incidence of difficulty caused by the pressure on the front of the neck [22]. The support was 27 cm long, 10 cm wide and 5 cm high.

Posterior displacement of the larynx by backward pressure on the thyroid or cricoid cartilage is frequently used during difficult intubations when the larynx is only partially seen. This enables a better view of the larynx to be obtained in some cases. This also can occasionally distort the anatomy and may require similar 'contra cricoid' pressure to the back of the neck. This may not always be effective in enabling the anaesthetist to visualize the cords.

Gum elastic catheter or bougie

A gum elastic catheter was first used as an aid to intubation by Macintosh in 1943 [34] when he found that the tracheal tube could obstruct his view of the cords. The lubricated gum elastic catheter was therefore first threaded through the tube and then gently placed into the trachea. The tube was pushed down into the trachea over the catheter and the catheter removed. The technique was also used when exposure of the larynx was inadequate. The technique is now commonly advocated when the cords cannot be seen at laryngoscopy (Figs 8–10). The catheter briefly retains the approximate shape into which it is bent. It is important to keep the catheter in the midline and to bend the distal end forward after it has been passed through the tracheal tube. The catheter can then be advanced blindly towards the cords and the tube then 'railroaded' over the catheter. It is necessary to check very carefully that the tube has passed into the trachea. In addition to

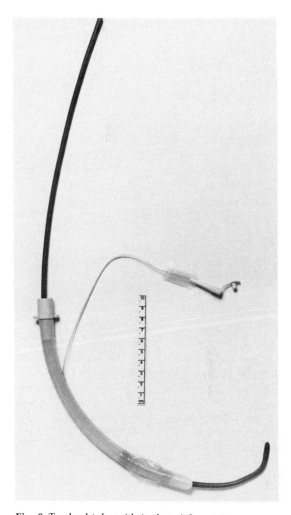

Fig. 8 Tracheal tube with 'catheter' (bougie).

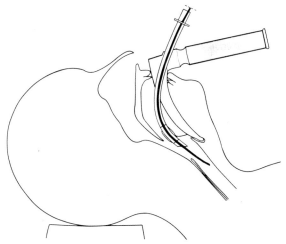

Fig. 9 Catheter threaded blindly into the trachea.

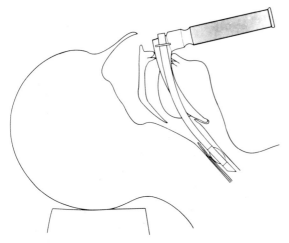

Fig. 10 Tube railroaded into trachea over catheter and catheter then removed.

listening to the chest and observing chest movement it is mandatory to listen over the stomach and if possible to measure expired carbon dioxide levels to exclude accidental oesophageal intubation. This technique is our first choice when the cords cannot be seen at intubation and a suitable catheter should therefore be available in every anaesthetic room.

Simulated difficult intubation and the gum elastic catheter

The trainee when faced with a difficult intubation with no view of the cords may panic and not have a clear idea of the correct way to solve the problem. This technique can be taught as part of a difficult intubation training programme [35, 154]. The larynx is first visualized and the laryngoscope blade then lowered so that the epiglottis drops back and conceals the cords. This simulated difficulty can then be managed using Macintosh's method [34]. An Oxford tube (a tube with a right angled bend) was preferred for training in simulated difficulty. Management of such a situation can be practised under controlled circumstances. This should boost confidence and decrease the incidence both of protracted and failed intubation. It was suggested that this programme should be taught in addition to the Tunstall failed intubation drill [3].

Introducers

Metal introducers or stylets have been used to facilitate placement of both tracheal catheters [26] and tracheal tubes [27–30]. Stylets have been made from a variety of materials including copper wire, coat hangers, knitting needles and brass rods. Unfortunately these are potentially traumatic and usually not sterile. Blunt ended disposable* and non-disposable†‡ introducers are commercially available and should be safer than the sharp ended metal in-house variety. Introducers are routinely used with flexible armoured tubes to help in advancing the tube. They are also helpful if a more rigid tube is deflected by irregular teeth. An introducer is most commonly required when visualization of the vocal cords is difficult. Occasionally the epiglottis can be seen but the cords are completely concealed or only their posterior portions are visible. Sometimes neither the epiglottis nor the cords are visible. Under these circumstances, a lubricated introducer is often bent into a J shape (Figs 11 and 12) and then passed into the tube; both are then directed in the midline towards the assumed position of the vocal cords. The tip of the rigid introducer is usually kept inside the tracheal tube to minimize the possibility of tracheal trauma. Alternatively the tip of the introducer can protrude past the end of the tube and then be passed blindly into the trachea. The tube is then 'railroaded' into position [31]. This technique is potentially traumatic even with a soft, blunt ended introducer.

An illuminated flexible stylet has been designed with a 2″ (5 cm) flexible distal end [32]. The stylet is placed inside the tracheal tube and flexion of the distal end is produced by a trigger at the proximal end. A light placed at the tip of the stylet, directly illuminates the pharynx and trachea. No data is available on the use of this stylet in cases of difficult intubation and the device is not commercially available. It may have been rendered obsolete by the development of fibreoptic direct vision techniques.

---

*Spick-stylette Polamedco, Inc 1625 17th St, Santa Monica, CA 90404, USA
†Flexiguide Division, Scientific Sales International Inc, PO Box 867, Ravina Station, Highlands Park, IL 60035, USA
‡Satinslip intubating stylet-Mallinckrodt.

The Salem/Resce intubation guide* (Flexi-guide) has a distal tip which can be flexed by operating the control on the proximal handle [33]. It is inserted through the tracheal tube then guided into the trachea.

A tracheal tube has been designed with a flexible distal end which can be directed towards the larynx.† This tube has a nylon line running along under the concave surface from distal to proximal end. The proximal end of the nylon line is fixed to a ring loop and when this is pulled the tip of the tube turns anteriorly (Fig. 13). In clinical use the tube is advanced through the nose or mouth and is placed in the pharynx. The tip is advanced towards the cords while traction is exerted on the ring loop to direct the tip of the tube. This device should be particularly useful for nasal intubation and reduce the need to use Magill intubating forceps.

Use of a smaller tracheal tube

A small diameter tube often facilitates intubation when intubation has been unsuccessful with a tube of an appropriate diameter. In the adult a 7 mm or even a 6 mm internal diameter tube may be chosen. It may then become necessary electively to ventilate the patient because there would be undue resistance to gas flow during spontaneous ventilation. Alternatively, if the smaller tube is unsatisfactory due to difficulty in effecting a seal with the cuff it can be changed using a polythene tube changer [23], stylet [24] or suction catheter [25]. This is not likely to be necessary for short procedures but would be appropriate when longer term ventilation is proposed. A technique employing a small tracheal tube and artificial ventilation is frequently used during operations on the larynx in order to allow good surgical access. Small tubes specially designed for microlaryngeal surgery with internal diameters of 4, 5 and 6 mm with a high volume large diameter cuff are commercially available‡ and could also be useful for cases of difficult intubation.

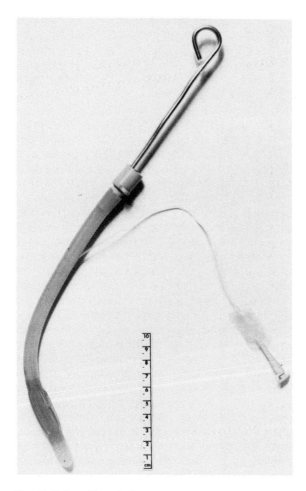

Fig. 11 Tube with stylet bent into a 'J' shape.

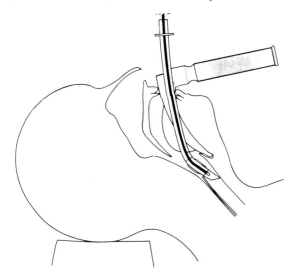

Fig. 12 Tube with bent stylet used to facilitate intubation.

*Flexiguide Division, PO Box 867, Ravinia Station, Highland Park, IL 60035, USA.
†Endotrol by Mallinckrodt. Obtained from American Hospital Supply (UK) Ltd, Station Road, Didcot, Oxon.
‡MLT endotracheal tube Mallinckrodt. Supplied by American Hospital Supply (UK) Ltd, Station Road, Didcot, Oxon.

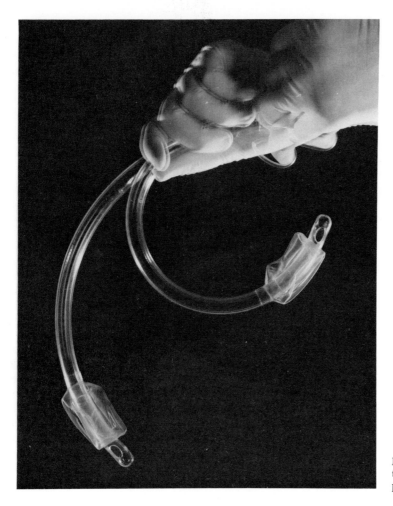

Fig. 13 Double exposure of 'endotrol' tube showing movement caused by pulling on ring loop.

Laryngoscope blades and handles

The standard curved blade described by Macintosh [36] in 1943 is usually satisfactory for revealing the larynx (Fig. 14). Occasionally a longer blade of the same design is required for tall patients. The laryngoscope was designed for intubation under spontaneous respiration when the larynx could be exposed at a lighter plane of anaesthesia. The tip of the blade in the vallecula (supplied by the glossopharyngeal nerve) did not touch the dorsal surface of the epiglottis (supplied by the superior laryngeal nerve, a branch of the vagal nerve). Almost exclusively Macintosh laryngoscope blades are used for intubating adults in the United Kingdom. The tip of the blade is lifted to expose the cords. Care should be taken to avoid exerting undue pressure on the upper teeth. It is important always to have available at least two working laryngoscopes for any intubation in case the light fails in one.

For difficult intubation most clinicians use an alternative technique rather than another type of laryngoscope blade. Over the years a large number of different designs of the blade have been described. In 1926 Magill described a straight blade laryngoscope used to pass a catheter with an accompanying expiratory tube into the larynx [37] (Fig. 15). The tip of the blade was placed behind the epiglottis. In 1941 this design was modified and improved by Miller [38]. The Miller blade was shallow with a curve 2″ back from the tip and had a round, narrow end. This shallow base decreased the risk of damage to the teeth and it was not necessary to open the mouth as widely as with the Magill blade. This type of blade is widely used in North America and is often employed for cases of difficult intubation.

A number of variations in design are available to facilitate intubation. The laryngoscope can be fitted with improved fibreoptic illumination [39, 40]. Most laryngoscopes are designed to intubate from the right side of the patient's mouth. A 'left sided entry' laryngoscope blade may be required for patients with deformities of the right side of the face and oropharynx [41]. This is a mirror image of the usual Miller or Macintosh blade and the tube can be introduced from the left side of the mouth. A shorter handle to the laryngoscope may be useful in obese or pregnant patients with large breasts when the usual laryngoscope handle may be impeded [42].

Other options are to detach the blade, pass it into the mouth and then reattach the handle or to use a 'polio' blade (Fig. 16). The handle of a 'polio' laryngoscope is arranged at an angle greater than 90° to the blade to enable easier insertion into the mouth. A ventilation device may be clipped to the standard laryngoscope handle enabling ventilation during intubation [43, 44] (Fig. 17) which would allow a more prolonged attempt at intubation and minimize the risk of hypoxia. A suction channel can also

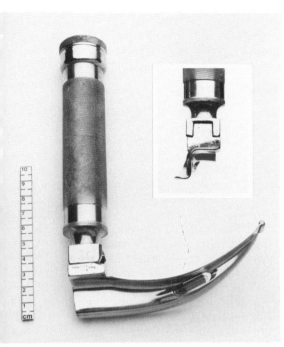

Fig. 14 Macintosh blade.

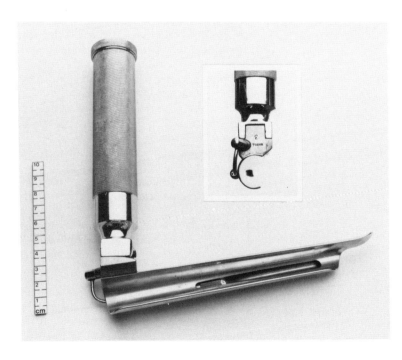

Fig. 15 Magill blade.

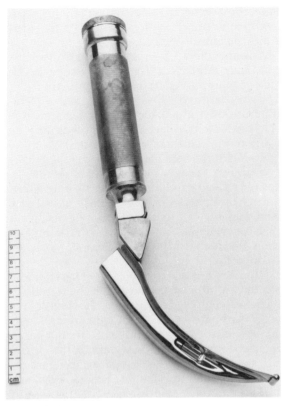

Fig. 16 Polio blade.

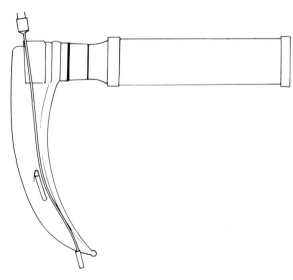

Fig. 17 The needle attached to the laryngoscope blade, showing the moulding to the shape of the blade. From Galloon [43].

be incorporated in the blade to facilitate immediate suction. Blades with mirrors and prisms are described elsewhere (p. 121).

Nasal intubation

The term 'blind nasal intubation' was first used by Rowbotham & Magill who utilized the technique during the First World War [45]. Accidentally they found that when working with dual insufflation tubes a larger bore tube passed nasally would frequently enter the glottis. The history of nasotracheal intubation has been reviewed by Elder [46], Gold & Buechel [47] and Pedersen [48]. By 1937 the most common method of intubation was with a laryngoscope under direct vision. Also widely used were blind nasal intubation, blind oral intubation through a divided airway, and blind oral intubation using the first two fingers of the left hand to palpate the epiglottis or larynx and then sliding the tube posteriorly down behind the epiglottis [49]. However Magill [50] and Lewis [51] still continued routinely to advocate blind nasal intubation rather than direct oral intubation. Anaesthetists of that era were skilled at atraumatic blind nasal intubation but with the advent of muscle relaxants the requirement for the technique largely vanished. In order to maintain the skill, some clinicians practise the technique where nasal intubation is required for elective surgical procedures such as tonsillectomy. Blind nasal intubation has been performed under general [52, 54], or local anaesthesia [47, 55, 56], and even without any form of anaesthesia [57].

Pederson has summarized some of the circumstances in which awake nasal intubation should be considered [48]:
1 decreased airway patency due to inflammation or neoplasm;
2 difficult laryngoscopy due to inability to open the mouth, mandibular agenesis, 'bull neck' or buck teeth;
3 maxillofacial deformities (after trauma);
4 when a mask can not be applied to the face;
5 cervical injuries limiting neck movement.

Before performing an awake intubation the anaesthetist should carefully explain the procedure to the patient. The patient is then lightly sedated, and the local anaesthetic administered (see chapter 6). The patient is positioned with the neck flexed and the head extended at the atlantoaxial joint in the 'sniffing the morning air' position described by Magill [50]. A well lubricated, curved, nasal tube is gently passed through the most patent nostril into the pharynx. The nasal mucous membranes can be constricted by the use of a phenylephrine spray. The opposite nostril should be occluded with the mouth shut and the chin lifted forwards. The patient is then asked to breathe in deeply and the tube advanced in the midline while listening for breath sounds. Gold & Buechel successfully intubated 48 out of 50 patients with

this method [47]. Confirmation of placement and monitoring of the progress of the tube is facilitated by monitoring carbon dioxide concentrations in the expired air.

Not all nasal intubations are performed so easily. A number of techniques have been described to facilitate the procedure (Table 10). If there is difficulty in passing the tube through the nose a smaller, well lubricated tube should be used and rotated as required (Figs 18 and 19). It is not uncommon to find that the tip of the tube is held up at the anterior tracheal wall and further movement is obstructed. When this happens the situation can usually be resolved by leaving the tube at the laryngeal inlet and flexing the neck when it usually easily passes into the trachea (Figs 20 and 21). The distal end

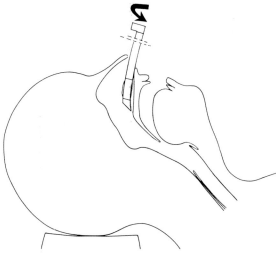

Fig. 18 Rotation of nasal tube may be required to facilitate passage through the nose (see also Fig. 19).

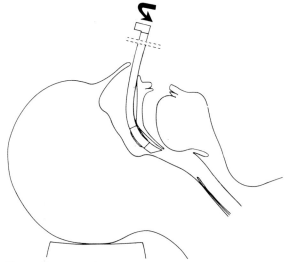

Fig. 19 Rotation of nasal tube may be required to facilitate passage through the nose.

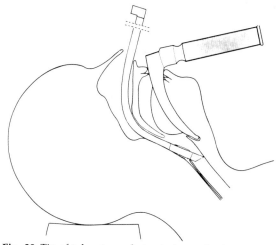

Fig. 20 Tip of tube stopped at anterior tracheal wall.

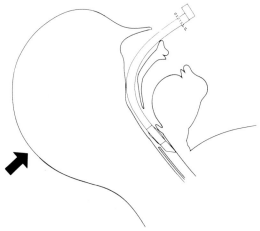

Fig. 21 Laryngoscope removed, neck flexed and tube then passed into the trachea.

Table 10 Techniques to facilitate nasotracheal intubation.

Reference	Used under local anaesthetic (LA) or general anaesthetic (GA)	Technique	Number of patients	Success rate (%)
Brodman & Duncalf (1981) [58]	LA or GA	A *soft thin suction catheter* was passed through the nose into the pharynx. The tracheal tube was then passed over the suction catheter. This avoided trauma to nose and pharynx	More than 20	100%
Mackinnon & Harrison (1979) [59]	Not stated	A *16FG Jacques rubber catheter* was placed on the end of the nasal tube. The Jacques catheter was passed through the nose into the mouth and the tracheal tube was then gently passed through the nose. The catheter was then disconnected from the tube. This was designed to prevent nasal and pharyngeal trauma	Not stated	Not stated
Nolan (1969) [60]	GA	A nasotracheal tube can get stuck in the nasopharynx in a patient with a prominent arch of the atlas vertebra. Traction on a *suction catheter* passed through the tube and out of the mouth lifted the tip of the tube into oropharynx. The catheter was then removed and the tube passed into the trachea	1	1(100)
Tahir (1970) [61]	LA or GA	Obstruction to the tube in the nasopharynx can occur at the base of the occipital bone the first cervical vertebra or from lymphoid tissue in children. *A suction catheter* is used as in Nolan's technique	Not stated	Not stated
Yamamura et al (1959) [62]	LA	A children's *laryngoscope bulb* on the end of a vinyl covered line was placed inside and just distal to the end of the nasotracheal tube. The room lights were dimmed. Intubation was then effected by observing the light transilluminating the neck in the midline and then advancing the tube	30	29 (96.7)
Schneiderman (1966) [63]	LA	A *clear plastic tube* was connected to the proximal end of the tracheal tube. Condensation of moisture on the tube occurred during expiration and cleared during inspiration. The tube was advanced into the larynx using this sign	Not stated	Not stated
Findlay & Gissen (1961) [64]	LA	A nasotracheal tube was advanced to the pharyngeal inlet where loud breath sounds indicated the tip was near the glottis. A *No. 12 nasogastric* tube was then advanced through the tube into the trachea. The tracheal tube was then advanced over the nasogastric tube into the trachea	11	11(100)
Dryden (1976) [65]	Not stated	On occasions the passage of the tube becomes obstructed near the introitus of the larynx despite neck flexion and changes in head position. *A suction catheter* was fed down the tube into the trachea and it was then possible to advance the tube into the trachea	Not stated	Not stated
Pedersen (1971) [48]	LA	A silk thread was firmly attached to the proximal end of a *suction catheter* which was then advanced through the nose and down to the laryngeal inlet. At this point, there were maximum breath sounds on auscultation. The patient was asked to breathe in deeply and the catheter advanced into the trachea. Local anaesthetic was then injected down the catheter into the trachea and the nasotracheal tube advanced over the taut silk thread and suction catheter	20	100%
Adams et al (1982) [66]		Tongue extrusion. When the tongue is extruded it shifts the supralaryngeal structures and provides a more favourable path for intubation	Not stated	Not stated
Waters (1963) [67]	GA	See retrograde technique (p. 122)		
Singh (1966) [68]	GA	See technique using a hook (p. 122)		

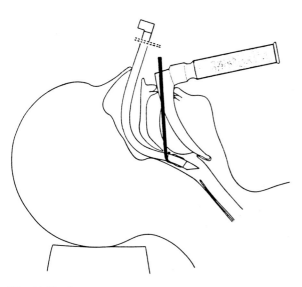

Fig. 22 Hook used to facilitate passage of nasal tube.

of the tube frequently needs to be manipulated through the cords either with Magill forceps or a hook (Fig. 22). Alternatively a suction catheter can be used to facilitate the passage of the tube into the trachea [65] (Figs 23–25).

Blind nasal intubation may be attempted under general anaesthesia following a failed oral intubation. The success rate is increased if the patient hyperventilates. Davies described a technique using nitrous oxide, oxygen, halothane and 7% carbon dioxide [54]. Ether and carbon dioxide are particularly effective in stimulating hyperventilation and facilitating the procedure.

Blind nasal intubation, although a simple procedure, has low reported success rates of 30% [47] and 28% [54] on the first attempt. Davies reported a final success rate of 93%. However, 40% of cases required between four and 12 attempts. It is clear that increased trauma, which may be disastrous, can result from prolonged and rough attempts.

A failure rate of 21% with blind nasal intubation was reported in 61 cases of ankylosis of the jaw [6]. In five cases (8.2%) considerable bleeding occurred and a fatality was reported in a 17-year-old man after hypoxia due to a severe epistaxis. In 60 similar cases the alternative technique of transtracheal ventilation was used without any problems [131].

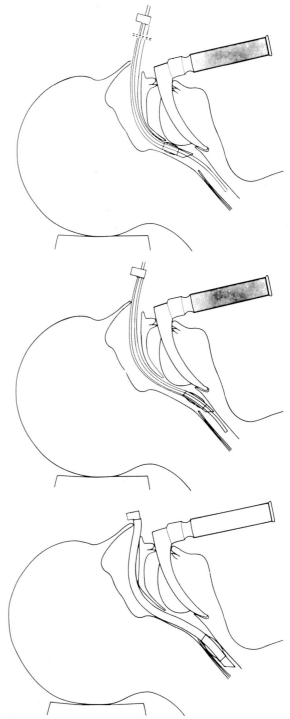

Figs 23-25. Use of suction catheter to facilitate passage of nasal tube through the cords. The suction catheter is passed through the tube into the trachea. The tube is then 'railroaded' over the suction catheter into the trachea and the catheter removed.

SPECIALIZED TECHNIQUES

Specialized techniques may be required if simple measures fail. The choice is determined by the availability of apparatus and the skill and experience of the operator. Although laryngoscope blades with prisms and mirrors are rarely used now they are included in this chapter for the sake of historical completeness.

Light wand

The lighted stylet or 'light wand'* has been used to facilitate intubation both under local and general anaesthesia. The light wand has a battery handle and a copper stylet covered in white plastic. There is a bulb on the distal end of the stylet (Fig. 26).

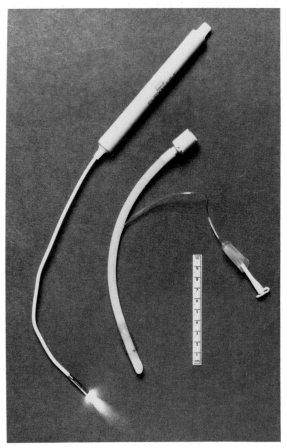

Fig. 26 The lighted stylet or 'light wand'.

---

*Flexi-Lum Surgical Light, Concept Inc, USA. Obtainable in the UK from Henleys Medical Supplies Ltd, London.

In Ducrow's original description intubation was performed with a red rubber tube [69]. The patient was given oxygen, anaesthetized and then given suxamethonium. The suitably curved, lubricated light wand was inserted into a 10″ (25 cm) length of size 22 suction catheter. The light wand was then passed in the midline towards the larynx. The neck was hyperextended and observed for the transilluminating light. When the light was manipulated into the trachea there was a bright patch of illumination in the midline below the cricoid cartilage. The light wand was then removed and a second 10″ length of size 18 suction catheter attached to the first piece of suction catheter. The tracheal tube was then threaded over the suction catheter guide into the trachea. The procedure was carried out in a darkened room and used electively on easy cases to gain experience.

Rayburn [70] later modified the method by inserting the light wand directly into a transparent plastic tracheal tube and used the technique under local anaesthesia for difficult intubations. The light wand was inserted just short of the end of the tube and both were bent into a J-shape (Fig. 27). When the tube was in the oesophagus no light was visible; light appeared as it was withdrawn into the pharynx, and was seen as the tip of the tube neared the laryngeal inlet. The tube was then slipped off the end of the light wand into the trachea. Alternatively

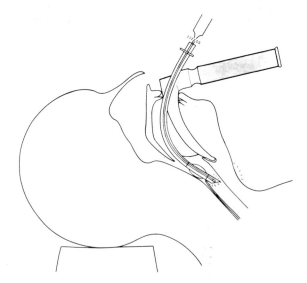

Fig. 27 The 'light wand' inside a transparent tracheal tube with light transilluminating the tissues of the neck.

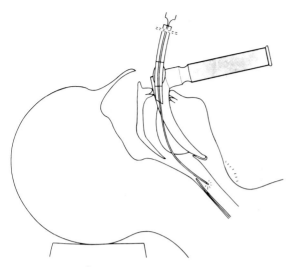

Fig. 28 The 'light wand' advanced distal to the tracheal tube.

the light wand could be passed through the tube and manipulated into the trachea prior to threading the tracheal tube into position (Fig. 28). The method was not recommended for children less than 2 years of age but it was successful for cases with a wide variety of causes of difficult intubation.

Despite Rayburn's difficulties in children, a thin fibreoptic bundle and light source have been used to aid intubation in children [71]. The specially designed fine 23.5 cm bundle will just pass through a 4 mm internal diameter tracheal tube and the light shining through the skin of the neck assists location of the larynx.

Mirrors and prisms

Siker in 1956 described a curved laryngoscope blade with an attached stainless steel mirror [72]. The laryngoscope was introduced in the

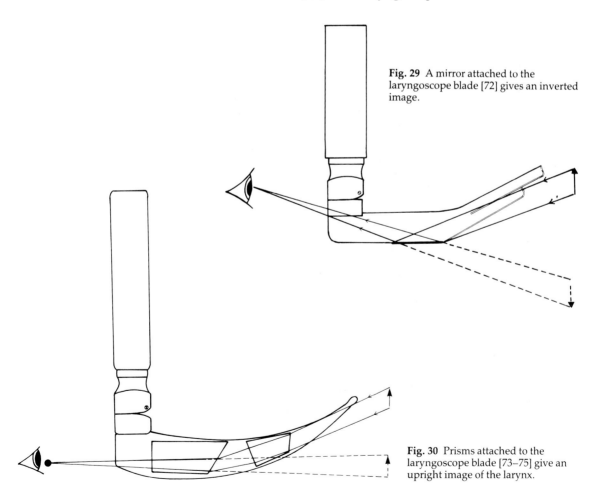

Fig. 29 A mirror attached to the laryngoscope blade [72] gives an inverted image.

Fig. 30 Prisms attached to the laryngoscope blade [73–75] give an upright image of the larynx.

usual way and the tube with stylet then directed towards the tip of the laryngoscope until the tip of the tube was seen through the mirror as it approached the vocal cords. It is essential to become accustomed to the inverted appearance of the image (Fig. 29) while manipulating the tube. Expertise should be gained by practising on elective cases. Siker reported successful intubation in three cases in which there had been previous failure with a curved Macintosh or a straight, U shaped cross sectional Guedel blade.

A modification enables one or two prisms to be applied to a laryngoscope blade [73–75]. Light can be refracted (Fig. 30) through as much as 80° and the view of the larynx is improved. Later versions of the prism were made of plastic and used with a fibreoptic light source. The image is then not inverted and thus the prism technique is easier to use.

Hooks

A hook, as an aid to nasotracheal intubation, was first described in 1962 [76]. It is particularly helpful in children where the larynx is placed anteriorly. The larynx is visualized with a laryngoscope and the nasal tube passed into the oropharynx. The tube is then advanced over the hook. An assistant advances the tube which is then guided into the larynx with the hook (Fig. 22). The method was claimed to be less traumatic and easier than using Magill forceps. A hook was used in 1965 [77] in an adult patient with a severe fixed flexion neck deformity. An awake blind nasotracheal intubation was attempted. The hook was introduced into the mouth and placed round the distal end of the nasotracheal tube. The tracheal tube was pulled forwards and guided into the trachea using the breath sounds to locate the laryngeal inlet. In 1966 a similar method was used after blind nasal intubation had failed in three patients with ankylosis of the jaw and micrognathia [68]. Specially designed less traumatic hooks are commercially available.

Waters [67] in 1963 used a retrograde method as an aid to intubation. An epidural catheter was passed into the oropharynx through a Tuohy needle inserted through the cricothyroid membrane. A hook was used to deliver the catheter from the mouth. The tracheal tube was then inserted using the catheter as a guide. It may be difficult or impossible to use a hook if the jaws are shut.

Rigid bronchoscope

Aro and his colleagues [2] used a rigid bronchoscope as an aid to intubation in 12 out of 3402 intubations (0.3%). In a further 68 difficult intubations (2%) an introducer in the tube produced a successful result. The bronchoscope was introduced into the trachea and then a thin atraumatic wire stylet introduced through the bronchoscope. The bronchoscope was then removed and the tube passed over the stylet into the trachea. In their hands the method was simple and safe. In a modification [78] the lubricated bronchoscope is passed inside the tracheal tube, and introduced into the trachea and then the tube slid down over the bronchoscope, which is then removed. These techniques can only be used in patients who are able to open their mouths.

A rigid bronchoscope may be required for the management of postintubation tracheal stenosis [159]. If the tracheal lumen was less than 5 mm in diameter Grillo dilated the airway under general anaesthesia with progressively larger paediatric bronchoscopes. This prevented the development of hypercarbia in these spontaneously breathing patients. Positive pressure ventilation was avoided both intra and postoperatively. If the diameter of the tracheal lumen was greater than 6 mm intubation was carried out above the lesion. Cardiopulmonary bypass was not required in any of the 208 patients. Neville in 1969, however, used cardiopulmonary bypass in 35 cases of tracheal disease [160]. He found that the technique was easy to use and did not result in complications.

Retrograde methods

Retrograde tracheal intubation was first described in a patient with a pre-existing tracheostomy [79]. The object was to avoid the tracheostomy tube obstructing surgical access during a cervical operation and to ensure an atraumatic and easy tracheal intubation. Following administration of topical analgesia a No. 16 French catheter was introduced through the tracheostomy, directed in a cephalad direction and delivered through the mouth. The catheter was then sutured to the tracheal tube and the

Table 11 Retrograde methods of tracheal intubation.

Reference	LA or GA	Oral nasotracheal	Needle used	Retrograde equipment	Other apparatus	Special instructions	Clinical indication	Number of patients	Success rate
Waters (1963) [67]	Thiopentone and LA in children	Oral	Tuohy with bevel facing cephalad	1 yard of sterile *vinyl plastic tube*	Hook to remove tube from mouth	Keep catheter taut. Do not use in cases of respiratory obstruction due to laryngeal pathology	Patients with trismus and cases of difficult intubation	Not given	Not given
Harmer & Vaughan (1980) [80]	LA	Oral	Tuohy needle	*Epidural catheter*	Large well greased suction catheter	Epidural catheter passed out of mouth. Suction catheter passed over epidural catheter until it reaches the cricothyroid membrane. Large bore armoured ET tube then passed over suction catheter and epidural catheter. Catheters then withdrawn. This avoids trauma of nasal intubation	Difficult intubation	Not stated	Not stated
Dhara (1980) [82]	LA	Nasal	Tuohy needle	*Epidural catheter*	14 FG suction catheter (hook *not required*)	Epidural catheter passed out of mouth. Suction catheter passed through nose and out of mouth. Epidural catheter then threaded through shortened catheter. Suction catheter then removed. (In two patients epidural catheter came straight out of nostril.) Soft red rubber tracheal tube then threaded over epidural catheter	Not stated	10 (in 6 years)	10
Bourke & Levesque (1974) [83]	Not stated	Oral and nasal	Large bore needle	*Catheter*	None	Catheter should be threaded through side hole of tracheal tube from outside and in through lumen of tube. This eliminates difficulties in threading tube into the trachea. Distance between cords and cricothyroid membrane is only 1 cm (Fig. 38)	Difficult intubation	Not stated	Not stated
Powell & Ozdil (1967) [84]	LA	Oral and nasal	17 gauge needle	Bardic intracath. (*central venous catheter*)	Rubber urethral catheter threaded through nose for nasal intubation	Catheter threaded either through lumen of tube or through hole near tip of tube. Keep catheter taut during intubation. Withdraw catheter from above	Ankylosis of the jaw tongue tumours cervical arthritis	15	15
Roberts (1981) [86]	Not stated	Oral or nasal	16 gauge catheter with stilette	120 cm teflon coated *Swan-Ganz introducer wire*	Laryngoscope and Magill forceps may be required to deliver the wire from the mouth	Often easy to pass into the nasopharynx and out of the nose	Difficult intubation	Not stated	Not stated

catheter pulled from below delivered the tube into the trachea. The catheter was then cut from the tube and the tracheostomy closed for the duration of the operation.

Subsequently a number of retrograde methods have been described employing guides passed percutaneously through the cricothyroid membrane [67, 80–87, 161]. Their main features are shown in Table 11.

Epidural catheters [67, 80–83], central venous catheters [84, 85], a Swan-Ganz wire [86], a Seldinger wire [87, 161] and silk or nylon thread have all been threaded in a retrograde direction through the cricothyroid membrane into the mouth. Techniques have included oral [80] and nasal routes [82] for tracheal intubation. If a patient is unable to open his mouth widely the chosen guide such as an epidural catheter should enable the patient readily to spit it out or to be delivered with a hook. A Seldinger wire may be unsuccessful if it cannot be delivered from the mouth and does not pass easily through the nose. Such wires, however, do sometimes pass without difficulty through the nose. A wire usually sits on the posterior pharyngeal wall and cannot be extruded easily by the patient unlike a non-rigid coiled epidural catheter. No comparison of the use of epidural catheters and flexible wire introducers has been made. It is possible that one particular method may be more successful in an individual patient. Therefore both types of guide should be available.

The technique used by the authors is a modification of that described by Harmer & Vaughan [80] (Figs 31–37). The patient is lightly sedated and has 2 ml of 4% lignocaine injected percutaneously through the cricothyroid membrane. The pharynx is sprayed with 4% lignocaine. The cricoid cartilage is palpated and a small horizontal incision made in the skin above the cartilage after subcutaneous infiltration with local anaesthetic. A Tuohy needle is inserted into the trachea and its presence confirmed by aspirating air into a syringe filled with sterile water. The syringe is then removed and an epidural catheter inserted into the pharynx. The patient then spits the catheter out of the mouth. The Tuohy needle is removed and a large lubricated suction catheter, which has been kept in a refrigerator to stiffen it, is passed over the epidural catheter into the trachea. Its presence in the trachea should be confirmed with a

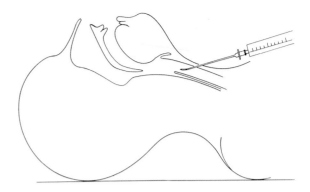

Fig. 31 Tuohy needle advanced through the cricothyroid membrane into the trachea. On aspiration into the fluid filled syringe air bubbles demonstrate that the end of the needle is in the trachea.

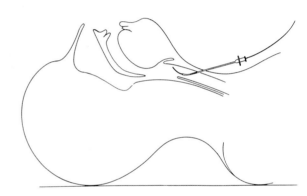

Fig. 32 Syringe removed and epidural catheter threaded cephalad.

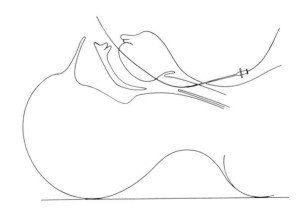

Fig. 33 Catheter delivered from mouth. Patient may spit it out or passage from the mouth may be facilitated with a hook.

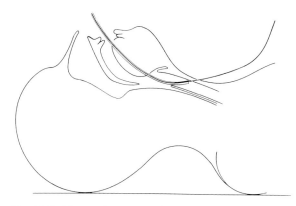

Fig. 34 Refrigerated suction catheter threaded over epidural catheter and position checked with a capnograph.

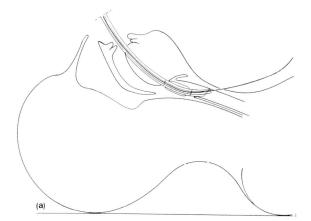

(a)

Fig. 35 (a) Tracheal tube threaded over suction catheter into the trachea. To facilitate passage of the tracheal tube, tension is applied by pulling on both ends of the epidural catheter. The final position of the tube is checked with a capnograph.

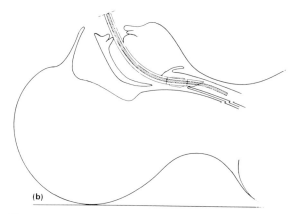

(b)

Fig. 35 (b) The epidural catheter is cut at the neck and pulled from above. The suction catheter is then pushed further into the trachea.

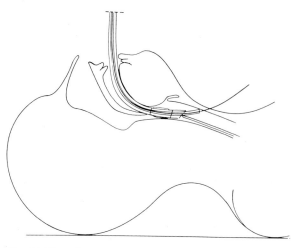

Fig. 36 The tube may get stuck at the glottis.

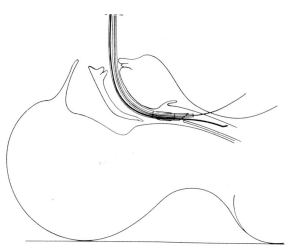

Fig. 37 Passage of a gum elastic catheter will facilitate passage of the tube.

capnograph. A small soft malleable tracheal tube is then passed over the suction catheter into the trachea and placement also confirmed with a capnograph. If the tube is held up at the laryngeal inlet a gum elastic catheter is passed into the trachea to facilitate its passage. The epidural catheter is then cut off near the skin entry site and the remaining catheter removed from above. The suction catheter should be inserted further into the trachea immediately after removal of the epidural catheter and before attempting to pass the tracheal tube to its final position. This technique can be used in awake

patients or under general anaesthesia in patients in whom failed intubation occurs unexpectedly. This technique is reasonably quick
and fairly easy even for the tyro.*

Success rates are high [81, 82, 84] with no
reported failures. Bourke & Levesque [83]
reported that the tube might not always pass
through the cords or could flip out of the
trachea as the epidural catheter was withdrawn.
They avoided this by passing the epidural
catheter through a side hole in the tracheal tube
(Fig. 38).

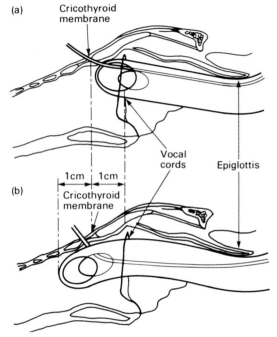

Fig. 38 Cross section of larynx and trachea with tracheal
tube and catheter guide passing through the cricothyroid
membrane. (a) Catheter passes through the end of the tube
and 1 cm of the tube passes through the cords. (b) Catheter
exits the side hole and 2 cm of the tube passes beyond the
cords. After Bourke and Levesque [83], with kind permission of the International Anesthesia Research Society.

Akinyemi [81] detailed complications occurring with a retrograde method in 12 patients
aged from 9 to 25 years with ankylosis of the jaw
secondary to cancrum oris. He first attempted
blind nasal intubation under general anaesthesia and if four attempts failed used a retrograde
technique [67] for nasotracheal intubation.

*A video showing a retrograde intubation will shortly be
available from the BMA film library.

Minor bleeding at the puncture site or from the
nose occurred five times, there was difficulty in
hooking the catheter through the nose three
times and airway problems occurred twice. He
concluded that these problems were minor and
the technique should be used more frequently.

The technique can be used both in adults and
in children [67, 87]. Retrograde techniques are
easy to learn and use and do not require
complex expensive apparatus. Many hospitals
in developed countries cannot afford fibreoptic
equipment and hospitals in third world countries are even less likely to have it available. In
contrast, the equipment for a retrograde technique should be readily available. It is not ethical
to practise on elective cases and in consequence
few clinicians have either seen or tried retrograde techniques.This situation can be remedied
by video or tape slide presentations and by
practice on training models or cadavers. All
trainees should receive formal teaching but only
16.5% of the clinicians in a retrospective survey
[5] had tried retrograde intubation techniques
(Table 3).

Fibreoptic endoscopy

The fibreoptic bronchoscope was introduced
into clinical practice in 1968 by Ikeda [88].
Fibreoptic bronchoscopy is commonly undertaken by physicians for diagnostic purposes and
therapeutic removal of secretions [89, 90]. The
technique is, however, not without hazards
including epistaxis, laryngospasm, hypoxia,
pulmonary bleeding, cardiac dysrhythmias and
vasovagal reactions [90–93].

Fibreoptic instruments have been used by
anaesthetists to facilitate tracheal intubation. In
1967 Murphy used a fibreoptic choledochoscope
for nasal intubation [94]. Taylor & Towey in
1972 [95] described the use of a fibreoptic
bronchoscope and there have been many other
descriptions of its use [96–102]. The fibreoptic
bronchoscope has a suction channel which is
invaluable for aspiration of secretions and
injection of local anaesthetic. The bronchoscope
is smaller in diameter than the laryngoscope
and gives a more intense light. It is an expensive
and delicate instrument but may be shared
between different departments in a large hospital, in which case it may only be available for
elective cases.

Table 12 Recommendations to facilitate fibreoptic intubation.

Reference	LA or GA	Oral (O) or nasal (N)	Comments and recommendations to facilitate intubation with fibreoptic scope	Number of patients	Success rate (%)
Sia & Edens (1981) [1]	LA	N	In the awake patient there is tonus of the tongue and the epiglottis. In an anaesthetized patient the tongue and epiglottis move posteriorly and fibreoptic intubation is more difficult. Also with the oral route the tip of the scope enters the glottis at an acute angle but by the nasal route at an oblique angle. Experience and frequent practice are required. 30 successful elective fibreoptic intubations should be performed before attempting a difficult intubation	Not stated	Not stated
Tahir (1972) [97]	GA or LA	N	Artificial ventilation can be performed during attempts at intubation. The tracheal tube is passed into the oropharynx and connected to the anaesthetic circuit. The scope is passed through a rubber diaphragm on the catheter mount. Ventilation can then be assisted or controlled thus preventing hypoxia	Not stated	Not stated
Davidson et al (1975) [98]	LA	N (10) and O (4)	All patients require atropine preoperatively. Aspiration channel on scope used to inject additional local anaesthetic. Secretions may be aspirated if necessary. This is a difficult procedure which may take 10–15 min. Bite block with oral intubations prevents patient biting the scope. Possible complications: overdose of local anaesthetic, regurgitation and aspiration with anaesthetized larynx	14	14 (100)
Messeter & Pettersson (1980) [100]	LA	N	Used safely and atraumatically in patients with rheumatoid arthritis. Less preoperative tracheostomies required than in a control group of 19 patients. If difficult intubation occurs unexpectedly patients should be woken up and later fibreoptic nasal intubation undertaken. If used after repeated attempts at intubation blood mucus and oedema reduced visibility	19 (23 nasal intubations)	23 (100)
Stiles et al (1972) [103]	LA and GA	Not stated	Preoperative tracheostomy avoided in 34 patients. With experience average time to intubate was less than 1 min. Spiral movement of the tube facilitated passage into the trachea when progress was impeded at the laryngeal inlet	104	100 (96) 4 failures due to copious secretions

Two fibreoptic laryngoscopes specifically designed to assist the placement of tracheal tubes were described in 1972 [103] and 1973 [104]. Other authors have documented their experience with the fibreoptic laryngoscope [105–109]. A number of authors have documented their experience with fibreoptic scopes [1, 95–108] and have made recommendations to facilitate the procedure (Table 12).

Although fibreoptic instruments have been available for many years only a small proportion of anaesthetists are trained to use them. Many try but abandon the technique after a few unsuccessful attempts. Only 16.5% of anaesthetists in one survey had tried the technique more than 25 times [110] (Table 13) and only 9%

Table 13 Survey of number of fibreoptic intubations performed by a group of clinicians. From Ovassapian & Dykes [110], with kind permission of the authors, the editor of *Anesthesiology* and the publishers, J.B. Lippincott Co.

No. of intubations	No. of clinicians performing intubations	%
None	51	30
1–5	55	32.4
6–10	22	12.9
11–25	13	7.6
>25	28	16.5
Not answered	1	0.6
Total	170	100

in another survey had tried more than 30 times [5]. Sia & Edens recommended that at least 30 successful elective intubations in conscious and anaesthetized patients should be undertaken before attempting a difficult intubation [1]. All agree that it takes a great deal of practice to become skilled with fibreoptic equipment.

Training programmes

In an attempt to improve training methods Ovassapian et al have developed a training programme [111–114]. After a careful demonstration of the instrument the programme was divided into three parts. Awake nasal fibreoptic intubations were performed on all patients presenting for elective nasal intubation.

Part 1: Practice on a training model

Trainees were given unlimited time to familiarize themselves with the anatomy and the manipulation and visual characteristics of the scope.

Part 2: Exposure of epiglottis and vocal cords in six patients

Written consent was obtained and the epiglottis and cords were then shown in six patients recovering from anaesthesia. The trainee learned the appearance of live moving laryngeal structures and how to recognize and correct problems caused by secretions. The scope was inserted through a nasopharyngeal airway. The instrument was kept well clear of the vocal cords in order to avoid the risk of laryngospasm. The trainee was formally evaluated on his sixth attempt. The mean time to demonstrate the epiglottis and cords by 12 trainees was 1.4 min (range 0.75–4 min)[113].

Part 3: Intubation in six awake sedated patients

Verbal consent was obtained and the procedure explained to patients requiring nasotracheal intubation for elective operations. Patients were premedicated with atropine and morphine. Further sedation was provided with approximately $0.15\,\mu g/kg$ i.v. of diazepam and $1.5\,\mu g/kg$ i.v. of fentanyl. Topical anaesthesia was achieved with 3 ml of 4% lignocaine injected by the translaryngeal route and application of 6%

cocaine to the nasal mucosa. The trainee followed a written step by step guide to the procedure. An 8 mm nasotracheal tube was inserted through the chosen nostril into the pharynx and after suctioning the fibrescope was passed through the tube into the pharynx. The epiglottis and cords were identified and the fibrescope passed into the trachea.

All intubations were closely supervised but advice given regarding sedation and topical analgesia only for the first case unless difficulty occurred in subsequent cases. The trainee was formally evaluated on the sixth attempt. The total time for intubation, that is from the start of application of the local anaesthetic, the actual time for intubation and the number of attempts (each removal of scope from nasal tube) were recorded. The mean total time was 17.7 min (range 9–25 min). The mean intubation time was 3.3 min (range 1–8 min) and only one trainee required two attempts at intubation [113].

The results of the formal training programme were compared with the results using the traditional approach in which the instrument was demonstrated and then one intubation was observed [112]. The formal programme yielded significantly better results; 88.9% of patients were successfully intubated compared to 54.2% in the control group ($P<0.001$) and a shorter mean time was required for intubation, 2.8 min and 4.5 min respectively.

Only nine out of 371 patients (1.6%) indicated at a postoperative interview that they would not like to have an awake intubation again. However, 27 patients (7.3%) remembered the procedure as being mildly unpleasant; 205 patients (55.3%) did not remember the procedure at all [114].

In patients with full stomachs topical anaesthesia was applied to the vocal cords through the suction channel of the scope just prior to intubation. Translaryngeal injection of local anaesthetic was avoided to minimize the risk of aspiration.

The technique can be performed under general anaesthesia. In some cases however the procedure will take a considerable time. It is important, therefore, to be able to ventilate during the attempts and this can be accomplished in a number of different ways [115] (Fig. 39). Experience with fibreoptic equipment can

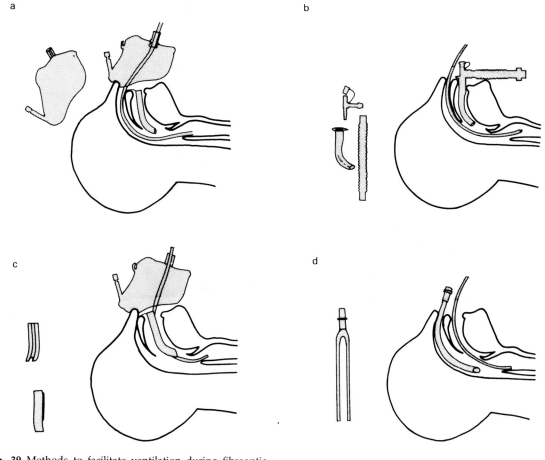

Fig. 39 Methods to facilitate ventilation during fibreoptic intubation: (a) mask with endoscopic port; (b) oral airway with Rowbotham connector and corrugated tubing; (c) oral airway with central groove for passage of endoscope and side ports for suction catheter; (d) binasal airway. From Patil et al [115], with kind permission of the authors, the editor of *Anesthesiology*, and the publishers, J.B. Lippincott Co.

be gained in patients ventilated by mask oesopharyngeal or nasopharyngeal airways and in spontaneously breathing patients through ports in the face mask. Most difficult cases should be intubated under local anaesthesia.

Causes and incidences of failure

Ovassapian and his colleagues have also investigated the incidence and causes of failure with fibreoptic nasal intubations [114]. In a few patients the scope could not be passed through narrowed nasal passages. Of the remainder there were five failures (1.2%) of 418 attempts.

In three the scope was passed into the trachea but the tube would not go through.

In 89% of cases visualization of the cords was classified as easy with a mean intubation time of 3 min (Table 14). These intubations were performed by trainees and the senior authors themselves were able to intubate in 20–30 s in patients in whom exposure of the cords was easy [114].

Intubation was easily accomplished in patients in whom there had been previous difficulty. Difficulties occurred when there was distorted airway anatomy, laryngeal pathology, or if there was decreased space between the

Table 14 Ease of laryngeal exposure in 353 intubations. From Ovassapian et al [114], with kind permission of the International Anaesthesia Research Society.

	Easy	Moderately difficult	Difficult
Visualization of vocal cords	315 (89.2%)	30 (8.5%)	8 (2.3%)
Mean intubation time (min)*	3.0	6.76	16.1
Mean total intubation time (min)†	16.4	19.6	28.1

*Time from insertion of fibrescope to completion of intubation.
†Time from beginning of sedation to completion of intubation.
Easy – on initial introduction the fibrescope was already aligned for good visualization of the vocal cords so that little or no manipulation of the tip of the scope was needed.
Moderately difficult – moderate manipulation of the fibrescope in all directions was necessary to locate the vocal cords.
Difficult – extensive manipulation of the fibrescope in all directions, often with changes in position of the operator, was necessary to identify the vocal cords.

edge of the epiglottis and the posterior pharyngeal wall and in the presence of bloody secretions. A suction channel is critically important if blood or secretions obscure the view. The causes of difficulty with this method are different from those when using a rigid laryngoscope.

The fibrescope, when used on anaesthetized patients, can be inserted through a mask with a diaphragm (Fig. 39) assuring a seal for positive pressure ventilation [115].

The fibrescope in children

Early scopes were of large external diameter and could only be used in adults. Improved technology has resulted in the availability of scopes with an external diameter as small as 3.2 mm which fit inside tubes with an internal diameter of 4.5 mm. A bronchoscope has been used to intubate a 3-year-old child with a cervical injury [116]. Fibreoptic bronchoscopes have been used in children for nasotracheal intubation [117] and in cases of upper airway obstruction [118].

Alternatively the bronchoscope can be positioned above the cords and a guide wire passed through its aspiration channel into the trachea. After removal of the bronchoscope a cardiac catheter can be passed over the guide wire. This

then acts as an introducer for the tracheal tube [119].

In a neonate with congenital fusion of the jaws a 3.2 mm fibreoptic bronchoscope was introduced through one nostril and a tracheal tube through the other [120]. The tracheal tube was then manipulated under direct vision into the trachea. It is clear that there is no place for the occasional operator when dealing with such demanding cases. Indeed in this case the intubation was carried out by a 'paediatric pulmonologist'. Two other experienced clinicians were also involved in the intubation.

Simplified oral intubation using a fibreoptic scope

Oral intubation was found to be much easier when using a special oral airway which also protected the instrument from the patients teeth [140]. The fibrescope was passed through the 'oral airway intubator' [141]. This is a clear plastic oropharyngeal airway (Fig. 40), originally designed for blind oral intubation. The distal end of the airway is positioned close to the laryngeal aperture. The technique was performed rapidly (in less than 2 min) and atraumatically in 25 difficult patients [140]. Intubation was performed under local anaesthesia in 16 patients and under general anaesthesia

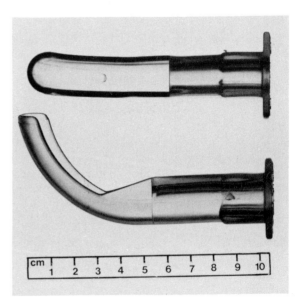

Fig. 40 The oral airway intubator. From Williams & Maltabey [141], with kind permission of the International Anaesthesia Research Society.

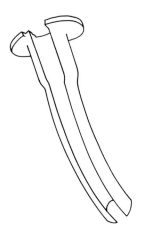

Fig. 41 Modified Guedel airway. Redrawn from Hogan et al [148], with kind permission of the authors and the editor of *Anaesthesia and Intensive Care*.

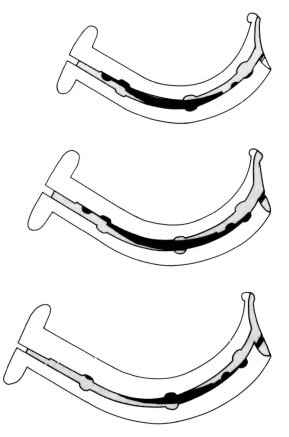

Fig. 42 Set of Berman II airways. Redrawn from Hogan et al [148], with kind permission of the authors and the editor of *Anaesthesia and Intensive Care*.

in the other nine patients using a mask with a diaphragm. Intubation was undertaken by clinicians who had previously performed only 0–3 fibreoptic intubations. The authors claimed the technique enabled fibreoptic intubation to be performed in difficult cases by clinicians with little or no previous experience.

A similar approach has been described using either a modified Guedel or Berman II airway (Figs 41 and 42) as a guide [148]. Excellent results were obtained by an inexperienced medical student (44 out of 50 successful intubations). Four of the failures were due to mucus obscuring the lens and were regarded as avoidable.

Flexible radiopaque directable catheter

A radiopaque catheter has been devised which can be manipulated in both an anteroposterior and a lateral direction by a proximal control handle [121]. This can be steered under direct vision into the trachea.

The procedure is carried out in the radiology department. A nasotracheal tube is first passed into the oropharynx under local anaesthesia. The 65 cm catheter is passed through the tracheal tube and steered under direct vision into the larynx using lateral screening. Rarely anteroposterior screening is required if the tip of

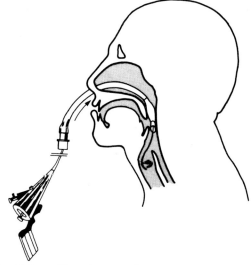

Fig. 43 Steerable catheter is advanced into the fluoroscopically visible trachea via the tracheal tube lumen. After Davidson et al. [121], with kind permission of the authors, the editor of *Anesthesiology*, and the publishers, J.B. Lippincott Co.

the catheter gets stuck in the pyriform fossa. The patient is asked to breathe slowly and deeply and not to cough as the catheter is advanced into the trachea. The tube is advanced into the trachea using the catheter as a guide (Fig. 43). The patient is then transferred to the operating theatre where general anaesthesia is administered.

The technique was used successfully in a number of patients where other techniques had failed. The small size of the catheter ensures it can also be used through paediatric tracheal tubes. The technique was used electively where difficult intubation was predicted preoperatively.

The cooperation of the radiology department is required for this procedure and some clinicians may be reluctant to induce anaesthesia away from the operating theatre.

Needle cricothyrotomy and transtracheal ventilation

Cricothyroid puncture has been used for many years for sputum sampling, bronchial lavage and for injection of local anaesthetic solutions before bronchoscopy or awake intubation. Percutaneous transtracheal ventilation was first described by Jacoby and his colleagues in 1951 [122] and there have been many other descriptions of the technique [123–129]. Cricothyroid ventilation has been used for resuscitation, during routine surgery [124], for oxygenation when intubation was difficult [127–129], for ventilation in patients with laryngeal pathology presenting for microlaryngeal surgery [130] and to ventilate patients with facial injuries or temporomandibular joint ankylosis during anaesthesia [131]. The technique was found to be a safe and simple alternative to blind nasal intubation [131].

In 1974 there were 13 deaths from upper respiratory tract obstruction per million of the population in England and Wales [139]. Hypoxic deaths occur regularly in anaesthetic practice due to failed intubation and subsequent inability to maintain an airway or prolonged laryngospasm [132]. In cases of complete airway obstruction from whatever cause a cricothyrotomy should be performed immediately with a wide bore needle [133]. Needle cricothyrotomy is usually quick to perform, easy and atraumatic. Needle cricothyrotomy can be performed

outside the hospital environment as an alternative to intubation.

Technique

The patient is positioned with the neck extended and both the cricoid and thyroid cartilage are identified. A large bore needle and cannula (14 or 16 gauge) are passed through the cricothyroid membrane into the trachea. The tip of the needle should point downwards towards the carina. Correct positioning is confirmed by aspiration of air, preferably though a liquid filled syringe. Trauma from the needle can be prevented by advancing only the cannula and keeping the needle stationary once the trachea is entered. The needle is then removed and the cannula sutured or taped in place ensuring secure fixation. The cannula is connected to a high pressure oxygen source for ventilation. During inspiration there is an upward flow of gas as soon as the pressure in the trachea is greater than atmospheric and during expiration gas also exits through the larynx. This upward flow of gas helps to prevent aspiration during surgery. The technique used on a typical patient by Layman [131] is shown in Figs 44 and 45.

Smith and his colleagues reviewed the complications that can occur with transtracheal ventilation [129]. No deaths were reported and there were few serious problems with the elective use of the procedure. Complications included subcutaneous and mediastinal emphysema; it is extremely important to check that the cannula is in the tracheal lumen before starting ventilation and to ensure that it remains securely in place. In cases of upper airway obstruction it is also vital to ensure that expiration is adequate as this may become obstructed. Since expiratory obstruction can occur during the introduction of the laryngoscope it has been recommended that ventilation be interrupted during that procedure. This can be resumed when the glottis is exposed.

Alternatively the patient may breathe air or oxygen enriched air spontaneously through the catheter [134, 135]. Oxygen can be delivered continuously at 3 l/min through the catheter while the patient breathes spontaneously [128]. The choice of spontaneous or artificial ventilation is determined by apparatus availability and clinical circumstances.

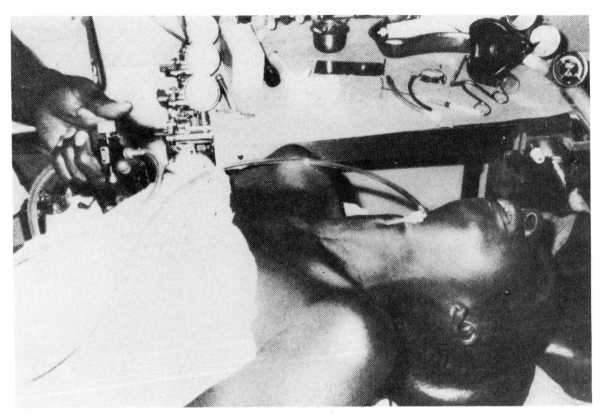

Fig. 44 Transtracheal cannula sutured in place with head and neck extended. From Layman [131], with kind permission of the editor of *Annals of the Royal College of Surgery of England.*

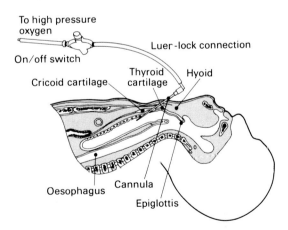

To high pressure oxygen

Luer-lock connection

On/off switch

Thyroid cartilage   Hyoid

Cricoid cartilage

Oesophagus   Cannula

Epiglottis

Fig. 45 Diagram to illustrate positioning of upper airway in relation to larynx and cannula. After Layman [131], with kind permission of the editor of *Annals of the Royal College of Surgery of England.*

Sometimes in an emergency it may be difficult to connect the needle to the oxygen supply or ventilator. Non-commercial connectors have been described with a tapered tracheal tube connector fitted into the barrel of a $2\,cm^3$ syringe [136], a catheter mount glued into the sawn off barrel of a $5\,cm^3$ syringe [137] and a needle connected to one end of a length of plastic intravenous tubing with a tracheal tube adapter on the other end of the tube [138]. The connector can then be connected to the anaesthetic machine and ventilation effected by intermittently switching on the emergency oxygen [138]. High frequency ventilation through a transtracheal cannula is effective in maintaining satisfactory blood gases and also minimizes the risk of aspiration [149]. A suitable connection should be available in each difficult intubation box ready for immediate use in cases of upper airway obstruction. In some centres this technique is used routinely for ventilation in cases for microlaryngoscopy. Such familiarity with the apparatus should enable the rare cases of upper airway obstruction to be managed more efficiently.

ALTERNATIVES TO TRACHEAL INTUBATION

A number of the following devices may be of value to the clinician. None of these, however, are commonly used in hospital practice at the present time.

Oesophageal obturator airway (OOA)*

In the hospital environment, the presence of an anaesthetist or other suitably trained doctor ensures that intubation can usually be carried out quickly and easily.

Outside the hospital alternative methods may be required for resuscitation especially where equipment for tracheal intubation or the required expertise are missing. In some countries paramedical personnel perform advanced resuscitation procedures in cases of prehospital cardiac arrest. Usually mouth-to-mouth ventilation is used initially for resuscitation. Some of the more highly trained paramedics are permitted to intubate the trachea [142]. It is important that they should be taught indications and contraindications to tracheal intubation.

A device that both blocks the oesophagus and aids pulmonary ventilation was described by Don Michael in 1968 [143] and can be used as an alternative to tracheal intubation. The oesophageal obturator airway (OOA) was introduced into clinical practice because mouth to mouth resuscitation was considered aesthetically displeasing, and to prevent gaseous distension of the stomach with subsequent pulmonary aspiration. The device has been in use since 1972 and had been used on an estimated 1.5 million patients by 1980 [144].

The OOA (Fig. 46) has an occluded distal end and multiple small holes in the portion situated in the pharynx. A special face mask is attached to the proximal end. The airway is inserted blindly into the mouth without the requirement for a laryngoscope. The operator's left thumb is placed behind the tongue and the lower jaw and tongue are lifted upwards. The middle and index fingers are placed on the chin. No force should be used during insertion of the airway. The tube sits on the posterior pharyngeal wall and should pass easily into the oesophagus

*Brunswick Mft. Co. Inc, North Quincy, MA 02171, USA.

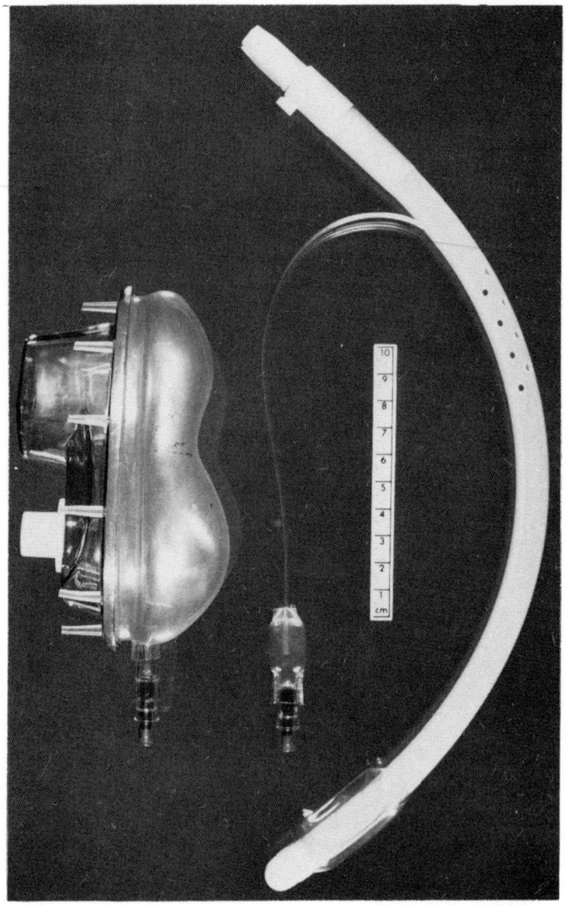

Fig. 46 The oesophageal obturator airway.

(Figs 47–49). Once the tube is in situ in the oesophagus a balloon is inflated. The mask is held firmly over the mouth and nose. Expired air can then be blown down the tube. The air escapes through the small holes and enters the trachea. Alternatively the patient can be ventilated with a self-inflating bag. The balloon and occluded distal end prevent air entering the stomach. The correct position of the tube should be checked by listening over the lungs for breath sounds and over the stomach to exclude the possibility of accidental tracheal intubation.

There have been a number of clinical studies with the OOA. Patients with prehospital cardiac arrest were initially resuscitated by paramedics using the OOA [145], and transferred to a hospital where a tracheal tube was inserted and the OOA removed. The paramedics had had a training programme totalling 16 h and an assessment before being allowed to use the

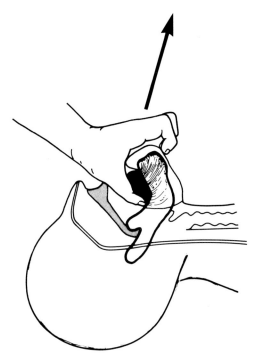

Fig. 47 Insertion of OOA. The thumb is inserted into the mouth and the chin lifted forwards.

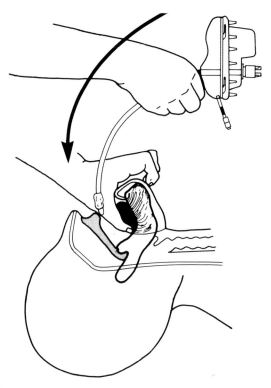

Fig. 48 The device is then inserted into the mouth.

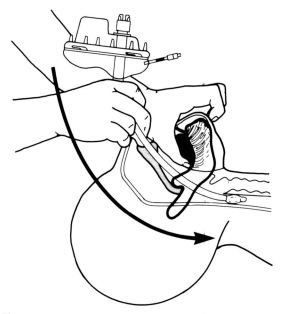

Fig. 49 The device is then pushed blindly into the oesophagus. Force should be avoided.

OOA in the field. The test of competence was when intubation of the oesophagus of a cadaver could be accomplished in less than 15 s.

The use of the OOA was carefully monitored in 300 cases of prehospital cardiac arrest. The results were compared with an earlier study using a mask and oral airway for resuscitation [146]. No important differences were observed in the incidence of resuscitation and subsequent transfer to an intensive care unit. Problems with the OOA occurred during insertion by the paramedics and later due to the unfamiliarity of physicians with the device when the patient arrived in the emergency room [145]. There were eight cases in which there was difficulty in using the apparatus, 13 cases of tracheal intubation and 11 cases in which the OOA could not be passed. Five of the 13 cases of tracheal intubation went unrecognized and all died (death in 1.7% of patients due to tracheal intubation and 4.3% tracheal intubations). Other authors have reported an inability to pass the OOA or tracheal intubation in 5–10% of cases [144]. Problems resulted from leaking balloons and difficulty in obtaining a good seal on the face with the mask. Oesophageal trauma was demonstrated in 10% of patients who had an autopsy. No case of oesophageal rupture occurred although this is a rare but well

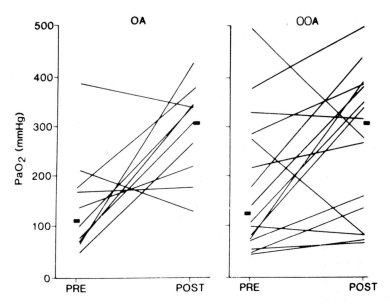

Fig. 50 Oxygenation before (pre) and after (post) tracheal intubation in two groups of patients. The first group initially had an oral airway (OA) in situ and the second had the oesophageal obturator (OOA) airway in situ prior to tracheal intubation. From Donen et al [145], with kind permission of the authors and the editor of the *Canadian Anaesthetists' Society Journal*.

recognized complication. The design of the tip of the OOA has been modified from an early bullet shape to a hemispherical shape in an attempt to prevent oesophageal rupture.

On arrival in the emergency room a tracheal tube was inserted and a marked improvement in arterial oxygen tension resulted (Fig. 50). In other studies oxygenation with the OOA was as effective as with tracheal intubation. When paramedical staff were trained both in tracheal intubation and in the use of the OOA and given a free choice, the OOA was used in approximately 35% of cases and the trachea was intubated in the other 65% [147].

The chief advantage of the OOA is that it reduces the incidence of vomitus in the upper airway at the time of tracheal intubation in the hospital; vomitus was present in the pharynx in 17% of the OOA group and 34% of the oral airway and mask group. In 56% of the patients in whom vomitus was present in the OOA group however, the material had already been noted in the pharynx *before* insertion of the OOA. It was concluded that the single advantage of the OOA over mask and airway was a reduction in the frequency of aspiration [145].

The place of the OOA in failed tracheal intubation in hospital practice is less certain. The OOA may be used in an attempt to minimize the risk of aspiration in an emergency if it is decided that the operation should not be cancelled. Most of such cases however can be

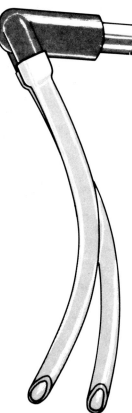

Fig. 51 Binasal pharyngeal airway assembly. Two Rusch nasopharyngeal tubes are attached to a Puritan rubber adaptor. Redrawn from Elam et al [150], with kind permission of the International Anaesthesia Research Society.

successfully intubated with specialized techniques.

Nasopharyngeal airways

Nasopharyngeal airways have been used in anaesthetic practice for many years. A binasal pharyngeal airway (BNPA) was described by Elam and his colleagues in 1969 [150, 151]. It consisted of two soft nasopharyngeal tubes connected to a suitable adaptor (Fig. 51). The BNPA was used both for elective surgery and for resuscitation in patients ranging in age from 2 to 92 years. Gastric dilatation was unlikely to occur with the BNPA because excess pressure could be vented through the mouth. The apparatus however should not be used in a patient with a full stomach. It was specifically recommended for patients in whom intubation was impossible or difficult and in the absence of personnel skilled at intubation.

The pharyngeal tracheal lumen airway (PTL)

This was designed as an alternative to the oesophageal obturator airway with the oesophageal tube functioning as a tracheal tube during accidental tracheal intubation [152]. It consisted of long and short tracheal tubes with a 150–200 ml proximal oropharyngeal cuff and a 30 ml distal cuff (Fig. 52). A preliminary study on 10 patients showed that effective ventilation could be maintained through the device. An advantage over the OOA is that the operator's second hand is free and is not required to maintain a seal with a face mask.

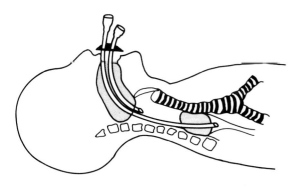

Fig. 52 The pharyngeal tracheal lumen airway in situ showing oral and oesophageal cuff. From Hooks et al [152], with kind permission of the International Anaesthesia Research Society.

The laryngeal mask

This consists of a shallow mask with an inflatable rubber cuff joined to a tube which connects with the lumen of the mask [153] (Fig. 53). The device is inserted facing backwards and rotated through 180 degrees as it is passed

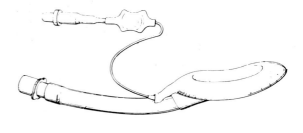

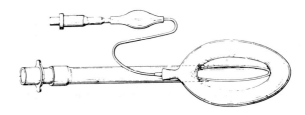

Fig. 53 Prototype of the laryngeal mask. From Brain [153].

downwards towards the larynx. The cuff is inflated when the mask is in place. The position of the mask is adjusted in patients in whom a good seal was not obtained. It offers an alternative both to tracheal intubation and the face mask and is considered valuable in cases of difficult intubation.

Oral, nasal anti-vomiting, anti-aspirating gastric tube (ONAT)*

This device protects the patient with a full stomach prior to intubation or when tracheal intubation is not possible. It consists of a three lumen tube that is passed into the stomach (Fig. 54). One lumen is used for suction to deflate the stomach, one to inflate a balloon which prevents regurgitation and another tube equalizes gastric and atmospheric pressure. This device is

---

*Rockway Enterprises, PO Box 8, St George, ME 04857, USA.

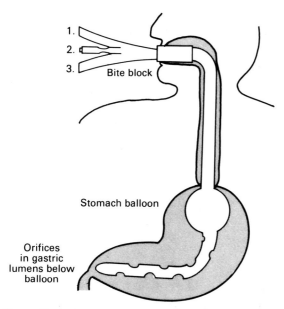

Fig. 54 The oral, nasal, anti-vomiting, anti-aspirating gastric tube (ONAT). A three lumen tube. 1 equalizes atmospheric and gastric pressure, 2 for balloon inflation with sterile water and 3 for suction.

compatible with tracheal tubes and could be particularly valuable in a patient with a full stomach in whom a difficult intubation is anticipated.

This device is used as an adjunct to the more conventional measures taken to protect the patient and minimizes the risk of aspiration in the presence of a full stomach. These may include drugs to speed gastric emptying and increase the gastro-oesophageal barrier pressure, preoxygenation, cricoid pressure and rapid sequence induction of anaesthesia.

CONCLUSION

It is important for every clinician to have a clear plan of action when dealing with a difficult or failed intubation. There is no easy totally risk free solution for every case. The risks to the patient should be reduced to a minimum.

Formal training programmes are essential if trainees are to become competent in simple and more complex techniques. Prospective comparison of different techniques to facilitate difficult intubation would be valuable in reaching rational decisions about choice of technique, although the design of studies is difficult due to the low incidence of difficult intubation. At present clinicians may have a real problem in choosing an appropriate technique from the many described in the literature. Clinicians who have a limited range of expertise may find that, if a simple technique fails, they are unable to intubate the patient. Changes in clinical practice are required to increase patient safety.

REFERENCES

1 Sia RL & Edens ET (1981) How to avoid problems when using the fiberoptic bronchoscope for difficult intubations. *Anaesthesia* 36: 74.

2 Aro L, Takki S & Aromaa U (1974) Technique for difficult intubation. *Br J Anaesth* 43: 1081.

3 Tunstall ME (1976) Failed intubation drill. *Anaesthesia* 31: 850.

4 Allen CTB (1976) Apparatus for emergency intubation in laryngeal obstruction. *Anaesthesia* 31: 263.

5 James W & Latto IP (1982) Retrospective Intubation Survey. Unpublished data Presented to Welsh Society of Anaesthetists.

6 Layman PR (1983) An alternative to blind nasal intubation. *Anaesthesia* 38: 165.

7 Kemthorne PM & Brown TCK (1983) Anaesthesia and the mucopolysaccharidoses: A survey of techniques and problems. *Anaesth Intensive Care* 11: 203.

8 Pollard BJ & Junius F (1980) Accidental intubation of the oesophagus. *Anaesth Intensive Care* 8: 183.

9 Howells TH & Riethmuller RJ (1980) Signs of endotracheal intubation. *Anaesthesia* 35: 984.

10 Cundy J (1981) Accidental intubation of the oesophagus. *Anaesth Intensive Care* 9: 76.

11 Stirt JA (1982) Endotracheal tube misplacement *Anaesth Intensive Care* 10: 274.

12 Chander S & Feldman E (1979) Correct placement of endotracheal tubes. *NY State J Med* 79: 1843.

13 Warden JC (1980) Accidental intubation of the oesophagus and preoxygenation. *Anaesth Intensive Care* 8: 377.

14 Ionescu T (1981) Signs of endotracheal intubation. *Anaesthesia* 36: 422.

15 Murray IP & Modell JH (1983) Early detection of endotracheal tube accidents by monitoring carbon dioxide concentration in respiratory gas. *Anesthesiology* 59: 344.

16 Linko K, Paloheimo M & Tammisto T (1983) Capnography for detection of accidental oesophageal intubation. *Acta Anaesthesiol Scand* 27: 199.

17 Utting JR, Gray TC & Shelley FC (1979) Human misadventure in Anaesthesia. *Can Anaesth Soc J* 26: 472.

18 Jackson C (1913) The technique of insertion of intratracheal insufflation tubes. *Surg Gynecol Obstet* 17: 507.

19 Sellick BA (1961) Cricoid pressure to control regurgitation of stomach contents during induction of anaesthesia. *Lancet* ii: 404.

20 Sellick BA (1982) Rupture of the oesophagus following cricoid pressure? *Anaesthesia* 37: 213.

21 Rosen M (1981) Deaths in obstetric anaesthesia (editorial). *Anaesthesia* 36: 145.

22 Crawford JS (1982) The 'contra cricoid' cuboid aid to tracheal intubation. *Anaesthesia* 37: 345.

23 Millen JE & Glauser FL (1978) A rapid simple technic for changing endotracheal tubes. *Anesth Analg* 57: 735.

24 Finucane BT & Kupshik HL (1978) A flexible stilette for replacing damaged tracheal tubes. *Can Anaesth Soc J* 25: 153.

25 Williams JH (1973) A method of changing tracheostomy tubes in small children. *Anaesthesia* 28: 343.

26 Rowbotham S (1920) Intratracheal anaesthesia by the nasal route for operations on the mouth and lips. *Br Med J* 2: 590.

27 Caine CW (1948) Endotracheal intubation. *Anesthesiology* 9: 553.

28 Ballantine RIW & Jackson I (1954) Anaesthesia for neurosurgical operations. *Anaesthesia* 9: 4.

29 Cass NM, James NR & Lines V (1956) Difficult direct laryngoscopy complicating intubation for anaesthesia. *Br Med J* ii: 488.

30 Bowen RA (1967) An introducer for difficult intubation. *Anaesthesia* 22: 150.

31 Edge WG & Whitman JG (1981) Chondro-calcinosis and difficult intubation in acromegaly. *Anaesthesia* 36: 677.

32 Henderson JB, Bontrager E & Morse HT (1970) An articulated stylet for endotracheal intubation. *Anesthesiology* 32: 71.

33 Salem MR, Mathrubhutham M & Bennett J (1976) Difficult intubation. *N Engl J Med* 295: 879.

34 Macintosh RR (1949) An aid to oral intubation. *Br Med J* 1: 28.

35 Cormack RS & Lehane J (1983) Simulating difficult intubation. *Br J Anaesth* 55: 1155p.

36 Macintosh RR (1943) A new laryngoscope. *Lancet* i: 205.

37 Magill IW (1926) An improved laryngoscope for anaesthetists. *Lancet* i: 500.

38 Miller RA (1941) A new laryngoscope. *Anesthesiology* 2: 317.

39 Lewis JJ (1975) Autoclavable Macintosh laryngoscope with high intensity fibreoptic illumination for routine anaesthesia use. *Anesthesiology* 43: 573.

40 Greenblatt GM (1981) Fiberoptic illuminating laryngoscope with remote light source—further development. *Anesth Analg* 60: 841.

41 Lagade MR (1983) Use of the Left-Entry laryngoscope blade in patients with right-sided oro-facial lesions. *Anesthesiology* 58: 300.

42 Datta S & Briwa J (1981) Modified laryngoscope for endotracheal intubation of obese patients. *Anesth Analg* 60: 120.

43 Galloon S (1973) The Toronto ventilating laryngoscope. *Br J Anaesth* 45: 912.

44 Lee ST (1972) A ventilating laryngoscope for inhalation anaesthesia and augmented ventilation during laryngoscopic procedures. *Br J Anaesth* 44: 874.

45 Rowbotham ES & Magill IW (1921) Anaesthetics in the plastic surgery of the face and jaws. *Proc R Soc Med* 14: 17.

46 Elder CK (1944) Naso-endotracheal intubation: advantages and technique of 'blind intubation'. *Anesthesiology* 5: 392.

47 Gold MI & Buechel DR (1960) A method of blind nasal intubation for the conscious patient. *Anesth Analg* 39: 257.

48 Pedersen B (1971) Blind nasotracheal intubation: A review and a new guided technique. *Acta Anaesthesiol Scand* 15: 107.

49 Sykes WS (1937) Oral endotracheal intubation without laryngoscopy: A plea for simplicity. *Anesth Analg* 16: 133.

50 Magill IW (1936) Endotracheal anaesthesia. *Am J Surg* 34: 450.

51 Lewis I (1937) Anaesthesia in general practice. Endotracheal anaesthesia. *Br Med J* 2: 630.

52 Chandra P (1966) Blind intubation. *Br J Anaesth* 38: 207.

53 Singh A (1966) Blind nasal intubation. *Anaesthesia* 21: 400.

54 Davies JAH (1972) Blind nasal intubation with propanidid. *Br J Anaesth* 44: 528.

55 Wycoff CC (1959) Aspiration during induction of anesthesia: its prevention. *Anesth Analg* 38: 5.

56 Thomas JL (1969) Awake intubation. *Anaesthesia* 24: 28.

57 Salem JE (1967) Intubation of conscious patients with combat wounds of upper respiratory passageway in Vietnam. *Oral Surg* 24: 701.

58 Brodman E & Duncalf D (1981) Avoiding the trauma of nasotracheal intubation. *Anesth Analg* 60: 618.

59 Mackinnon AG & Harrison MJ (1979) Nasotracheal intubation: an atraumatic technique. *Anaesthesia* 34: 910.

60 Nolan RT (1969) Nasal intubation: an anatomical difficulty with Portex tubes. *Anaesthesia* 24: 447.

61 Tahir AH (1970) A simple manoeuvre to aid the passage of a nasotracheal tube into the oropharynx. *Br J Anaesth* 42: 631.

62 Yamamura H, Yamamoto T & Kamiyama M (1959) Device for blind nasal intubation. *Anesthesiology* 20: 221.

63 Schneiderman BI (1966) An aid for blind naso-endotracheal intubation. *Anesthesiology* 27: 93.

64 Findlay CW & Gissen AJ (1961) A guided nasotracheal method for insertion of an endotracheal tube. *Anesth Analg* 40: 640.

65 Dryden GE (1976) Use of a suction catheter to assist blind nasal intubation. *Anesthesiology* 45: 260.

66 Adams AL, Cane RD & Shapiro BA (1982) Tongue extension as an aid to blind nasal intubation. *Crit Care Med* 10: 335.

67 Waters DJ (1963) Guided blind endotracheal intubation. *Anaesthesia* 18: 158.

68 Singh A (1966) Blind nasal intubation A report of the use of a hook in three cases of ankylosis of the jaw. *Anaesthesia* 21: 400.

69 Ducrow M (1973) Throwing light on blind intubation. *Anaesthesia* 33: 827.

70 Rayburn RL (1979) Light wand intubation. *Anaesthesia* 34: 667.

71 Foster CA (1977) An aid to blind nasal intubation in children. *Anaesthesia* 32: 1038.

72 Siker ES (1956) A mirror laryngoscope. *Anesthesiology* 17: 38.

73 Huffman JP & Elam JO (1971) Laryngoscopy. *Anesth Analg* 50: 64.

74 Huffman JP (1968) The application of prisms to curved

laryngoscopes: a preliminary study. *J Am Assoc Nurs Anesth* 36: 138.

75 Huffman JP (1970) The development of optical prism instruments to view and study the human larynx. *J Am Assoc Nurs Anesth* 38: 197.

76 Bearman AJ (1962) Device for nasotracheal intubation. *Anesthesiology* 23: 130.

77 Munson ES & Cullen SC (1965) Endotracheal intubation in a patient with ankylosing spondylitis of the cervical spine. *Anesthesiology* 26: 365.

78 Mirakhur RK (1972) Technique for difficult intubation. *Br J Anaesth* 44: 632.

79 Butler FS & Cirillo AA (1960) Retrograde tracheal intubation. *Anesth Analg* 39: 333.

80 Harmer M & Vaughan RS (1980) Guided blind oral intubation. *Anaesthesia* 35: 921.

81 Akinyemi OO (1979) Complications of guided blind endotracheal intubation. *Anaesthesia* 34: 590.

82 Dhara SS (1980) Guided blind endotracheal intubation. *Anaesthesia* 35: 81.

83 Bourke D & Levesque PR (1974) Modification of retrograde guide for endotracheal intubation. *Anesth Analg* 53: 1013.

84 Powell WF & Ozdil T (1967) A translaryngeal guide for tracheal intubation. *Anesth Analg* 46: 231.

85 Graham WP & Kilgore ES (1975) Endotracheal intubation in complicated cases. *Hospital Physician* 3: 60.

86 Roberts KW (1981) New use for Swan-Ganz introducer wire. *Anesth Analg* 60: 67.

87 Borland LM, Swan DM & Leff S (1981) Difficult pediatric intubation: a new approach to the retrograde technique. *Anesthesiology* 55: 577.

88 Ideka S (1968) The flexible bronchofiberoscope. *Keio J Med* 17: 1.

89 Sackner MA, Wanner A & Landa J (1972) Applications of bronchofiberscopy. *Chest* 62: 70S.

90 Editorial (1979) Hazards of fibreoptic bronchoscopy. *Br Med J* 1: 212.

91 Dubrawsky C, Awe RJ & Jenkins DE (1975) The effect of bronchofiberscopic examination on oxygenation status. *Chest* 67: 137.

92 Britton, RM & Nelson KG (1974) Improper oxygenation during bronchofiberoscopy. *Anesthesiology* 40: 87.

93 Albertini R, Harrel JH & Moser KM (1974) Hypoxemia during fiberoptic bronchoscopy. *Chest* 65: 117.

94 Murphy P (1967) A fibreoptic endoscope used for nasal intubation. *Anaesthesia* 22: 489.

95 Taylor PA & Towey RM (1972) The broncho-fiberscope as an aid to endotracheal intubation. *Anaesthesia* 44: 611.

96 Conyers AB, Wallace DH & Mulder DS (1972) Use of the fiberoptic bronchoscope for nasotracheal intubation. *Can Anaesth Soc J* 19: 654.

97 Tahir AH (1972) The bronchofiberscope as an aid to endotracheal intubation. *Br J Anaesth* 44: 1118.

98 Davidson TM, Bone RC & Nahum AM (1975) Endotracheal intubation with the flexible fiberoptic bronchoscope. *Eye Ear Nose Throat* 54: 346.

99 Mulder DS, Wallace DH & Woolhouse FM (1975) The use of the fibreoptic bronchoscope to facilitate endo - tracheal intubation following head and neck trauma *Trauma* 15: 638.

100 Messeter KH & Pettersson KI (1980) Endotracheal intubation with the flexible fiberoptic bronchoscope. *Anaesthesia* 35: 294.

101 Aps C & Towey RM (1981) Experiences with fibre-optic bronchoscopic positioning of single-lumen endobronchial tubes. *Anaesthesia* 36: 415.

102 Vredevoe LA (1981) New techniques for fiberoptic intubation and laryngeal examination. *Anaesth Analg* 60: 617.

103 Stiles CM, Stiles QR & Denson JS (1972) A flexible fiber optic laryngoscope. *JAMA* 221: 1246.

104 Davis NJ (1973) A new fiberoptic laryngoscope for nasal intubation. *Anesth Analg* 52: 807.

105 Raj PP, Forestner J, Watson TD, Morris RE & Jenkins MT (1974) Techniques for fiberoptic laryngoscopy in anaesthesia. *Anesth Analg* 53: 708.

106 Dennison PH (1978) Four experiences in intubation of one patient with Still's disease. *Br J Anaesth* 50: 636.

107 Davies JR (1978) The fiberoptic laryngoscope in the management of cut throat injuries. *Br J Anaesth* 50: 511.

108 Anderton JM (1978) The use of the flexible fiberoptic laryngoscope. *Br J Anaesth* 50: 1267.

109 Lloyd EEl (1980) Fiberoptic laryngoscopy for difficult intubation. *Anaesthesia* 35: 719.

110 Ovassapian A & Dykes MH (1982) Difficult pediatric intubation–an indication for the fiberoptic bronchoscope. *Anesthesiology* 56: 412.

111 Ovassapian A, Dykes MHM & Golman ME (1980) Fiberoptic nasotracheal intubation: a training program. *Anesthesiology* 54: S352.

112 Ovassapian A, Yelich S, Dykes MHM & Golman ME (1981) Fiberoptic nasotracheal intubation: Stepwise training versus traditional teaching. *Anesthesiology* 55: A347.

113 Ovassapian A, Yelich SJ, Dykes MHM & Golman ME (1983) A training programme for fiberoptic nasotracheal intubation. Use of model and live patients. *Anaesthesia* 38: 795.

114 Ovassapian A, Yelich SJ, Dykes MHM & Brunner EE (1983) Fiberoptic nasotracheal intubation—incidence and causes of failure. *Anesth Analg* 62: 692.

115 Patil V, Stehling LC, Zauder HL & Koch JP (1982) Mechanical aids for fiberoptic endoscopy. *Anesthesiology* 57: 69.

116 Hemmer D, Tai-Shoin L & Wright BD (1982) Intubation of a child with a cervical spinal injury with the aid of a fiberoptic bronchoscope. *Anaesth Intensive Care* X: 163.

117 Rucker RW, Silva WJ & Worcester CC (1979) Fiberoptic bronchoscopic nasotracheal intubation in children. *Chest* 76: 56.

118 Vauthy PA & Reddy R (1980) Acute upper airway obstruction in infants and children. Evaluation by the fiberoptic bronchoscope. *Ann Otologica* 89: 417.

119 Stiles CM (1974) A flexible fiberoptic bronchoscope for endotracheal intubation in infants. *Anesth Analg* 53: 1017.

120 Alferey DD, Ward CF, Harwood IR & Mannino FL (1979) Airway management for a neonate with congenital fusion of the jaws. *Anesthesiology* 51: 340.

121 Davidson AJ, Reynolds AC & Stewart ET (1981) Use of a flexible radiopaque directable catheter for difficult tracheal intubation. *Anesthesiology* 55: 605.

122 Jacoby JJ, Hemelberg W, Reed JP & Gillespie B (1951) A simple method of artificial respiration (demonstration). *Am J Physiol* 167: 798.

123 Spoerel WE, Narayanan PS & Singh NP (1971) Transtracheal ventilation. *Br J Anaesth* 43: 932.

124 Jacobs HB (1972) Needle-catheter brings oxygen to the trachea. *JAMA* 222: 1231.

125 Smith RB (1973) Transtracheal ventilation during anesthesia. *Anesth Analg* 53: 225.

126 Chakravarty K, Narayanan PS & Spoerel WE (1973) Further studies on transtracheal ventilation: the influence of upper airway obstruction on the patterns of pressure and volume. *Br J Anaesth* 45: 733.

127 Smith RB, Myers EN & Sherman H (1974) Transtracheal ventilation in paediatric patients. *Br J Anaesth* 46: 313.

128 Attia RR, Battit GE & Murphy JD (1975) Transtracheal ventilation. *JAMA* 234: 1152.

129 Smith RB, Schaer WB & Pfaeffle H (1975) Percutaneous transtracheal ventilation for anaesthesia and resuscitation: a review and report of complications. *Can Anaesth Soc J* 22: 607.

130 Carden E, Becker G & Hamood H (1977) An improved percutaneous jetting system for use during microlaryngeal operations. *Can Anaesth Soc J* 24: 118.

131 Layman PR (1983) Transtracheal ventilation in oral surgery *Ann R Coll Surg Engl* 65: 318.

132 Report on Confidential Enquiry into Maternal Deaths in England and Wales 1973–75 (1979) HMSO, London.

133 Atkinson RS, Rushman GB & Lee JA (1977) *A Synopsis of Anaesthesia*. 8th edn, p. 856. John Wright, Bristol.

134 Lee TH (1978) Needle tracheostomy for acute upper airway obstruction. *Br Med J* 1: 281.

135 Clarke SW & Cochrane GM (1975) Emergency tracheostomy. *Practitioner* 215: 340.

136 Stinson TW (1977) A simple connector for transtracheal ventilation. *Anesthesiology* 47: 232.

137 Hilton PJ (1982) A simple connector for cricothyroid cannulation. *Anaesthesia* 37: 220.

138 DeLisser EA & Muravchick S (1981) Emergency transtracheal ventilation. *Anesthesiology* 55: 607.

139 *Mortality Statistics England and Wales 1974* (1977) Office of Population Censuses and Surveys London. HMSO, London.

140 Rogers SN & Benumof JL (1983) New and Easy techniques for fiberoptic endoscopy—aided tracheal intubation. *Anesthesiology* 59: 569.

141 Williams RT & Maltabey JR (1982) Airway intubator. *Anesth Analg* 61: 309.

142 Cobb IA, Alvarez H & Medic I (1973) In: *Proceedings of Third Conference on National Standard for Emergency Care*, pp. 179–182. American Heart Association, New York.

143 Don Michael TA, Lambert EH & Mehran A (1968) Mouth to lung airway for cardiac resuscitation. *Lancet* ii: 1329.

144 Don Michael TA & Gordon AS (1980) The oesophageal obturator airway: a new device in emergency cardiopulmonary resuscitation. *Br Med J* 281: 1531.

145 Donen M, Tweed WA, Dashfsky S & Guttormson B (1983) The esophageal obturator airway: An appraisal. *Can Anaesth Soc J* 30: 194.

146 Tweed WA, Bristow G & Donen N (1980) Resuscitation from cardiac arrest: assessment of a system providing only basic life support outside of hospital. *Can Med Ass J* 122: 297.

147 Williams JH (1979) The oesophageal airway. *Br Med J* ii: 798.

148 Hogan K, Harpur MH & Pollard BJ (1984) Use of a pharyngeal guide to aid intubation with the fibreoptic laryngoscope. *Anaesth Intensive Care* 12: 18.

149 Klain M, Keszler H & Stool S (1983) Transtracheal high frequency jet ventilation prevents aspiration. *Crit Care Med* 11: 170.

150 Elam JO, Titel JH, Feingold A, Weisman H & Bauer R (1969) Simplified airway management during anaesthesia or resuscitation: a binasal pharyngeal system. *Anesth Analg* 48: 307.

151 Weisman H, Weis TW, Elam JO, Bethune RM & Bauer R (1969) Use of double nasopharyngeal airways in anaesthesia. *Anesth Analg* 48: 356.

152 Hooks PJ, Scarberry EH & Bryan-Brown CW (1984) The pharyngeal tracheal lumen (PTL) airway: a one handed emergency resuscitation tube. *Anesth Analg* 63: 229.

153 Brain AIJ (1983) The laryngeal mask—a new concept in airway management. *Br J Anaesth* 55: 801.

154 Cormack RS & Lehane J (1984) Difficult tracheal intubation in obstetrics. *Anaesthesia* 39: 1105.

155 Ford RWJ (1983) Confirming tracheal intubation in a simple manoeuvre. *Can Anaesth Soc J* 30: 191.

156 Eastley R, Latto IP, Ng WS, Vaughan RS, James W & Draper M (1984) Prospective survey of incidence causes and management of difficult intubation in 1200 patients (unpublished data).

157 Wilson RF, Steiger Z, Jacobs J, Sison OS & Holsey C (1984) Temporary partial cardiopulmonary bypass during emergency operative management of near total tracheal obstruction. *Anesthesiology* 61: 103.

158 Maharaj RJ, Whitton I & Blyth D (1983) Emergency extracorporeal oxygenation for an intratracheal foreign body. *Anaesthesia* 38: 471.

159 Grillo HC (1979) Surgical treatment of postintubation injuries. *J Thorac Cardiovasc Surg* 78: 860.

160 Neville W (1969) Discussion of Grillo HC. *J Thorac Cardiovasc Surg* 57: 52.

161 McLean (1982) Guided blind oral intubation. *Anaesthesia* 37: 605.

CHAPTER 8 Case reports

Plans should be prepared for dealing efficiently with cases of difficult intubation. Even so in some cases problems develop quickly and unexpectedly and the clinician may have to modify the plan and deal with the situation to the best of his ability. These cases illustrate difficulties in maintaining the airway or in inserting a tracheal tube which have been managed in a practical manner.

A major airway problem during anaesthesia with a facemask requiring a fibreoptic intubation

Examination and assessment

A 48-year-old man was admitted to hospital for removal of bladder stones by the transurethral approach. The patient had multiple skeletal abnormalities and those of particular relevance to the anaesthetist were a short neck and marked upper dorsal kyphoscoliosis (Fig. 1). A chest X-ray showed a number of hemivertebrae in the upper dorsal region causing kyphoscoliosis; while in the neck there was fusion of C1/2, C3/4 and C4/5. There was a functioning joint at C2/3, C5/6 and C6/7. On examination it was clear that he had very limited neck extension. Jaw opening was also limited. In addition, he was hypertensive and when seen by an anaesthetic registrar his blood pressure was 205/115 mmHg. He also had an aortic systolic murmur. Treatment was instituted and the surgery postponed.

Method chosen

The patient, one of many presenting on a busy urology list, was first seen by a consultant anaesthetist on the day before surgery. He was premedicated with atropine (0.6 mg) and pethidine (50 mg) and also given 500 mg of ampicillin 1 h preoperatively as a prophylactic measure. Oxygen was administered and an intravenous injection of 4 ml of althesin was followed by inhalation of nitrous oxide, oxygen and enflurane. After about 5 min sudden

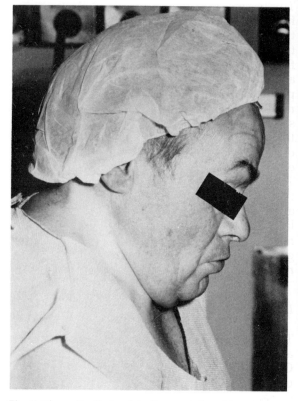

Fig. 1 The patient's head in the neutral position showing the short neck.

airway obstruction developed and he became markedly cyanosed. Attempts to inflate the chest were unsuccessful and insertion of an oral airway did not help. Suxamethonium (100 mg) was administered intravenously and careful attempts made to inflate the lungs with oxygen. Fasciculation was noted after about 2 min probably due to a prolonged circulation time. Oxygenation improved after development of muscle relaxation but the airway could only be maintained with great difficulty. Attempts to visualize the larynx and intubate the patient were unsuccessful due to limited mouth opening, a short neck and abnormal airway. Not even the epiglottis could be seen. The anaesthetic was discontinued and the operation deferred.

The patient was transferred to the University Hospital of Wales and the operation planned for the following day. It was decided to try a retrograde intubation and if this failed a fibreoptic intubation. A retrograde technique was attempted under local anaesthesia, but the Tuohy needle could not be placed properly; however a 16 gauge Venflon was inserted into the trachea. A nylon thread passed easily through the venflon but could not be delivered from the mouth. The retrograde attempt was abandoned and a fibreoptic technique employed. Local anaesthesia was instilled into the nose and pharynx and the bronchoscope inserted through the nostril and down through the larynx into the trachea. The larynx was deformed and oedematous and there was evidence of bleeding and clots in the trachea. The tracheal tube was then threaded down over the bronchoscope into the trachea. A balanced anaesthetic technique was used and the patient later extubated when awake. He was transferred to the high dependency unit and blood gases were monitored at regular intervals. He recovered without complications.

Discussion

This case clearly illustrates the danger of anaesthetizing such a patient with a mask. Critical airway problems developed quickly and unexpectedly. The patient's life was therefore threatened.

It is possible that a nasopharyngeal airway might have remedied the obstruction but this was not attempted. The use of suxamethonium was clearly not without risk but did enable manual ventilation to be accomplished with some improvement in oxygenation. Needle ventilation during the emergency would have been difficult.

In this patient with a fixed flexion neck deformity a retrograde technique was very difficult even under elective conditions and would have been impossible in an emergency. We were inexperienced with the retrograde technique at that time, but believe that the intubation would have been successful had an epidural catheter been threaded through the cannula. This case history shows the value of having available a clinician competent in the use of a fibreoptic bronchoscope.

An impossible intubation emergency presentation for a tracheostomy

Examination and assessment

A 37-year-old woman was admitted for exploration of a thyroglossal sinus. She first presented 6 months earlier with a submental mass which had become painful, red and swollen and had been drained twice by the general surgeons before referral to the ENT Department. On admission she was fit and there was no significant past medical history.

Method chosen

She had a general anaesthetic and tracheal intubation at 10 a.m. An ellipse of scar tissue was removed through a transverse skin incision and the thyroglossal cyst remnant was removed together with the central portion of the hyoid bone. The dissection extended almost to the base of the tongue. The wound was closed with a subcuticular stitch. She returned to the recovery room at 12 midday. She made an uneventful recovery and was returned to the ward at 1 p.m. At approximately 6 p.m. she complained of discomfort in the neck. At 8 p.m. she was given aspirin for neck pain and had prominent upper neck swelling and bruising. By 10 p.m. she complained of difficulty in swallowing and the swelling was more marked. It was decided that the wound should be explored.

When seen by the duty anaesthetist she had difficulty talking, was unable to swallow and dribbled blood-stained saliva. She complained of pain in the region of the surgical incision. There was swelling across the anterior aspect of the neck extending around up to the temporomandibular joints. She was distressed, sitting upright, and using her accessory respiratory muscles. She felt dizzy and her systolic blood pressure rose from 125 mmHg when she was sitting to 140 mmHg when she was supine.

She had very limited jaw movement and could only open her mouth about 2 cm. Her tongue was severely swollen and was pressed up against the roof of her mouth. A consultant anaesthetist was called.

In the anaesthetic room after venous cannulation, attachment of an electrocardiogram and preoxygenation, thiopentone (150 mg) was injected slowly intravenously. She was ventilated with 6 1/min oxygen with 1% halothane while remaining in a sitting position. Ventilation, although difficult, was initially adequate. She was lowered to the supine position and immediately developed a partial airway obstruction. Cyanosis and bradycardia developed. Cricothyroid puncture with a 14 G Medicut was attempted but due to swelling and anatomical distortion this was not successful. An ENT surgeon started to perform an emergency tracheostomy which proved very difficult but the airway was eventually restored with the insertion of a tracheostomy tube. Surgery proceeded, the bleeding point was found and a large clot evacuated. Laryngoscopy performed after tracheostomy and clot evacuation showed gross oedema of the floor of the mouth with the epiglottis pushed backward and the vocal cords could not be seen.

She made a good recovery and her tracheostomy was closed 5 days later. At that time indirect laryngoscopy showed some oedema in the supraglottic region, but the vocal cords were visible.

Discussion

The clinicians looking after this lady were not familiar with either fibreoptic or retrograde techniques. In any case due to the extreme urgency and blood in the pharynx, fibreoptic intubation would not have been easy. Due to swelling of the neck and anatomical distortion a retrograde technique would also have been extremely difficult. Indeed attempted needle ventilation and insertion of a cannula through the cricothyroid membrane into the trachea proved impossible. A tracheostomy under local anaesthesia might have been feasible but even under general anaesthesia this proved very difficult. The option chosen was hazardous: to preoxygenate and administer halothane in oxygen proceeding to tracheostomy as quickly as possible, although this seemed the most appropriate choice at the time.

Failed fibreoptic intubation: a spinal anaesthetic

Examination and assessment

A 22-year-old female with severe rheumatoid arthritis presented for total hip replacement surgery. She had a fixed flexion neck deformity (Fig. 2). The trachea was palpable for a distance of only 1 cm above the sternal notch; the mandible prevented access to the upper portion of the trachea and the cricothyroid membrane. Temporomandibular disease severely limited mouth opening.

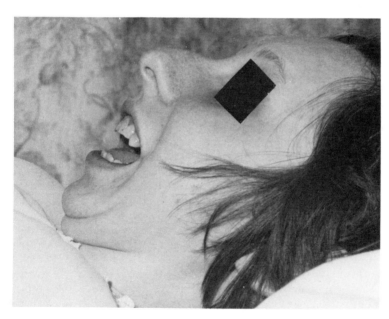

Fig. 2 Maximum mouth and neck extension.

Anaesthetic management

Preoperatively, the procedure was discussed in detail with the patient to allay anxiety and to gain the patient's cooperation. Premedication consisted of diazepam (10 mg orally) 2 h preoperatively and hyoscine (0.4 mg i.m.) 1 h preoperatively. An amethocaine lozenge (60 mg) was administered 30 min preoperatively. An 'awake' intubation was initially attempted using the fibreoptic bronchoscope. Sedation with diazemuls (5 mg i.v.) and fentanyl (50 μg) was administered slowly to prevent respiratory depression. A 21 s.w.g. 'Butterfly' needle was inserted through the anterior aspect of the trachea, above the sternal notch, with the patient in the supine position. Local anaesthetic was injected into the trachea. This produced a bout of violent coughing which spread the local anaesthetic agent towards the larynx. The chosen nasal cavity was sprayed with 4% lignocaine, after testing nasal patency.

A fibreoptic bronchoscope was then passed through the nose into the pharynx; utilizing the suction port to spray 4% topical lignocaine solution when necessary. Unfortunately, although the vocal cords could be visualized, the bronchoscope could not be introduced through them. The anaesthetist had performed 20 successful attempts at intubation using this technique 1 year previously.

The patient was then placed in the lateral position and a successful spinal anaesthetic was administered. The resultant block was unilateral possibly because of anatomical problems associated with the rheumatoid arthritis.

Discussion

Prolonged general anaesthesia administered by a mask should only be employed when all other methods have failed. Inadequate depth of anaesthesia could lead to laryngospasm; maintenance of the airway can be difficult and sometimes impossible; there is a risk of aspiration unless the patient can be placed in the lateral position with a Trendelenburg tilt. In the anaesthetized subject attempts at blind nasal intubation or fibreoptic instrumentation increase the risks of laryngospasm and vomiting.

Local anaesthetic techniques are preferable provided that they do not produce a situation which demands emergency intubation. Inadvertent total spinal blockage, associated with attempted epidural administration, favours the use of deliberate intrathecal injection with a dose of local anaesthetic agent appropriate for that route. Systemic toxicity associated with absorption of local anaesthetic agents must be avoided; a convulsive episode could be fatal in association with management of a difficult airway.

'Awake' intubation seemed a reasonable choice. Retrograde catheterization of the trachea would have been virtually impossible because of the inability to gain access to the cricothyroid membrane. Blind nasal intubation was considered but would have been impossible because of the fixed flexion deformity of the cervical vertebrae. The fibreoptic method failed possibly because of the acute angle between the pharynx and larynx.

The experience of the anaesthetist was limited to 20 cases which was probably inadequate to successfully manipulate the bronchoscope in the required direction as a 'one-off' procedure. Regular practice with routine cases is essential to enable successful intubation to be accomplished in the difficult case.

Anaesthesia with a facemask for Caesarean section: elective presentation

Examination and assessment

The patient had Still's disease and was confined to a wheelchair. She had previously undergone a hip operation at which attempts at fibreoptic intubation by a skilled anaesthetist failed (see previous case). A subsequent spinal anaesthetic gave rise to a unilateral block. She became pregnant, refused an abortion, and was referred to the obstetric unit at 20 weeks gestation.

She was 130 cm tall and weighed 60 kg. She had practically no movement at the neck, limited mouth opening, and fixed shoulders with only slight movements at the left elbow and both hands. There was no movement of the hips or knees. Her respiratory function showed restrictive airways disease with a peak flow rate of 120 l/min. It was decided that she would be delivered electively by Caesarean section at 36 weeks. She refused both local infiltration, and a repeat attempt at fibreoptic intubation. This was therefore a rare clinical situation and the options for the anaesthetist were limited. She had accepted an invitation to appear on national television in a programme related to her decision to go on with the pregnancy; it was proposed that her anaesthetic and elective section were filmed.

Method

Premedication was with atropine (0.6 mg i.m.), ranitidine (150 mg orally) 1 h preoperatively and magnesium trisilicate (30 ml) half an hour preoperatively. After 10 min, preoxygenation (in the semi-lateral position) she was induced with thiopentone (125 mg, given in 25 mg increments). Nitrous oxide 50% and additional carbon dioxide (10%) were inspired until ether was introduced after about 3 min when she was breathing smoothly. A well lubricated 32F latex nasopharyngeal tube was inserted and cricoid pressure was applied during induction. The Caesarean section was uneventful and there was no difficulty in maintaining a clear airway. Ergometrine (0.25 mg, i.v.) was administered after the delivery of the baby. Anaesthesia was maintained until the end of surgery and during recovery she was turned into a head down position on the left side, being postured with many pillows (this was practised preoperatively!) and oxygen administered. She awoke without nausea or vomiting, and was sitting up in her room within 1 h conversing with her husband and nursing their baby.

Discussion

This courageous mother realized the risks involved in continuing with the pregnancy. A previous attempt at an awake fibreoptic bronchoscopy had been unsuccessful and she was unwilling for this to be tried again. Spinal anaesthesia resulted in a unilateral block, possibly indicating unusual anatomy, and suggesting that epidural anaesthesia was also unlikely to be successful. She absolutely refused infiltration anaesthesia which would have been a reasonable and safe alternative. She was also unwilling for other attempts at awake intubation to be made. Intubation under general anaesthesia was considered either directly or by the retrograde route. The former would have

been difficult, and the latter was precluded by inadequate access to the cricothyroid membrane due to neck flexion. Therefore general anaesthesia without a tube seemed the only choice. The risk of aspiration was reduced by an H_2 antagonist and antacid therapy. The choice of inhalation anaesthetic was governed by previous wide experience with nitrous oxide and diethyl ether. It is important with this technique not to administer too much thiopentone or breathing during induction will be depressed. There is then great difficulty in introducing ether. Added carbon dioxide speeds up the induction. Cricoid pressure was maintained until diethyl ether induction was complete. No additional uterine haemorrhage occurred but if it had it would have been treated with syntocinon, lightening of the ether anaesthesia and administration of intravenous pethidine increments (5–10 mg). Halothane 1% would have been a reasonable substitute for an anaesthetist unfamiliar with ether.

The televised version was criticized by anaesthetists unfamiliar with diethyl ether because phonation was interpreted as respiratory obstruction. Postoperative vomiting did not occur and is only seen in a minority of mothers. However, anaesthesia should be maintained until surgery is complete, and the dressing applied to avoid vomiting in the semi-lateral position. Recovery should then be in the head down lateral position. It would be easier to conduct similar cases again, but without being filmed!

Elective use of the retrograde intubation technique

Examination and assessment

A 40-year-old man was scheduled for a hip joint replacement. The upper third of the femoral shaft also needed resection and replacement with a modified long stem prosthesis. The patient had 'burnt out' Still's disease and severe ankylosing spondylitis.

On examination he was able to open his mouth only 2 cm due to temporomandibular joint involvement (Fig. 3). He also had a deviated nasal septum with bilateral nasal polypi. There was severe limitation of neck extension. There were no other major problems.

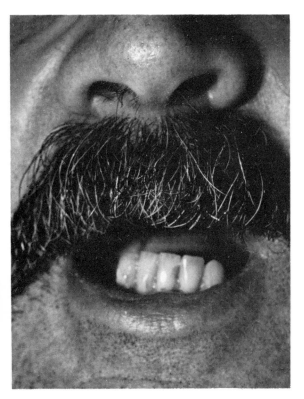

Fig. 3 Limited mouth opening.

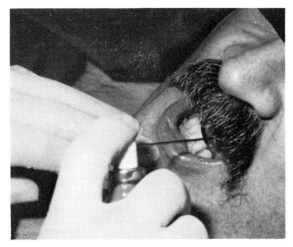

Fig. 4 Spraying buccal cavity.

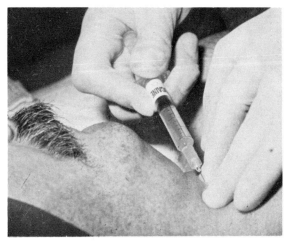

Fig. 5 The skin wheal over the cricothyroid membrane.

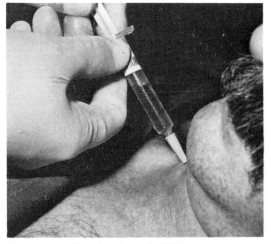

Fig. 6 Aspiration of air into a fluid filled syringe.

Method chosen

It was decided to use a modification of Water's retrograde technique (see p. 122). The patient was premedicated with 5 mg of diazepam orally 1 h preoperatively and given an amethocaine lozenge (60 mg) half an hour preoperatively. In the anaesthetic room the electrocardiogram was attached, the blood pressure measured and an intravenous cannula inserted. Fentanyl (100 μg) and droperidol (5.0 mg) were administered intravenously. The procedure was as follows:

1 The buccal cavity was sprayed with topical lignocaine (Fig. 4).

2 A skin wheal was raised over the cricothyroid region with 1% plain lignocaine and a small incision made in the skin (Fig. 5).

3 A 23 gauge needle was advanced through the cricothyroid membrane into the trachea (Fig. 6). Confirmation of correct needle position was confirmed by aspirating air into the syringe filled with saline. Four millilitres of 4% lignocaine were injected into the trachea at the end of expiration.

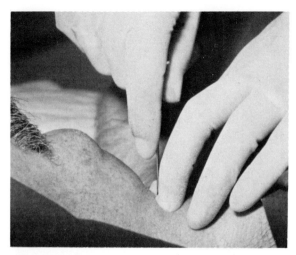

Fig. 7 Insertion of the Tuohy needle.

4 A 16 gauge Tuohy needle was advanced through the cricothyroid membrane into the trachea with the bevel pointing cephalad (Fig. 7).

5 The trocar was removed and an epidural catheter introduced through the needle (Fig. 8).

6 As the catheter entered the pharynx the patient was asked to spit it out and at least 20 cm pulled outside the mouth (Fig. 9).

7 The Tuohy needle was withdrawn. A sterile 16 gauge suction catheter, which had been stored in the freezing compartment of a refrigerator for 1 h, was then pushed over the epidural catheter from the mouth into the trachea (Fig. 10).

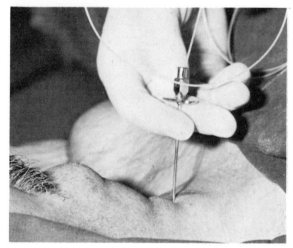

Fig. 8 Insertion of the epidural catheter.

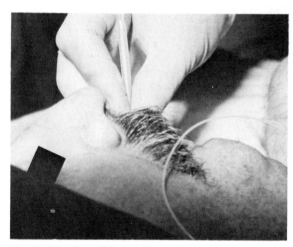

Fig. 10 Insertion of the suction catheter. Position checked by capnography.

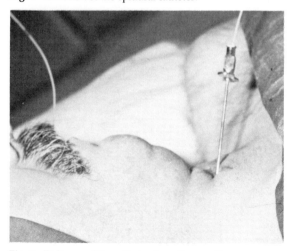

Fig. 9 Delivery of the catheter from the mouth.

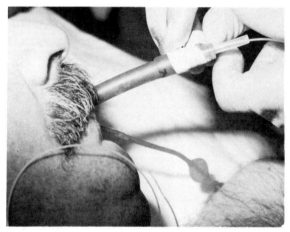

Fig. 11 Insertion of the tracheal tube. Position checked by capnography.

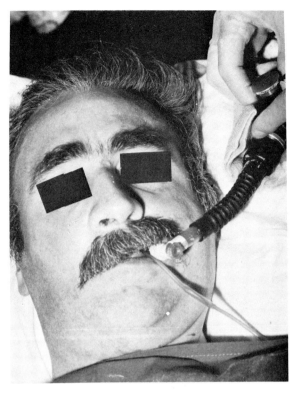

Fig. 12 Final tube position after removal of epidural and suction catheters. Position checked by capnography.

8 An armoured tracheal tube was then passed over the suction catheter into the trachea, gentle pressure being applied to the catheter to make it bend back towards the posterior pharyngeal wall (Fig. 11). This prevents the tip of the tracheal tube from catching onto the epiglottis. A capnograph confirmed tracheal placement of the tube.

9 The epidural catheter was cut off near the skin and pulled out from above. Simultaneously the suction catheter was pushed further into the trachea.

10 The tube was then guided further into the trachea. The suction catheter was removed and the tracheal tube connected to the anaesthetic circuit (Fig. 12). Placement was confirmed by auscultation and capnography.

A balanced anaesthetic technique was used. This enabled the patient to be easily awakened at the end of the procedure. With the patient awake and able to maintain his airway self extubation was allowed.

Discussion

Epidural or spinal block was impossible as the spine was completely ankylosed. Spontaneous respiration using a mask and a volatile agent were a last resort as there was no guarantee of maintaining a clear airway. A tracheostomy would have been extremely difficult due to the

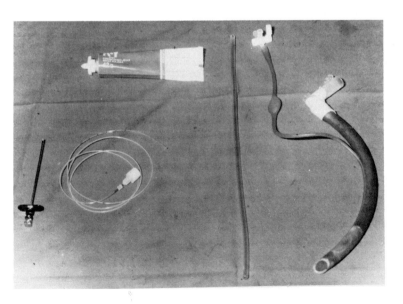

Fig. 13 The equipment required: tracheal tube, suction catheter, epidural catheter and Tuohy needle.

flexion deformity of the neck, and the patient was reluctant to agree to the procedure. The nasal route was impossible due to anatomical and pathological problems mentioned earlier. Fibreoptic intubation was possible but the apparatus was not available at that time in the hospital where surgery was planned.

We believe that such situations are not uncommon in hospitals, in developed and underdeveloped countries. The retrograde technique is ideal in such circumstances, had been used successfully several times before and the apparatus was readily available (Fig. 13).

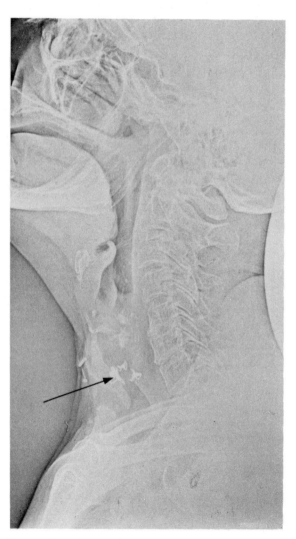

Fig. 14 Lateral xeroradiogram showing marked tracheal narrowing at the site of the stainless steel sutures.

Transtracheal ventilation in a case of tracheal stenosis

Examination and assessment

This patient was a 50-year-old woman who had been involved in a serious traffic accident some years earlier. Following this she required a prolonged period of intubation, initially with an oral tube but later she had a tracheostomy. She had developed tracheal fibrosis and stenosis at the site of the cuff. Following recovery she underwent resection of the stenosed portion of the trachea and the tracheal ends were sutured using stainless steel wire. She made an uneventful recovery.

Later she developed further tracheal narrowing at the site of the resection due to granuloma formation. The patient presented for endoscopic removal of the stainless steel wires and curetting of the granuloma.

On clinical examination she was thin and very nervous. She had scars on her neck from past surgery. There was no cyanosis or stridor at rest but severe stridor on exertion. Her trachea was central though surrounded with scar tissue. Lateral and anteroposterior radiograph of the neck showed the position of the wires but did not clearly demonstrate the area of stenosis. A xeroradiogram showed marked narrowing at the site of the anastomosis (Fig. 14). The tracheal diameter at the site of the stricture was approximately 5 mm. At indirect laryngoscopy the larynx was easily visualized and there were bilateral cord movements.

Method employed

Lorazepam (2 mg) was administered on the evening prior to and 2 h preoperatively. An intravenous cannula was inserted into a forearm vein and the patient was positioned with the neck extended in a position similar to that employed for thyroid surgery. A skin wheal was raised over the lowest palpable part of the trachea using 1% lignocaine and the deeper tissues infiltrated with 1% lignocaine. A 14 g teflon intravenous cannula was carefully inserted through the skin weal and into the trachea below the site of the stenosis. The position of the cannula was confirmed by attaching it to a capnograph and it was then securely sutured in place.

With the patient breathing 100% oxygen, anaesthesia was induced with an infusion of etomidate and a bolus dose of 0.3 mg fentanyl. When consciousness was lost the tracheal cannula was connected to oxygen at 60 lb/in^2 and the lungs intermittently inflated. When it was clear that the lungs could be easily inflated pancuronium (5 mg) was administered. In order to allow adequate expiration an I:E ratio of approximately 1:4 was employed. To ensure expired gas could freely flow out, an oropharyngeal airway was inserted until an operating endoscope was in position.

Anaesthesia was maintained throughout the procedure with a continuous infusion of etomidate with supplements of fentanyl. At the end of the procedure residual neuromuscular blockade was antagonized with atropine and neostigmine. Transtracheal ventilation was stopped when adequate spontaneous ventilation returned. Cardiovascular monitoring showed no abnormality throughout the procedure. On recovery of consciousness the tracheal cannula was removed and the patient made an uneventful recovery.

Discussion

Transtracheal ventilation seemed the optimum choice which would allow free access to the larynx and the area of surgery and avoid another tracheostomy. Alternative techniques were rejected. The patient was adamant that she did not want another tracheostomy. The tracheostomy site would have been very low and the procedure technically difficult due to scar tissue, and might result in further stenosis. The trachea was 5 mm in diameter at its narrowest portion so that a maximum size tube would have been only 2.5–3.0 mm in internal diameter, and would have disturbed access. A suction catheter could have been inserted past the stenosis and ventilation then effected with a high pressure inflation technique, but the catheter would have obstructed the surgery. Cardiopulmonary bypass would have been an option reserved as a last resort.

If transtracheal ventilation is used the technique must be meticulous. The cannula must be confirmed in position in the trachea and fixed securely in place. High pressure ventilation into the tissues can cause massive surgical emphysema making urgent tracheotomy difficult. It is essential to ensure free flow of gases during expiration, especially before and after surgery when an oro or nasopharyngeal airway should be inserted. During surgery it is important that blood is sucked clear before it clots and causes a restriction to expiration.

CHAPTER 9

Difficult and failed intubation in obstetrics

INTRODUCTION

In the triennial Confidential Enquiry into maternal deaths of 1975–78 [1], 30 cases were classified as avoidable and associated with anaesthesia. In 16 cases difficult tracheal intubation was the factor leading to death; in seven this difficulty was associated with inhalation of gastric contents. This is a mortality rate of about 1 per 6000 Caesarean sections. Probably therefore, some difficulty in intubation may be expected many times more often than death and a figure of 1 in 300 has been estimated for failed intubation at Caesarean section [2]. So preparation for such a problem must be made before every Caesarean section.

Preoperative examination will prepare the anaesthetist for obvious pathological or anatomical difficulties. In that case, the most skilled person available can be called and special equipment made immediately available. A detailed assessment may not always be possible, but even a brief examination of the patient before induction can warn the anaesthetist and enable him to prepare more adequately. However, many incidents of difficult intubation in obstetric patients will remain unanticipated. Laryngeal oedema secondary to pregnancy toxaemia is a possibility [3–7].

The priorities for the anaesthetist should be to maintain oxygenation, intermittently ventilating the patient so long as she is paralysed: to continue cricoid pressure; to avoid trauma (bleeding will make the situation even more serious); and to limit the duration of any periods of attempted intubation. An adequately trained assistant is essential.

EQUIPMENT

The basic equipment available at every anaesthetizing site should be:

1 Macintosh standard laryngoscopes (2) with large adult blades;

2 polio blade (blade at 135° to handle);
3 malleable stilette to place inside a tracheal tube;
4 gum elastic bougie or malleable stilette sufficiently long for 'railroad' technique;
5 tracheal tubes (5–8 mm);
6 soft (latex rubber) naso-pharyngeal tubes;
7 equipment for percutaneous tracheal ventilation (see p. 122).

PROBLEMS DURING INTUBATION

The difficulties during tracheal intubation are threefold; an inability to put the laryngoscope into the mouth, failure to visualize the vocal cords and failure to maintain ventilation during the process. Intubation should be limited to two attempts for 1 min each, separated by 30 s of ventilation.

The laryngoscope cannot be placed in the mouth

This may be a problem if the patient has large breasts and a short neck, or if her mouth will not open fully, or her neck is fixed in flexion. Each deformity or combination may cause this difficulty.

The laryngoscope blade should be separated from the handle, put into the mouth, and then re-attached to the handle. Sometimes only the polio or a similar blade is effective and should usually be used in the first instance.

The vocal cords cannot be visualized; or are only just in view; or only the tip of the epiglottis is visible

It is important to avoid trauma, and subsequent haemorrhage by gentle management of laryngoscopy. It is wise to time the events so as to ventilate the patient with 100% oxygen for about 30 s after each minute of trial intubation.

First, test the effects of manipulating the position of the head and check whether the cricoid pressure is correctly applied. Then try to intubate with a stylet inside the tracheal tube using a tube of smaller diameter than intended. If this fails, lubricate the whole length and flex the tip of a long malleable gum-elastic bougie into a J-shape. Gently pass the tip behind the epiglottis towards the vocal cords. When it is assumed to be in the trachea (it can often be felt by palpating the larynx and trachea externally), pass the tracheal tube into place on the outer surface of the stilette ('railroad') and remove the stilette. Compress the chest and feel whether the expiration is warm. Then inflate ausculating for air entry over the trachea, the apices of both lungs and over the epigastrium. If the patient cannot be intubated after 2 min, further attempts should be abandoned.

Difficulty in maintaining an airway

An oropharyngeal or nasopharyngeal airway may be required in this case. If that fails then percutaneous tracheal ventilation will be necessary, or even tracheostomy.

FAILED INTUBATION

It is essential to have a plan of action prepared if tracheal intubation is not possible.

If the operation can be postponed even temporarily the patient should be ventilated until spontaneous respiration returns, then turned into the semi-prone, head down position until she recovers. There are then the choices, additional to general anaesthesia, of regional block or local anaesthetic infiltration. There may also be time to find someone more skilled and who may also be trained to use a more sophisticated method of intubation such as fibreoptic bronchoscopy (p. 126).

In some emergency situations, such as major maternal haemorrhage or urgent fetal distress, it may be essential to continue with a general anaesthetic. In estimating the alternative risks it should be noted that before 1950, general anaesthetics for Caesarean section were mainly carried out without a tracheal tube. The resultant mortality is not known with certainty but was not more than a single percentage

figure (i.e. < 10%) and almost certainly much less. It is therefore statistically unlikely *in a specific case* that maintaining the airway without a tracheal tube should result in disaster or death. This observation is not intended to encourage complacency but to emphasize that whatever method of management is used for this uncommon emergency it should be within the capacity and experience of the anaesthetist rather than being an attempt at a 'perfect' theoretical approach. It is therefore an important safety measure that the anaesthetist should use a familiar technique.

Plan

1 Maintain the patient's position (semi-lateral to prevent aortocaval compression).
2 Ventilate if the patient is not breathing and maintain cricoid pressure (at least while artificial ventilation is being used).
3 Administer 50% nitrous oxide and 50% oxygen with 1% halothane or 2% enflurane or forane. When spontaneous respiration returns continue with that mixture (or increase the vapour concentration if necessary).
4 Commence the operation. If there is time, ask the surgeon to infiltrate the incision with 0.5% lignocaine (50–75 ml).
5 If in any doubt about the possibility of inducing vomiting (too light anaesthesia) do *not* pass a gastric tube. Do not pass a gastric tube if spontaneous respiration is returning until the patient is much more deeply anaesthetized— usually after the baby has been delivered. If paralysis is prolonged a gastric tube can be passed safely and the stomach emptied. Remove the gastric tube if it prevents the facemask making an airtight seal with the face even after partly deflating the cuff around the mask.
6 When the baby has been delivered, administer diluted pethidine (20 mg i.v.) over 1 min, repeated at 5 min intervals until the respiratory rate is reduced to 15–25 per min. The inspired concentration can then be lowered to halothane 0.5% or enflurane 1% or forane 1% which would reduce any effect on uterine contractility. At the same time the nitrous oxide concentration can be increased to 70%.
7 If there is still undue bleeding, after consulting the obstetrician, additional syntocinon (10 units) or ergometrine (0.25 mg) should be administered.

8 Anaesthesia is maintained until the operation is completed and the patient placed in the semi-prone, head down position.

This plan differs from another (Tunstall, 1976) in that:

a The patient is not initially turned into the lateral position, which may often be impractical and in which it is difficult to ventilate a patient.

b Cricoid pressure is continued, at least as long as the patient is ventilated.

c Gastric intubation is avoided if there is a possibility of inducing vomiting due to active reflexes.

d Halothane is used in preference to ether or methoxyflurane.

These are practical plans to deal with mortal situations in obstetrics. Various other emergency apparatus such as oesophageal intubation and gastric decompression have been used. None have been validated or tested by anaesthetists in training. They may be useful in an emergency if all else fails, but should not be 'first line' approaches at present.

ADDITIONAL METHODS

Deliberate oesophageal intubation with tracheal tube

The oesophagus is deliberately intubated, the cuff inflated and the open end of the tube placed at the corner of the mouth under the mask. This provides a pathway for gastric emptying spontaneously or after passing a nasogastric tube. Usually ventilation can be successfully accomplished [8], and cricoid pressure relieved [9]. The technique may be

made even more effective by preparing a face mask with a 15 mm male tracheal connector fixed in place at the lower part of the mask onto which a tracheal tube can be attached. This reduces leakage around the face mask.

Oesophageal gastric tube airway [11,12]

This tube, designed for cardiopulmonary resuscitation, has been used successfully for an obese patient having a Caesarean section in whom

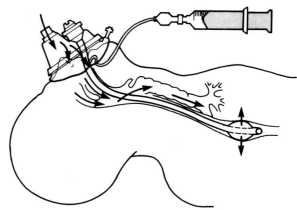

Fig. 1 The oesophageal gastric tube airway (EGTA). Inspired air reaches the pharynx via the nose and mouth and enters the larynx by flowing around the outside of the tube of the EGTA. The inside of the tube will accommodate the passage of a smaller lubricated tube for gastric aspiration.

intubation could not be performed and ventilation was difficult [13] (Fig. 1). This is an oesophageal tube which passes through a holder in a special face mask, through which gastric contents can pass or be aspirated. A cuff is inflated with 35 ml of air. The shape of the tube helps to push the larynx forward away from the posterior pharyngeal wall [13]. A flaccid or anaesthetized patient is essential for its use or it may lacerate the oesophagus or pass into the trachea.

REFERENCES

1 Department of Health and Social Security. Report on Confidential Enquiries into Maternal Deaths in England and Wales 1976–1978. HMSO, London.

2 Evans R & Cormack RS (1984) Difficult intubation. *Anaesthesia Points West* 17: 79.

3 Brocke-Utne JG, Downing AJW & Seedat I (1977) Laryngeal oedema associated with pre-eclamptic toxaemia. *Anaesthesia* 32: 556.

4 Mackenzie AI (1978) Laryngeal oedema complicating obstetric anaesthesia, three cases. *Anaesthesia* 33: 271.

5 Keeri-Szanto M. (1978) Laryngeal oedema complicating obstetric anaesthesia, yet another case. *Anaesthesia* 33: 272.

6 Jouppila R, Jouppila P & Hollmen A (1980) Laryngeal oedema as an obstetric anaesthesia complication. *Acta Anaesthesiol Scand* 24: 97.

7 Tillmann Hein HA (1984) Cardiorespiratory arrest with laryngeal oedema in pregnancy-induced hypertension. *Can Anaesth Soc J* 31: 210.

8 Cucchiari RF (1976) A simple technique to minimise tracheal aspiration. *Anaesth Analg* 55: 815.

9 Boys JE (1983) Failed intubation in obstetric anaesthesia. *Br J Anaesth* 55: 187.

10 Sivaneswaran N & McGuinness JJ (1984) Modified mask for failed intubation at emergency Caesarean section. *Anaesth Intensive Care* 12: 279.

11 Gordon AS (1983) Improved esophageal obturator airway (EOA) and new esophageal gastric tube (EGTA). In: Schtar P (ed) *Advances in Cardiopulmonary Resuscitation*, p. 58. Springer Verlag, New York.

12 Campbell WI (1983) Failed intubation in obstetric anaesthesia. *Br J Anaesth* 55: 1040.

13 Tunstall ME & Geddes C (1984) 'Failed Intubation' in obstetric anaesthesia: An indication for use of the 'Esophageal Gastric Tube Airway'. *Br J Anaesth* 56: 659.

CHAPTER 10

Endobronchial intubation

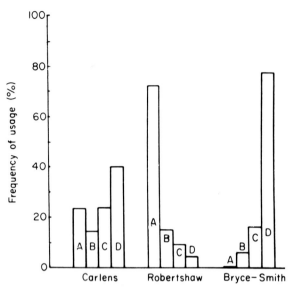

Fig. 1 The frequency of usage of double lumen endobronchial tubes. A: frequent (66–100%); B: sometimes (33–65%); C: rare (1–32%); D: never. From Pappin [3], with kind permission of the author and Academic Press, publishers of *Anaesthesia*.

The history and evolution of thoracic anaesthesia, and endobronchial intubation in particular, have been elegantly reviewed by White [1] and Rendell-Baker [2]. Both articles deal with various influences that eventually led to the development of present day skills, techniques and equipment.

The practice of endobronchial intubation in the United Kingdom was reviewed by Pappin in 1979 [3]. He showed that the use of double-lumen endobronchial tubes had increased over the last few years. In current practice, the most popular double-lumen tube was the Robertshaw [4] used by 72% of anaesthetists practising thoracic anaesthesia (Fig. 1).

The use of single lumen endobronchial tubes had, however, decreased over the same period. Indeed, 'the majority of anaesthetists never use single lumen endobronchial tubes' (Fig. 2). The most popular single lumen endobronchial tubes used were the Gordon Green [5] and the Brompton Pallister [6]. Furthermore, the use of these tubes was limited to cases in which there were secretions, a 'wet lung', or when a bronchopleural fistula was present. This decline

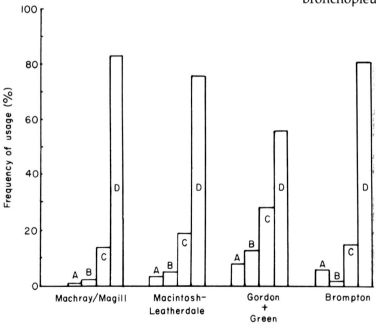

Fig. 2 The frequency of usage of single lumen endobronchial tubes. Key as for Fig. 1. From Pappin [3], with kind permission of the author and Academic Press, publishers of *Anaesthesia*.

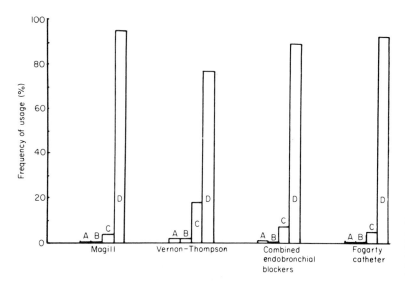

Fig. 3 The frequency of usage of endobronchial blockers. Key as for Fig. 1. From Pappin [3], with kind permission of the author and Academic Press, publishers of *Anaesthesia*.

in use has been associated with improved living conditions for the population and the considerable advances made in antibiotic therapy with a resultant decline in the incidence of tuberculosis. These factors have also contributed to a much improved preoperative condition of the cases for pulmonary surgery.

Bronchial blockers are 'rarely to never' used (Fig. 3). The Magill [7] blocker was no longer in use while the Vernon-Thompson [8] was only occasionally required. The main indication for a blocker was for teaching purposes. The Fogarty catheter [9], occasionally used in children, is not used in adult patients.

Naturally, hand-in-hand with the decline in use of blockers has been the decline in the use of intubating bronchoscopes. The uses of the Magill [10], and the modification described by Mansfield [11], are rarely taught. The increasing use of fibreoptic instruments makes it possible that they will replace the intubating bronchoscopes which may well disappear from the armamentarium of the thoracic anaesthetist.

Thus, endobronchial intubation in advanced countries is achieved as follows:
1 in the majority of cases with double lumen tubes;
2 in a small minority with single lumen tubes;
3 bronchus blockers are rarely used except in children.
Therefore, this review of endobronchial intubation concentrates on the indications for use, equipment available in current practice, the methods of intubation and possible complications.

INDICATIONS FOR DOUBLE LUMEN TUBES

No double lumen tubes are specifically designed for children. In adults, indications can be classified in conjunction with the surgical pathology.

Cardiac

1 Closure of patent ductus arteriosus;
2 repair of coarctation of the aorta;
3 resection of intrathoracic aneurysm;
4 closed mitral valvotomy;
5 pericardectomy;
6 insertion of cardiac pacemakers.

Pulmonary

1 Pulmonary resection;
2 pleurectomy;
3 pleuropneumonectomy [12];
4 surgical correction of unilateral pneumothorax;
5 surgery associated with the diaphragm.

Oesophageal

1 Repair of hiatus hernia;

2 repair of oesophageal pouches;
3 Heller's operation;
4 resection of tumours.

Others

1 Chest wall surgery;
2 gastric and hepatic surgery;
3 correction of vertebral column deformities.

In all these surgical conditions, the anaesthetist could use a tracheal tube but most anaesthetists and surgeons prefer the greater control of the lung and increased safety particularly in the presence of pus or a fistula.

EQUIPMENT

The available equipment includes endobronchial tubes and allied aids.

Endobronchial tubes

These are divided into double and single lumen tubes.

1. Double lumen tubes

There are a variety of tubes available which are usually named after the designer (e.g. Robertshaw [4]). Regardless of the type of tube, there are fundamental characteristics in design, common to all, which are illustrated in Fig. 4.

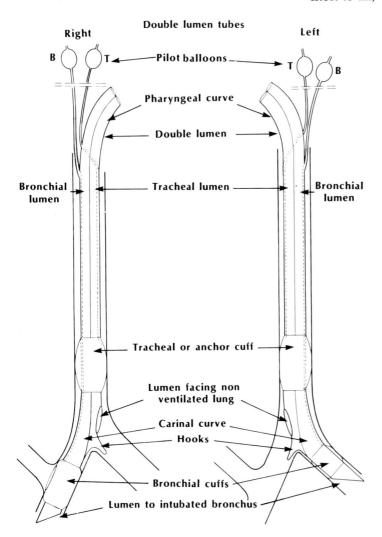

Fig. 4 Characteristics in design of double lumen endobronchial tubes.

Pilot balloons. There are two pilot balloons linked with the tracheal or bronchial cuffs. The linkage is either colour coded or the pilot balloon has a capital T (tracheal) or B (bronchial) marked on it. These balloons indicate that the cuffs are expanding but do not indicate the volume of gas required nor the resultant pressure necessary for an airtight fit. Excessive inflating pressure may cause rupture of the balloon or bronchus.

Curves. All double lumen tubes have two curves. The proximal curve is shaped to the pharynx and the distal curve is designed to assist entry into the appropriate bronchus.

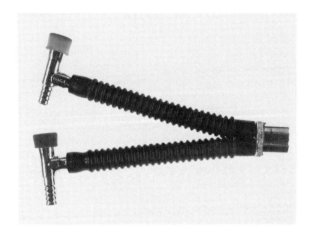

Fig. 5 Purpose designed catheter mount for double lumen tube.

Double lumen. Each lumen is hemispherical (D) in shape and can be separately connected to a purpose-designed catheter mount (Fig. 5). Each lumen can also be labelled as the tracheal or bronchial component of the double lumen tube (Fig. 6). The individual catheter mountings assist with the correct placing of the tube and allow both individual lung ventilation and suction as and when required.

Tracheal cuff. The tracheal cuff not only seals off the trachea but also acts as the 'anchor cuff' fixing the endobronchial tube in the trachea.

Lumen to non-intubated bronchus. This is nearly always placed 'blind'. Ideally it should completely face the bronchus to the lung which requires surgery.

Hooks. The first endobronchial double lumen tube, introduced by Carlens [13] for differential bronchospirometry, had a hook attached to it so that the tube would arrest at the carina. However, in the newer versions of endobronchial tubes, there are no hooks as they have caused difficulty with intubation and occasionally, considerable trauma.

Bronchial cuff. This cuff is inflated to attain an airtight seal in the appropriate main bronchus so that one lung ventilation can be maintained, if required, during surgery. Excessive inflating

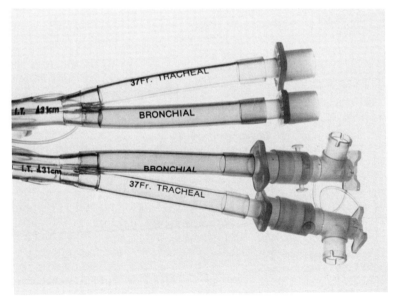

Fig. 6 Individual labelling of tracheal and bronchial components of two double lumen tubes.

pressure may rupture the cuff, damage the bronchus or cause the cuff to herniate and block the open end of the distal lumen.

Lumen in the intubated bronchus. This is the furthest point of the endobronchial tube and allows inflation of the isolated lung. This lung usually, but not always, is the lower lung during surgery and is known as the 'dependent lung'. In addition, the tip of the tube may sometimes have several perforations to allow ventilation if the distal lumen becomes obstructed [14] (Fig. 7).

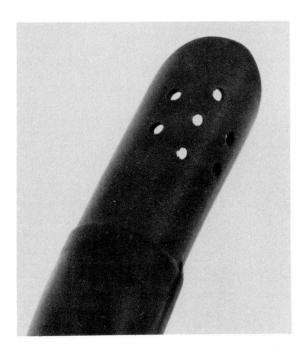

Fig. 7 Perforations at the distal end of an endobronchial tube.

Slit for the right upper lobe bronchus. The anatomy of the bronchi differ (chapter 1). The bronchus to the right upper lobe usually arises about 2.5 cm from the carina. It is essential that the position of this bronchus is noted initially at bronchoscopy. After right sided endobronchial intubation, the position of the slit relative to the bronchus is checked by auscultation over the right upper lobe.

2. Single lumen tubes

Although ordinary tracheal tubes can enter either the right or left main bronchus, they are not used as endobronchial tubes. Indeed, on the right side, they could be positively dangerous since there is no slit for the upper lobe orifice. The Machray tube [15] was designed for this purpose but is not now used. Some single lumen tubes are designed to be introduced blindly into the appropriate bronchus while others have a curve similar to a tracheal tube so that they may be placed over an intubating bronchoscope. There are fundamental characteristics in design regardless of the type of tube and they are illustrated in Fig. 8.

Pilot balloons. There are always a minimum of two balloons, one each for the tracheal and bronchial cuffs. Each is marked T or B as appropriate or is colour coded. However, with left sided tubes there is a 'spare' pilot balloon for the 'spare' cuff. This is underneath the bronchial cuff. This concept was originally introduced by Pallister [6] to contend with a sudden leak if the bronchial cuff was surgically damaged and collapsed during sleeve resection of the right upper lobe bronchus.

Single lumen. This lumen runs the length of the endobronchial tube and may vary in shape from above down.

Tracheal cuff. This is generally longer but otherwise similar to those seen on tracheal and double lumen endobronchial tubes.

Hooks. These were designed to fit over the carina but are usually removed (anaesthetic surgery!) or are no longer included in modern designs.

Bronchial cuff. This is usually shorter than the tracheal cuff and isolates the lung distal to the intubated bronchus. Single and double lumen right sided endobronchial tubes have similar cuffs with a special slit for the right upper lobe bronchus. Left sided tubes have two cuffs while some have perforated distal tips [14].

No double or single lumen tubes similar to adult tubes are available for children. In rare circumstances where an endobronchial tube is required, small tracheal tubes have been adapted for selective main bronchus intubation,

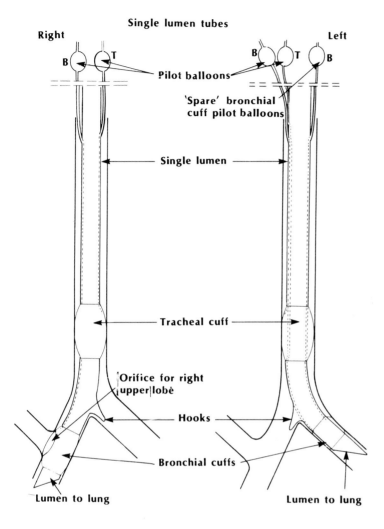

Fig. 8 Characteristics in design of single lumen endobronchial tubes.

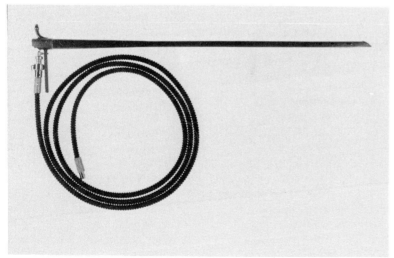

Fig. 9 Adult Negus bronchoscope with fibreoptic attachment.

placing them using X-ray, fibreoptic and auscultation methods [16].

Bronchoscopes

Three types of bronchoscopes are utilized by anaesthetists: the straight Negus, the intubating and fibreoptic varieties.

Negus and Storz bronchoscopes (diagnostic)

These are widely available for diagnostic purposes. The anaesthetist should use them to examine both trachea and main bronchi to see if there is an obstruction which would prevent endobronchial intubation. The position of the right upper lobe bronchus should also be identified when the right lung only is to be ventilated. The Negus bronchoscopes range from suckling to adult sizes (Fig. 9). Modern bronchoscopes, such as the Storz, utilize a fibreoptic light source and have quite excellent optics. Artificial ventilation can be performed with the Storz bronchoscope using the Sanders injector [17] (Fig. 10) or an adaptation of a standard breathing circuit (Fig. 11).

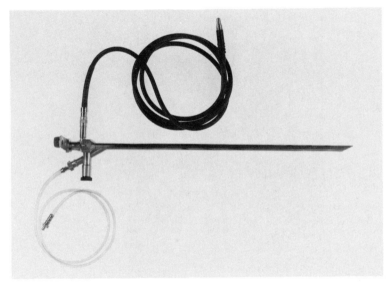

Fig. 10 Storz adult bronchoscope with Sanders injector attachment.

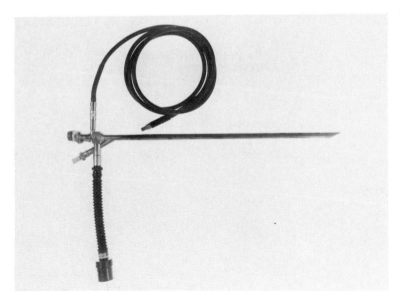

Fig. 11 Storz adult bronchoscope adapted to connect with a breathing circuit.

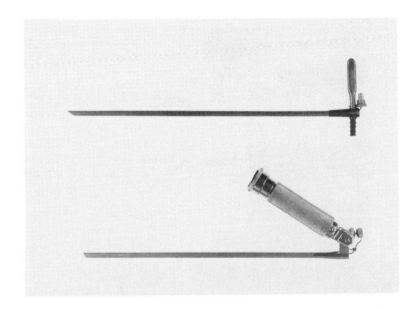

Fig. 12 Intubating bronchoscopes—
Mansfield above and Magill below.

Intubating bronchoscope

The Magill [10] (Fig. 12) intubating bronchoscope is used for endobronchial intubation with
single lumen tubes under direct vision. There
are two major differences compared with a
Negus or Storz bronchoscope:
1 The diameter is smaller than the diagnostic
bronchoscope and remains constant from end to
end.
2 The bevels of each bronchoscope are illustrated below (Fig. 13). The Mansfield [11] (Fig.
12) is used for the same purpose as the Magill
bronchoscope.

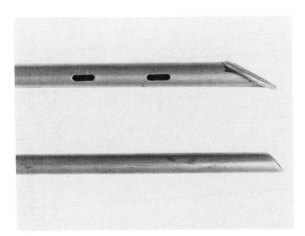

Fig. 13 Comparison of the end of a diagnostic bronchoscope (above) and an intubating bronchoscope (below).

Fibreoptic bronchoscope (Fig. 14)

These are increasingly used for diagnostic
purposes. A narrower external diameter, su-
perb optics, plus the ability easily to obtain a
suitable biopsy has made bronchoscopy under
local anaesthesia and sedation a very acceptable
technique. They are also used to facilitate
endobronchial intubation.

Endobronchial intubation

Before intubation is attempted, the anaesthetist
should perform a preliminary bronchoscopy
usually under general anaesthesia or occasionally using local analgesia. Bronchoscopy must be
practised before an anaesthetist can become an
expert. The following are instructions in this
skill.

The patient's neck is partially flexed. A rigid
bronchoscope is introduced into the mouth in
the midline or laterally through a suitable gap in
the teeth. A fibreoptic bronchoscope can also be
introduced through the nasal or oral route.

There are two possible approaches to the
laryngeal aperture:
1 The bronchoscope is passed over the tongue
until the tip of the epiglottis is seen. The
bronchoscope is then eased over the surface of
the epiglottis and the cords visualized.
2 The bronchoscope is 'dropped' onto the
posterior wall of the pharynx and moved slowly

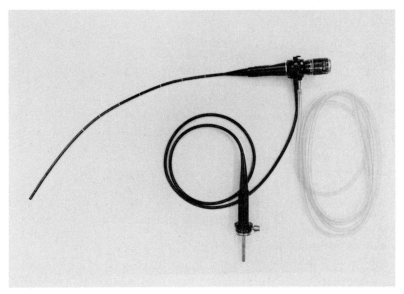

Fig. 14 A fibreoptic bronchoscope.

anteriorly. It may be useful to look for transillumination through the anterior aspect of the neck at this point. As the bronchoscope is brought forward, the larynx appears and the vocal cords are visualized.

The bronchoscope is passed through the vocal cords into the trachea which appears as a series of glistening whitish ridges in between red troughs. The bronchoscope is advanced to the carina. The angle of the carina is noted and the bronchoscope 'tapped' against the carina to give some indication as to the texture (e.g. rigid or soft). The orifice of the right upper lobe bronchus should be found particularly if the right lung is to be electively ventilated. Any abnormality seen is noted, especially those that may cause difficulty during intubation, for example, external compression causing bronchial narrowing.

Endobronchial intubation with a double lumen tube

1. Blind method

The patient's head should be correctly positioned for laryngoscopy. The double lumen tube, occasionally with its connectors attached, is held so that the protruding tip is in the anteroposterior plane (Fig. 15). The tube is passed through the cords under direct vision

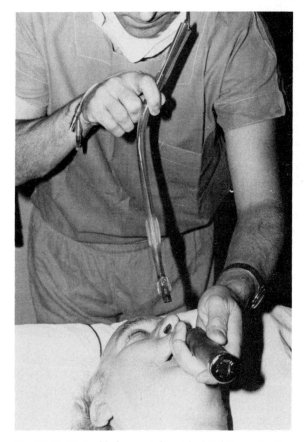

Fig. 15 Right double lumen tube with distal tip protruding in anteroposterior plane.

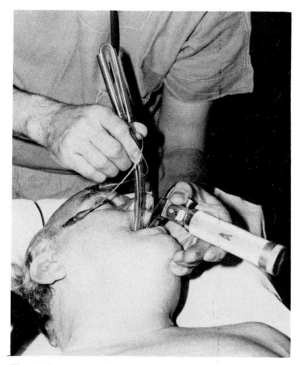

Fig. 16 Insertion of a right double lumen tube. Note the head and neck turned to the opposite side.

In addition, the same bronchoscope can be passed through the tracheal lumen to check the positions of both the bronchial cuff and the opening of the tracheal lumen relative to the main bronchus leading to the non-dependent lung. Indeed, in a recent letter [21], it was recommended that teaching this use of the flexible fibreoptic bronchoscope should be incorporated into all departmental training programmes.

Whichever method is used to place a double lumen tube, the tube has to be checked to ensure it is in the correct position. This is usually performed by first inflating the tracheal cuff to make an air tight seal and checking the air entry to both lungs with a stethoscope. The bronchial cuff is inflated until the pilot balloon expands (2–5 ml); again the air entry to the lungs is checked with the stethoscope. The connection which allows ventilation to the lung where surgery is planned (i.e. the non-dependent lung) is clamped and the bung removed (Fig. 17).

into the trachea and the laryngoscope, usually but not always, removed. The tube is then rotated through 90° either to enter the left or right main bronchus as appropriate. It may be helpful to turn the head and neck to the opposite side (Fig. 16).

The distal part of the tube is advanced until it enters the appropriate bronchus. It is usually accompanied by an increased resistance as the main part of the tube abuts against the carina.

2. Fibreoptic method

The blind method has been associated with a 25% failure rate while attempting to correctly place a double lumen tube [18]. To achieve a more accurate placement percentage, a flexible fibreoptic bronchoscope has been used [19,20].

After the double lumen tube has been introduced into the trachea and the ventilation checked, the flexible bronchoscope is passed through the bronchial lumen of the endobronchial tube. The bronchoscope is advanced into the appropriate bronchus and the endobronchial tube guided into the same bronchus.

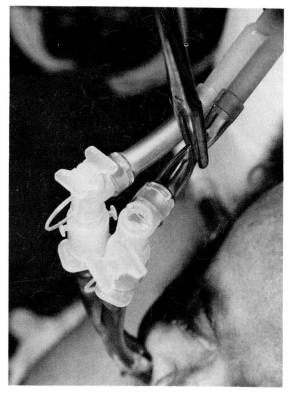

Fig. 17 Right sided double lumen tube. Note clamping of the connection to the left lung and the bung which is open to air.

Gas inflating the dependent lung can only enter the non-dependent lung by 'leaking' around the bronchial cuff. This leak results in an audible gas flow through the open ended tube to the atmosphere. The bronchial cuff is gradually inflated until this audible leak disappears and an air tight seal achieved. It is imperative to check air entry to the isolated lung with a stethoscope, particularly when the right side is intubated. When the position of the tube is satisfactory, the bung is replaced, the clamp removed and the tube firmly secured with bandage or adhesive tape. The patient is turned onto the side and the position of the tube is again carefully checked as before. Both lungs are inflated until the chest is opened.

Some difficulties may be encountered:
1 There may be a difficulty in introducing the tube into the larynx. The Magill intubating forceps may be useful to guide the tip of the tube into the larynx. A long elastic gum bougie passed through the bronchial lumen of the tube can also be used as a guide. More recently, fibreoptic bronchoscopes have been used to counter this difficulty.
2 There may be difficulty in placing the tube in the correct position in the bronchus. In which case, either substitute a smaller tube (medium for large, small for medium) or use a tracheal tube with or without a bronchial blocker.

Before the chest is opened it is important to note:
1 the fresh gas flow;
2 percentage oxygen in the fresh gas flow;
3 the tidal volume;
4 the pressure required to deliver that tidal volume;
5 the respiratory rate;
6 an arterial blood sample should be taken for measurement of blood gases.
Most of these parameters will require adjustment as soon as one lung anaesthesia is instituted.
During the operative procedure secretions and blood may accumulate in the bronchi above the cuff particularly from the non-dependent lung. Both bronchi should be sucked out before deflating either cuff or re-expanding part of a lung after a lobectomy. Suction should also be applied before extubation. Some anaesthetists

will also perform a post extubation bronchoscopy with bronchial toilet.

Endobronchial intubation with a single lumen tube

A single lumen tube can be introduced 'blindly' or with the aid of an intubating or fibreoptic bronchoscope [22].

1. Blind method

This is unsatisfactory and takes advantage of the natural curves of some endobronchial tubes. Intubation is checked by auscultating each lung with the cuffs first inflated and then deflated.

2. Intubating bronchoscope method

The endobronchial tube with its catheter mount attached is slipped over the intubating bronchoscope (Fig. 18) which has had the external surface very well lubricated. The tip of the tube and the end of the bronchoscope should be in line (Fig. 19). The catheter mount is usually set at 90° to the main axis of the intubating bronchoscope so that, following a successful intubation, the connections will lie comfortably alongside the cheek. The optic systems are checked and the patient's head placed in the classic intubating position.
The bronchoscope and endobronchial tube can be introduced into the larynx either by visualizing the laryngeal aperture with a laryngoscope or in a similar fashion to conventional bronchoscopy. As the tube and bronchoscope are advanced into the trachea the patient's head is extended. The head may also be rotated to the opposite side similar to the technique described earlier for double lumen intubation. When the carina is seen, the handle of the bronchoscope is rotated through 90°, right or left and advanced into the appropriate bronchus. The tube is held firmly with the left hand at the mouth and the bronchoscope smoothly withdrawn with the right hand. It may be difficult to withdraw the bronchoscope without moving the endobronchial tube unless the external surface of the bronchoscope has been well lubricated.

3. Fibreoptic bronchoscope method

The fibreoptic bronchoscope is passed through an endobronchial tube until the end protrudes

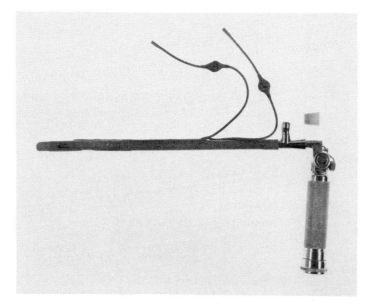

Fig. 18 Intubating bronchoscope inside a right sided single lumen tube. Note angle made by connector.

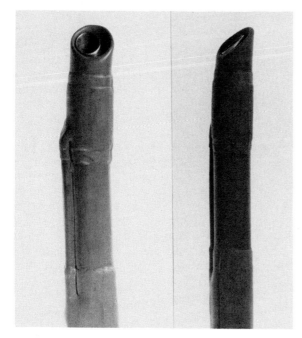

Fig. 19 The ends of the single lumen tube and intubating bronchoscope lying in the same place.

through the tube by about 3–6 cm. This allows the tip of the bronchoscope to move freely. The bronchoscope and tube are introduced into the larynx using a laryngoscope (which is then removed) and the bronchoscope advanced to the carina.

Alternatively, the endobronchial tube can be introduced into the larynx using a laryngoscope. The latter is then removed. The bronchoscope is passed through the endobronchial tube and advanced until the carina is seen.

The bronchus is entered under direct vision and the endobronchial tube guided over the bronchoscope into that bronchus. The endobronchial tube is held firmly with the left hand and the bronchoscope withdrawn with the right hand.

The main disadvantage of the fibreoptic method is that the endobronchial tube is not fully supported by the bronchoscope so it can bend and twist. Such movements may make it more difficult to place these tubes. However, if the tube is not correctly placed at the first attempt or slips, the fibreoptic bronchoscope can easily be reintroduced and the position of the tube adjusted. With an intubating broncho-scope under similar conditions, the patient would need to be extubated and the total procedure repeated from scratch.

Whichever method is used, the *tip* of the endobronchial tube *must not* pass beyond the origin of the upper lobe bronchus on the left, but *must* pass beyond the upper lobe orifice but no further than the middle lobe orifice on the right.

The bronchial cuff is inflated so that an airtight seal is just achieved and the air entry to the appropriate lung checked with a stethoscope. Excessive inflating pressures must be avoided as the bronchial cuff may herniate over the lumen of the tube, become displaced or even rupture the bronchus.

The tracheal cuff is inflated to achieve an airtight seal and anchors the endobronchial tube in the trachea. The endobronchial tube can easily be converted into a tracheal tube by deflating the bronchial cuff. Both cuffs remain inflated while the patient is turned into the lateral position and the checking process repeated.

Although single lumen tubes are similar in length to the double lumen varieties, they do not have the same structural strength and consequently tend to kink. This tendency is augmented by the natural anatomical curves of the respiratory pathway.

At the carinal curve, malalignment and kinking are strong possibilities and can present as 'bronchospasm'. This can be treated by correct realignment and anchoring the tube with the tracheal cuff. At the pharyngeal curve, kinking will occur if the neck is allowed to flex excessively, particularly in the lateral position. Lastly, it is also possible that excessive neck flexion will cause kinking in the roof of the mouth or at the tube connection interface just proximal to the lips.

Consequently, when a single lumen tube has been correctly placed and anchored at a tracheal level, it should be firmly secured at the mouth. This prevents the tube slipping or being pulled out either accidentally or by the weight of the anaesthetic connections. Again, in the lateral position, the neck should be extended and the position of the tube checked once more before surgery is allowed to commence.

Before extubation, the patient should be placed in the head down position and 100% oxygen administered for several minutes. The tracheal cuff is deflated so any secretions can run down towards the larynx. A suction catheter is passed beyond the end of the endobronchial tube and bronchial toilet performed. The bronchial cuff is deflated and the endobronchial tube slowly withdrawn. The suction catheter should be left beyond the end of the tube and suction applied continuously during extubation. All the debris from the bronchus and trachea is sucked out as the endobronchial tube and suction catheter are withdrawn together. Some anaesthetists always perform a bronchoscopy following extubation.

Endobronchial intubation in infants and children

This is a difficult procedure but can be accomplished blindly or by using direct vision.

1. Blind method

A technique using a suitably sized Portex tracheal tube was originally described by Callum et al [17]. A lateral chest X-ray is taken and the distance from the mouth to the carina measured. One centimetre is added to that length so that the tube, when correctly placed, will enter either main bronchus. If the right side

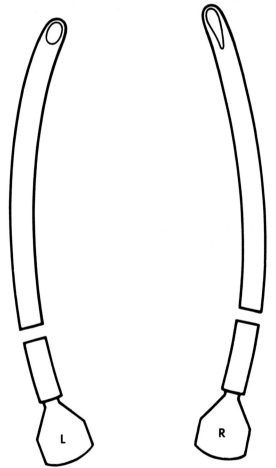

Fig. 20 Tracheal tubes used for endobronchial intubation in infants. Note the lengthened bevel for the right side. From Cullum et al [16], with kind permission of the authors and Academic Press, publishers of *Anaesthesia*.

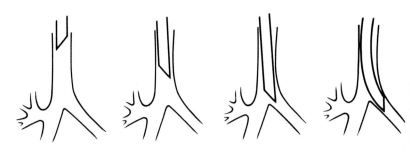

Fig. 21 Rotations of tracheal tube to accomplish endobronchial intubation. From Cullum et al [16], with kind permission of the authors and Academic Press, publishers of *Anaesthesia*.

is to be intubated, the bevel of the Portex tube must be lengthened under sterile conditions (Fig. 20). The tube is introduced into the trachea with the open bevel pointing to the side where intubation is required. The tracheal tube is then rotated through 180° and the head of the infant is moved away from the side where intubation is planned. As the anaesthetist advances the tube, the tip passes along the lateral tracheal wall towards the appropriate main brochus. When the full extent of the tube is in place with the connector at the mouth, the tube is rotated back through 180° so that the bevel now faces the lateral wall of the appropriate bronchus (Fig. 21). The position is confirmed with a stethoscope.

2. Direct vision methods

Bronchoscopic method. A Fogerty catheter [9] can be passed through a suitably sized broncho- scope into the main bronchus to block off the diseased lung or lobe bronchus. It is inflated under direct vision to just fill the bronchial lumen. Excessive pressure may cause damage to the bronchus and force the balloon proximal- ly. The bronchoscope is carefully removed so that the catheter is not displaced. A tracheal tube is inserted (cuffed or uncuffed depending on the age of the child) and the lungs inflated.

Fibreoptic method. Flexible paediatric fibreoptic bronchoscopes have been used to achieve both selective endobronchial blocking and intuba- tion.

In one study [23], a Swan-Ganz catheter was introduced into the trachea under direct vision. The tip was guided using the bronchoscope into the diseased pulmonary lobe. When the tip is in the correct place, the balloon is inflated. A tracheal tube is introduced and the chest auscultated to confirm that both the balloon and tracheal tube are correctly placed.

Others have used both flexible [24] and rigid [25] fibreoptic bronchoscopes to accurately place suitably sized tracheal tubes in the appropriate bronchus to act as endobronchial tubes. These methods have also found a place in the management of critical care patients [26].

However, whichever methods are chosen, correct placement is always carefully confirmed clinically by auscultation and occasionally with chest radiography.

Before extubation, the operating table is tilted into the head down position and secretions sucked out. The tube is then removed. If this is not feasible, the child should be placed in a steep head down position so that secretions can run down the trachea to be expectorated or removed by suction from the pharynx. A post extubation bronchoscopy may be performed if required.

Complications

Complications associated with endobronchial tubes are predominantly traumatic, positional and physiological.

Traumatic

An endobronchial tube is longer and thicker than a tracheal tube. Most double lumen tubes are still passed 'blind' while some tubes still possess hooks, for example the Carlens [13] tube, which can cause trauma to the respiratory tract. It is sometimes forgotten that such tubes can also cause damage at extubation. The trauma varies from mild ecchymosis of mucous membranes to arytenoid dislocation. Vocal cords and tracheal mucosa have also been torn by the tips of tubes and attached hooks.

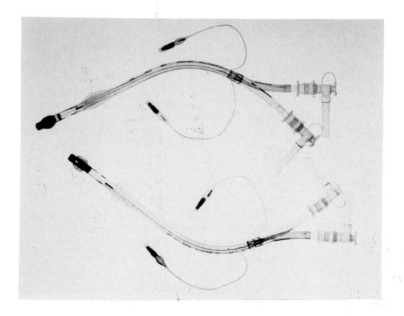

Fig. 22 Polyvinyl chloride (PVC) double lumen endobronchial tube.

The most serious complication however is tracheobronchial rupture [27,28]. Such injuries are usually associated with a large tube forcefully passed or a hook caught at the vocal cords. The tip of the tube may pass into the mediastinum or the bronchus may rupture following the very rapid overinflation of the cuffs.

The diagnosis depends on visual haemorrhage or a pneumothorax with surgical emphysema presenting as the 'Michelin man syndrome' with inadequate gas exchange. The diagnosis is confirmed by rapid bronchoscopy and any laceration found should be repaired immediately.

Modern double lumen tubes made from polyvinyl chloride (PVC) (Fig. 22) have a much smoother surface, specific introducers and no hooks. When compared with red rubber tubes [29,30] it was found that the PVC tubes were easier to pass with a high percentage of 'first time' correct placements. In addition, the time taken from beginning of intubation to correct placing was much reduced (3 min for PVC as against 10 min for red rubber). Furthermore, when the respiratory tract was inspected before intubation and after extubation, there was considerably less damage following the use of PVC endobronchial tubes. These types of results, and a recent cost effective survey which supported the general use of PVC tubes, may well see the eventual demise of the red rubber tube [31].

Positional

Difficulties in correctly positioning an endobronchial tube are usually due to the tube being too large. Reduction in size usually overcomes the problem. However, an extensive tumour causing anatomical abnormality may prevent any endobronchial tube being correctly placed. The bronchoscopy performed before intubation should have alerted the anaesthetist to this possibility.

Any endobronchial tube incorrectly placed will cause impaired ventilation. Sometimes, neither lung can be isolated nor ventilated. This is usually associated with the endobronchial tube failing to pass beyond the carina and subsequent inflation of the bronchial cuff obstructing the distal lumen of the tube. Further, an incorrectly placed tube with an inflated cuff can also cause serious problems as some of the inflating volume remains in the lung at the end of each respiratory cycle. This can eventually increase the intra-alveolar pressure, cause lung rupture and a pneumothorax. If unrecognized, a tension pneumothorax may result.

Occasionally, the lung may not deflate after the chest is opened. If the surgeon is unable to proceed easily, deflating the appropriate cuff may deal with the problem. Adjustments can also be achieved by advancing or withdrawing the tube and reinflating the cuffs. During these manoeuvres, the ventilation of the upper lung can be observed through the thoracotomy wound but the dependent lung should be checked by auscultation and mediastinal movement observed at each subsequent inflation.

Another method [32] has been described to help overcome difficulties in positioning when the non-dependent lung will not collapse during the operation. A Foley catheter has been passed down the lumen which supplies that lung. It is introduced 'blindly' into the appropriate bronchus and its balloon inflated. The balloon then acts as a bronchus blocker and the distal lung collapses as alveolar gas passes through the tip and up the catheter to the atmosphere. The position of the balloon is confirmed by observing the lung collapse, the movements of the mediastinum and auscultation over the dependent lung.

If this fails, the endobronchial tube can be converted into a tracheal tube by withdrawing it slowly, observing the lung in the open chest and checking the dependent lung by auscultation.

A major danger exists if malposition occurs when the right lung is the dependent lung as it is imperative that the right upper lobe remains ventilated. This lobe should be checked after intubation, turning and at frequent intervals during the procedure. Failure to ensure right upper lobe ventilation can lead to severe hypoxaemia as the total ventilation will have to occur within the right middle and lower lobes. This type of problem is seldom seen on the left side as the tip of any endobronchial tube rarely passes beyond the orifice of the upper lobe bronchus.

It is also as well to remember that lung operations were successfully performed before endobronchial tubes became common place and indeed continue to be so when endobronchial tubes cannot be utilized.

Physiological [33,34]

The most common and dangerous complication associated with endobronchial intubation is hypoxaemia. There are several reasons for the hypoxaemia.

Ventilation perfusion. The blood continues to flow through both pulmonary arteries after one lung has collapsed. Any volatile anaesthetic agents will increase this shunt due to pulmonary vasodilation. There is also increased shunting in the dependent lung which receives all the minute volume. Hence, there is a considerable increase in venous admixture.

Pressure. When one lung is ventilated preferentially and the tidal volume delivered remains the same as it was originally for both lungs, the intra-alveolar pressure in that lung inevitably increases. This increase in pressure decreases venous return, cardiac output and increases the resistance to blood flow through the dependent lung. More of the cardiac output is then diverted through the collapsed lung thus increasing venous shunting.

Treatment. Before commencing one lung ventilation, the parameters referred to earlier should have been measured (p. 166). Hypoxia, suspected or measured, associated with one lung anaesthesia should be treated as follows:

1 Increase the inspired oxygen concentration to at least 0.5 and, if necessary, to 1.0.
2 The intra-alveolar pressure in the dependent lung should be kept as low as possible. The minute volume should remain the same but the respiratory rate increased and the tidal volume decreased. High frequency ventilation may be valuable in achieving such a pattern of ventilation.
3 The use of volatile agents may have to be discontinued if severe hypoxia or hypotension develop. However, this can lead to awareness and haemodynamic stimulation so that additional intravenous analgesia will be required. This may lead to delay in the onset of spontaneous ventilation at the end of the operation although Alfentanil, as a short acting analgesic agent, may be useful.
4 Surgical clamping of the pulmonary artery to the non-ventilated lung will help but is only performed preceding pneumonectomy. Snaring the arterial supply to the non-dependent lung may be useful temporarily in difficult circumstances.
5 Ensure that carbon dioxide tension remains within normal limits for efficient myocardial contraction.
6 Decrease body oxygen consumption by total muscle relaxation and profound analgesia.
7 Arterial blood gases should be measured to

monitor progress. Occasionally a metabolic acidosis will develop which may need treatment.

8 Finally, two lung anaesthesia may be reintroduced and surgery performed on a moving target and not on a 'quiet' lung.

REFERENCES

1 White GMJ (1960) Evolution of endotracheal and endobronchial intubation. *Br J Anaesth* 32: 235.

2 Mushin WW (1963) *Thoracic Anaesthesia*, Ch 20. Blackwell Scientific Publications, Oxford.

3 Pappin JC (1979) The current practice of endobronchial intubation. *Anaesthesia* 34: 57.

4 Robertshaw FL (1962) Low resistance double lumen endobronchial tubes. *Br J Anaesth* 34: 576.

5 Green R & Gordon W (1957) Right lung anaesthesia. Anaesthesia for left lung surgery using a new right endobronchial tube. *Anaesthesia* 12: 86.

6 Pallister WK (1959) A new endobronchial tube for left lung surgery with specific reference to reconstructive pulmonary surgery. *Thorax* 14: 55.

7 Magill IW (1934) Anaesthesia for thoracic surgery. *Newcastle Medical Journal* 14: 67.

8 Rusby LN & Thompson VC (1943) Carcinoma of the lung: diagnosis and surgical treatment. *Postgrad Med J* 19: 44.

9 Vale R (1969) Selective bronchial blocking in a small child. Case Report. *Br J Anaesth* 41: 453.

10 Magill IW (1936) Anaesthesia in thoracic surgery with special reference to lobectomy. *Proc R Soc Med* 29: 643.

11 Mansfield RE (1957) Modified bronchoscope for endobronchial intubation. *Anaesthesia* 12: 477.

12 Butchart EG, Ashcroft T, Barnsley WC & Holden MP (1981) The role of surgery in diffuse malignant mesothelioma of the pleura. *Semin Oncol* 8: 321.

13 Bjork VO, Carlens E & Freiberg O (1953) Endobronchial anaesthesia. *J Thorac Cardiovasc Surg* 14: 60.

14 Macintosh R & Leatherdale RAL (1955) Bronchus tube and bronchus blocker. *Br J Anaesth* 27: 556.

15 Machray R (1958) Anaesthesia for surgical treatment of chest diseases. *Tuberculosis Index* 13: 172.

16 Cullum AR, English ICW & Branthwaite MA (1973) Endobronchial intubation in infancy. *Anaesthesia* 28: 66.

17 Sanders RD (1967) Two ventilating attachments for bronchoscopes. *Del Med J* 39: 170.

18 Read RC, Friday CD & Eason CN (1977) Prospective study of the Robertshaw endobronchial catheter in thoracic surgery. *Ann Thorac Surg* 24: 156.

19 Ovassapian A, Braunschweig R & Joshi CW (1983) Endobronchial intubation using a flexible fiberoptic bronchoscope. *Anesthesiology* 59: 501.

20 Shinnick JP & Freedman AP (1982) Bronchofiberscopic placement of a double-lumen endotracheal tube. *Crit Care Med* 10: 544.

21 Ovassapian A (1983) Fiberoptic bronchoscope and double-lumen tracheal tubes. *Anaesthesia* 38: 1104.

22 Aps C & Towey RM (1981) Experiences with fibreoptic bronchoscopic positioning of single lumen endobronchial tubes. *Anaesthesia* 36: 415.

23 Dalers E, Labbe A & Haberer JP (1982) Selective endobronchial blocking vs selective intubation. *Anesthesiology* 57: 55.

24 Watson CB, Bowe EA & Bunk W (1982) One lung anesthesia for pediatric thoracic surgery: a new use for the fiberoptic bronchoscope. *Anesthesiology* 56: 314.

25 Rao CC, Krishna P & Grosfeld JL (1981) One lung pediatric anesthesia. *Anesth Analg* 60: 450.

26 Cay DL, Csenderitz LE, Lines V, Lomaz JP & Overton JH (1975) Selective bronchial blocking in children. *Anaesth Intensive Care* 3: 127.

27 Guernelli N, Bragagha RB, Briccoli A et al (1979) Tracheobronchial ruptures due to cuffed Carlens tubes. *Ann Thorac Surg* 28: 66.

28 Heiser M, Steinberg JJ, Macvaugh H et al (1979) Bronchial rupture, a complication of use of the Robertshaw double lumen tube. *Anaesthesia* 51: 88.

29 Clapham MC & Vaughan RS (1985) Endobronchial intubation. A comparison between polyvinyl chloride and red rubber double lumen tubes. In press.

30 Watson CB, Kasik LR, Battaglini J et al (1984) A functional comparison of polyvinyl chloride and red rubber double lumen endobronchial tubes. Society of Cardiovascular Anesthesiologists, Boston, Massachusetts, May 1984.

31 Linter SPK (1985) Disposable double lumen bronchial tubes. *Anaesthesia* 40:

32 Conacher ID (1983) The urinary catheter as a bronchial blocker. *Anaesthesia* 38: 475.

33 Gothard JWW & Branthwaite MA (1982) *Anaesthesia for Thoracic Surgery*, Ch. 4. Blackwell Scientific Publications, Oxford

34 Kaplan JA (1983) *Thoracic Anesthesia. Part III. Cardiopulmonary Physiology.* Churchill Livingstone, Edinburgh.

CHAPTER 11 Teaching intubation

INTRODUCTION

All practising anaesthetists will at some time have been taught how to perform laryngoscopy and intubation. The methods used may have been largely trial and error or some form of organized teaching programme may have been employed. In general terms there are three groups to whom intubation is taught and each group will require a slightly different approach as each will be expected to utilize the learnt skills in different ways. Medical student teaching of intubation is an important part of general training and should be designed to generate awareness of airway management in all fields of practice. Teaching of anaesthetists should aim to allow skills to develop in order that complex intubation problems may be overcome with confidence. The paramedical group require sound training in airway management with a stress on the problems of performing intubation and guidelines on its usage.

MEDICAL STUDENTS

Aims of teaching

Medical students are seldom seconded to anaesthetics for very long, the normal attachment being for 1–2 weeks only. It is clearly accepted that this does not allow enough time to teach the subject of anaesthesia in any depth. Most clinicians faced with this short attachment period choose in their teaching to highlight certain aspects of anaesthetic practice that will be of value to the student after qualification irrespective of the speciality he chooses to follow. Our own stress in Cardiff has been towards an understanding of basic applied physiology, the technique of intravenous cannulation and cardiopulmonary resuscitation.

Although intubation is a part of cardiopulmonary resuscitation in the hospital situation, it is important to point out to undergraduates that intubation is not absolutely essential in order to perform adequate ventilation of the lungs and it is not always as simple as it looks. As Lunn points out [1]: 'the technique often appears to be very easy, and indeed it usually is to an expert, but sometimes it can be very difficult. The worst situation in which to have to perform tracheal intubation is when the patient is lying on the floor and in receipt of closed cardiac massage at the same time'. Airway management and lung inflation by means of mask and self-inflating bag are simple and important techniques that should be mastered before intubation training is introduced. It must be made quite clear that attempts at tracheal intubation by inexperienced personnel may cause unnecessary delays in implementing adequate ventilation and oxygenation.

Once students have mastered the technique of artificial ventilation using a mask and bag, the teaching of tracheal intubation should proceed in a gradual ordered manner. The process of teaching may be split into lectures, films, demonstrations and practice on teaching aids and finally experience in the operating theatre.

Lectures

These preliminary lectures should be used to point out the indications for intubation both electively and in emergencies, to introduce the equipment used and its mode of usage and to describe the anatomy of the area with particular reference to the positioning of the head and neck prior to intubation. Regional anatomy is often difficult to illustrate as the three dimensional structure of the larynx is hard to visualize with simple drawings.

Films

A short film, of which there are several available, is very useful to illustrate the anatomical considerations of intubation. It can clearly demonstrate the position in which to place the head and neck for optimal intubating conditions. In addition most of these films give a view of the larynx as seen by the operating anaesthetist. They should also highlight the importance of checking tube position following intubation.

The particular film used in Cardiff is entitled 'Tracheal Intubation' and is a product from Medical Electronic Educational Services Inc, California, USA. It initially describes the anatomy of the area and stresses the different axes present in mouth, pharynx and trachea. It shows how these different axes may be altered to a common axis for intubation. It then shows the equipment involved in intubation and the actual technique of intubation in anaesthetized patients. The film shows intubation as seen by the onlooker from the side as well as giving an 'anaesthetist's eye view' of the intubation.

Demonstration and practice of teaching aids

Teaching aids to intubation have been available for some time. The three most commonly used aids are manufactured by Vitalograph, Laerdal and Ambu.

1. Vitalograph Royal Free Hospital System

This consists of an intubation trainer which has a fixed head position but has interchangeable teeth, a movable trachea and a separate laryngeal model to aid anatomical understanding. Excessive pressure on the upper teeth causes a buzzer to sound.

In addition to the trainer the system includes teaching cards and a slide/cassette audio-visual collection.

2. Laerdal Intubation Simulator

This model has the features of a large male head, neck and upper thorax. The anatomy of the pharynx and larynx are lifelike. The tongue size and consistency may be adjusted by inflation with air. Excessive pressure on the upper teeth is signalled by a red light.

3. Ambu Intubation Trainer

This model has a cutaway section showing the larynx, trachea and cervical spine and so aids the appreciation of correct positioning prior to intubation. It also allows nasotracheal intubation to be practised. There is a buzzer to indicate excessive pressure on the upper teeth.

Unfortunately none of the teaching aids are exactly equivalent to human intubation, the largest problem being the design of the tongue and epiglottic attachments. However, they are sturdily made and so tolerate the rough handling associated with inexperienced attempts at intubation.

In order to obtain the best from such aids it is important to allow plenty of time for practice. The instructor should demonstrate firstly to the group and then to individuals the technique of laryngoscopy which is usually the hardest part to master, followed by the more easily performed act of intubation. The control of the laryngoscope and minimization of trauma should be stressed. Students should then be allowed to practise on the teaching aid with no restriction on the time taken to achieve intubation. Once able to intubate with a degree of confidence a time limit should be imposed of, say, 30 s and the students allowed to practise again.

Safar [2] recommends the use of a checklist with strict criteria of intubation competence as in Fig. 1. The advantage of using training aids was realized in 1973 by Hilary Howells [3] who pointed out that such aids allow unlimited time to acquire manipulative expertise and this results in subsequent experience on the human subject being gained confidently, safely and quickly.

Practice in the operating theatre

Once students are confident in their ability to intubate a teaching aid they may be allowed to intubate patients in the operating theatre but this must always be done under the direct supervision of a qualified anaesthetist. It is important to point out the delicacy of pharyngeal and laryngeal tissues and the possibility of causing injuries to eyes by careless technique and hand positioning. Laryngoscopy and demonstration of the anatomy is difficult for students to master quickly and this is often related to a hurried approach to laryngoscope placement. Tube placement is usually simple once the larynx has been clearly displayed. Another common mistake made by students is to place their eyes too close to the mouth thus preventing binocular vision. If the operator's head is held approximately 1 foot from the mouth this problem should be avoided. All students should aim to perform 10 intubations in the operating theatre during their attachment.

Although intubation is an important part of medical student education it must be stressed

Student's name   Date   Evaluator's name

☐ Passed
☐ Failed

Measures   Technique   Time

☑ Check if correct performance   ☑ Check if within
                                      correct time lapse

Tracheal intubation of *adult* manikin	☐ Checked laryngoscope light before use	sec.
	☐ Checked tube patency before use	
	☐ Held laryngoscope correctly	
	☐ Used no grossly traumatic manoeuvre during intubation attempt	
	☐ Inserted tube into trachea rapidly................	☐ <30
	☐ Gave first lung inflation rapidly via tube by bag-valve or mouth..................	☐ <60
	☐ Inflated cuff of tube correctly (with helper)	
	☐ Used bite-block, secured tube and connected ventilation device correctly	
	☐ Checked to rule out bronchial intubation	
Tracheal intubation of *infant* manikin	☐ Checked laryngoscope light before use	
	☐ Checked tube patency before use	
	☐ Held laryngoscope correctly	
	☐ Used no grossly traumatic manoeuvre during intubation attempt	
	☐ Inserted tube into trachea rapidly................	☐ <30
	☐ Gave first lung inflation rapidly via tube (by mouth)	☐ <60
	☐ Used bite-block, secured tube and connected ventilation device correctly	
	☐ Checked to rule out bronchial intubation	
Tracheal suctioning (curved-tipped catheter)	☐ Used correct technique to suction each lung separately	☐ <60

Fig. 1. A checklist for intubation competence (as recommended by Safar [2]).

that students are taught electively under ideal conditions on preoxygenated patients who are not vomiting; this may not be the case during cardiopulmonary resuscitation. For this reason it cannot be overstressed that valuable time should not be wasted in futile attempts at intubation in difficult situations when ventilation of the lungs may be perfectly feasible by the use of a mask and self-inflating bag.

Student competence

The degree to which medical student training in tracheal intubation is successful is hard to assess. One article evaluating medical students'

practical experience upon qualification showed that in a group of 89 students studied, 7% had never undertaken tracheal intubation whilst a further 40% had only done so on one occasion. The remaining 53% had undertaken intubation on more than three occasions. Of the whole group only 30% perceived themselves competent at tracheal intubation[4].

A very short introduction to the technique of tracheal intubation does not make the medical student an expert. Further exposure to intubation may occur during house officer appointments and a survey of preregistration house officers showed that all those interviewed had performed tracheal intubation on more than three occasions and 89% of them considered themselves competent at the skill[5].

It is probable that there is a difference between perceived and actual competence in an emergency situation and this has been highlighted by Casey [6] who tested junior hospital doctors' theoretical and practical skills at single-handed cardiopulmonary resuscitation using a mannikin. Only 8% were able to manage a cardiopulmonary arrest adequately. Similar disappointing findings were reported by Skinner [7] where the intubation skills of house-officers were assessed on training manikins. Only 34% were able to intubate the manikin at all and none were able to intubate in less than 35 seconds (the upper limit of time allowed for pass grade in advance cardiac life support examination in the USA). There must be a need for organized programmes of training for all medical staff and this may include the appointment of permanent resuscitation officers [8] and the availability of adequate resuscitation training areas such as described by Baskett [9].

ANAESTHETISTS

Initial training

Intubation is normally undertaken by the anaesthetist to facilitate the management of general anaesthesia rather than for cardiopulmonary resuscitation. The trainee undergoes an initial induction period during which he is taught the principles governing the running of the department. When starting clinical duties he works closely with one consultant for at least a month. The consultant demontrates the technique and teaches the principles of intubation and also the principles of elective and emergency anaesthesia. The trainee then learns to intubate under close supervision. He is first taught to demonstrate the anatomy at laryngoscopy and secondarily to insert the tracheal tube. At a later stage which varies widely between departments and trainees, he is allowed to undertake the management of anaesthetics without direct supervision. Help should be readily and immediately available at this transition stage as difficult intubations and other problems can present unexpectedly and quickly. Every trainee should have a simple efficient method of dealing with a difficult intubation. The transition can be stressful to trainees and potentially

harmful to patients; acute airway problems, difficult or failed intubation and aspiration of gastric contents are hazards which may trap the unwary trainee. The Obstetric Anaesthetists' Association, mindful of the occurrence in obstetric practice of the unexpectedly difficult intubation with accompanying airway problems, has recommended that trainees should have at least 1 year's anaesthetic experience before working without direct supervision in this area.

The time for the trainee to achieve competence depends on the number of intubations he is able to undertake. There may, in addition, be variations in speed of learning and manual dexterity between individuals. It is therefore not appropriate to have rigid rules indicating when the trainee should be allowed to work without supervision for the first time.

The trainee needs 'hands on' experience and it is important that he be allowed to attempt intubation when difficult cases occur. The duration of his attempt must be a matter for the judgement of the teacher. Some clinicians find delegation difficult under these circumstances and may hastily take over the procedure.

The apprentice system in operation in the United Kingdom means that the types of intubation procedure taught may vary widely. This will depend on the number of difficult cases encountered, the common techniques chosen to facilitate the procedure and the experience of the teacher with complex techniques. Techniques taught should include rapid sequence induction and intubation together with preoxygenation and cricoid pressure; the management of a difficult intubation with a gum elastic bougie or stylet; simulated difficult intubation (see p. 112) to gain experience and confidence for the unexpected case when the cords cannot be visualized and a failed intubation drill for obstetric anaesthesia which is also applicable in any patient with a full stomach.

The UK system of training is in marked contrast to that in operation in the USA. There all residents are supervised during the induction of anaesthesia and intubation for the duration of their residency. This has the advantage of offering extra protection to the patient. Its disadvantage is that the trainee is never put in a position where he has unexpectedly to manage single-handed a problem airway or difficult intubation. The adoption of such a staffing pattern in the UK clearly would have major implications on the deployment of medical manpower.

Complex techniques

The weakness of the system in operation in the UK is that advanced techniques are rarely taught on a formal basis. In many centres skills in fibreoptic and retrograde techniques for intubation are not available. It is clear that these techniques are not required on a regular basis and that many clinicians seem able to manage the majority of cases without them. In larger teaching centres, however, it is important that juniors are thoroughly taught the principles and practice of such techniques.

Since suitable cases present only rarely, and it is not ethical to practise retrograde techniques electively on normal patients, 'hands on' experience in patients is difficult to come by. This difficulty may be solved largely by a combination of theoretical teaching, practice on cadavers or models and training films. The technique is usually quick and easy to perform (see p. 122). It is certainly ethical to perform this technique electively in the patient judged to be very difficult preoperatively or in a patient with a previous failed intubation.

Fibreoptic intubation is intrinsically more difficult and it has been clearly shown that formal training procedures are helpful in gaining expertise (see p. 128). The limiting factors in gaining such expertise are discouragement after a few initial failures, poor training programmes and financial restrictions limiting the availability of equipment. It is clear that only a small percentage of clinicians are skilled at fibreoptic intubation (see Table 13, Chapter 7) and there is considerable scope for improving this figure. It is also important to remember that the equipment needs to be used on a regular basis in order to maintain a high level of expertise.

PARAMEDICAL STAFF

The need for paramedical training

There can be little doubt that the technique of tracheal intubation is an important part of every medical person's training, but there is some controversy as to the value of teaching this technique to paramedical staff. Safar [2] suggests that intubation should be taught to intensive care unit staff and a selected group of paramedics. In the United Kingdom the paramedical group is represented by selected ambulancemen. Many health authorities have started training groups of ambulance staff to be proficient in the insertion of intravenous cannulae and tracheal intubation in addition to basic airway management. However what evidence is there that such training is beneficial to the patient?

There is a good deal of information on the effect that such trained staff have on survival following cardiac arrest in the non-hospital situation. Vertesi [10] reported the experience of using 'paramedic' ambulances over a 27 month period. There were 227 cases of cardiac arrest in this period of which 198 (87.2%) were intubated. The number surviving to hospital admission was 58 (25.6% of cases) but of these only 21 (9.25%) were discharged alive. The authors concluded from this experience that 'sudden death from cardiac disease can be prevented in a considerable proportion of instances and that early circulatory and ventilatory support may prevent deterioration in a variety of other disorders'. However, set alongside this is the fact that survival figures following cardiac arrest can be greatly improved by widespread training in basic resuscitation as has been shown by Lund & Skulberg [11] where 36% of cardiac arrest victims given prompt attention by bystanders survived and were subsequently discharged from hospital. The ideal situation would seem to be a combination of widespread education of the general public in the basic skills of resuscitation (mouth to mouth ventilation and external cardiac massage) in combination with a small group of highly trained 'paramedics' skilled at more complex resuscitation techniques.

Indications for 'field' intubation

The main occasion when intubation by paramedical staff may be deemed necessary is at cardiac arrest following myocardial infarction. Comatose patients and those with extensive trauma where intubation may be necessary to provide an adequate airway are further examples.

If one considers the management of cardiac arrest it is clear that intubation is not an essential part of resuscitation. The lungs can be adequately ventilated using a bag and mask but if intubation can be performed rapidly and correctly this aids both lung inflation and protects the airway from soiling. There is very little literature available to evaluate the performance of intubation by 'paramedics'. Stewart et al [12] presented the results of attempted intubation by paramedics in 779 patients. A total of 701 (90%) were successfully intubated. The majority of these (57.9%) were intubated at the first attempt, whilst 26.1% and 5.3% were intubated at the second and third attempts respectively. There was a complication rate of 9.5% of which the major part was prolonged attempts at intubation (>45 s). However, there were three unrecognized oesophageal intubations. Of the patients intubated, 224 (28.8%) were reported to have vomited prior to attempts at intubation whilst seven (0.9%) vomited during intubation. Intubation in these situations would be advantageous in protecting the airway.

The value of early 'field' intubation following major trauma is even harder to assess. The type of case where this is likely to be most beneficial, apart from trauma induced cardiac arrest, would be in head and neck and chest injuries. However, it is these very cases that can pose intubation problems for even the most skilled of anaesthetists. In addition, unless intubation is performed with great care it may aggravate the injuries. Unlike the situation of managing cardiac arrest following myocardial infarction there may not be such a strong argument for 'paramedics' performing tracheal intubation on trauma victims.

One major problem would seem to be that it is not difficult to train a group of people to be proficient at intubation, but it is difficult to specify when not to intubate patients. Guidelines for training should include the categories of patients in which intubation should be attempted, the number and duration of attempts, the route to be utilized and a list of conditions in which intubation is contraindicated.

Training programmes

The method of training such personnel varies between the UK and North America. From experience in Brighton, where a coronary ambulance service has been in existence since 1969, the training of ambulancemen for such duties is extensive. Initial selection there is by the ambulance service training officer in combination with a pre-course examination. The main course is hospital based and comprises over twenty-four lectures of 90 min each, plus 1 month full time attachment to the Cardiac Care Unit. After passing the course examination, a further 6 months on the road experience is completed before a further week's training in airway management is undertaken. A 5 day refresher course is taken annually covering all areas of resuscitation and emergency care [13]. Training in the USA is even more extensive and a typical programme would be similar to that employed in Seattle. Training consists of 1000 h of intensive theoretical and clinical training covering all aspects of resuscitation as well as emergency operative procedures such as tracheostomy and thoracotomy [14].

In so far as tracheal intubation is part of this extensive training programme for paramedics, some thought must be given to how best to train these people. It is reasonable to set about teaching in a similar manner to that advocated for medical students. As there is no substitute for 'hands on' practice, as much time as possible should be spent in the operating theatre with anaesthetized patients.

CONCLUSION

It is unfortunate that intubation is frequently not well taught. If a structured training programme is not employed this is hardly surprising. Even if such a programme is used and the initial training is of good quality with a high degree of success in skill acquisition, the skills learnt will soon deteriorate to a dangerous level. It is essential that all medical and paramedical staff who may be called upon to perform intubation have regular reinforcement of their initial training.

The major shortcomings of training are different in each group. The anaesthetist's training may be deficient in the ability to cope with problems or utilize complex techniques. The shortcoming for the paramedic is in the need for patient selection as intubation may be dangerous in certain circumstances. The medical student training is normally somewhat fundamental but the aim should be to impress the value of the skill in their future career especially if this is in hospital practice.

Although in the hospital situation emergency intubations are usually performed by an anaesthetist, it is important that other staff be able to perform intubation and ventilation if the anaesthetist is unavailable. For this reason, intubation should be one of the skills acquired and regularly reinforced for all medical staff involved in the acute hospital care of patients.

REFERENCES

1 Lunn JL (1982) *Lecture Notes on Anaesthetics*, 2nd edn. Blackwell Scientific Publications, Oxford.
2 Safar P (1981) *Cardiopulmonary Cerebral Resuscitation*. W.B. Saunders, Philadelphia.
3 Hilary Howells T, Emery FM & Twentyman JEC (1973) Endotracheal intubation training using a simulator. *Br J Anaesth* 45:400.
4 Wakeford R & Roberts S (1982) An evaluation of medical students' practical experience upon qualification. *Medical Teacher* 4:140.
5 Evans I & Wakeford R (1983) House officers' perceptions of their experience and competence. *Medical Teacher* 5:68.
6 Casey WF (1984) Cardiopulmonary resuscitation: a survey of standards among junior hospital doctors. *J Roy Soc Med* 77:921.
7 Skinner DV, Camm AJ & Miles S (1985) Cardiopulmonary resuscitation skills of preregistration house officers. *Br Med J* 290:1549.
8 Baskett PJF (1985) Resuscitation needed for the curriculum? *Br Med J* 290:1531.
9 Baskett PJF, Lawler PGP, Hudson RBS, Makepeace APW & Cooper C (1976) Resuscitation teaching room in a district general hospital: concept and practice. *Br Med J* i:568.
10 Vertesi L (1978) The paramedic ambulance: a Canadian experience. *Can Med Assoc J* 119:25.
11 Lund I & Skulberg A (1976) Cardiopulmonary resuscitation by lay people. *Lancet* ii:702.
12 Stewart RD, Paris PM, Winter PM, Pelton GH & Cannon GM (1984) Field endotracheal intubation by paramedical personnel. *Chest* 85:341.
13 Studd C (1982) Abstract from *International Conference on Cardiac Arrest and Resuscitation*.
14 Mayer JD (1979) Seattle's paramedic program: geographical distribution, response times, and mortality. *Soc Sci Med* 13D:45.

Index